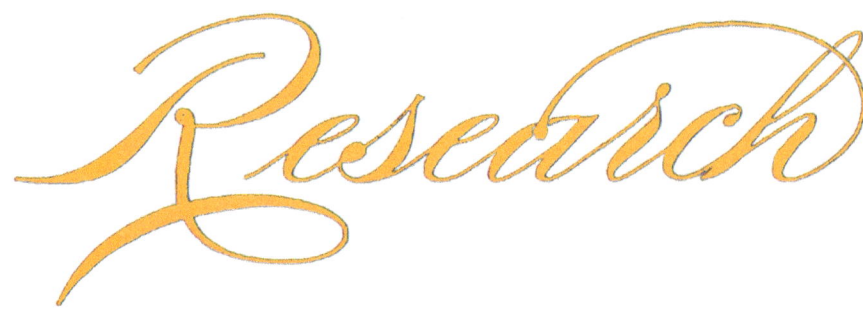

INCLUDING

STUDIES
REPORTS
LECTURES
AND
CASE REPORTS

REGARDING

BEMER* THERAPY

FROM

CLINICS
SCIENTISTS
RESEARCHERS
AND
PHYSICIANS

---

* BEMER is the registered trademark of Bemer International AG

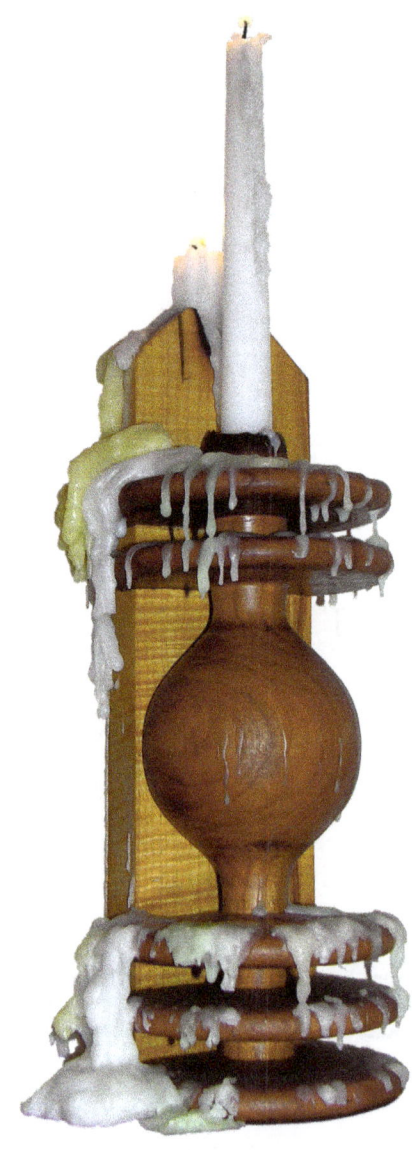

Publishing Rights Reserved © 2018 by Mark Vedder. This publication may not be reproduced for publishing without written permission of the Editor or Publisher. Individual articles hold additional rights per author and/or publication. Use of material in quotes, extracts, & etc. to credit this publication as well as sources referenced herein.

                Research / Various Authors / Edited by Mark Vedder
        300 pp   2 cm
ISBN 978-1-941776-35-3
Medical research on a specific signal carried by magetic waves—Studies—Reports—Lectures
Contains both original and redrawn illustrations.

                                                          2018
                                        ISBN 978-1-941776-35-3
                                      Publishing rights reserved
                                                  by
                                            Mark Vedder
                                   sufferingduckman@gmail.com

Quick Table of Contents

General Medical Practice	Page 1
Cardiology and Hematology	Page 18
Ophthalmology	Page 35
Surgery	Page 40
Dermatology	Page 48
Oncology	Page 57
Gynaecology	Page 84
Otorhinolaryngology	Page 95
Endocrinology	Page 127
Internal Medicine	Page 131
Pain Therapy	Page 139
Neurology	Page 170
Orthopedics	Page 172
Physiology	Page 189
Rehabilitation	Page 248
Sports Medicine	Page 258
Dentistry	Page 281
Veterinary medicine	Page 282
History	Page 291

Full Table of Contents

Page	Category / Specialty	Doctor / Researcher	Year	Subjects	Type
1	**General Medical Practice**				
1	ad hoc applicants	Schönfeld, Rolf	2000	201	Lec of St
8	General	Michaelis Horst	2002	1,116	Study
10	General	Michaelis Horst	2003	2,031	Study
12	General, Questionnaire	Wolfgang Bohn	2013	658	Abstract
13	Wound Care	Leizi Naude	2013	8 Cases	Report
18	**Cardiology and Hematology** (see also Physiology)				
18	Diabetic Polyneuropothy	R Klopp	2008		Study
24	Necrotizing Fasciitis	Zsófia Borbély	2007	5 Cases	Lecture
25	Lower Limb Circulatory Disorders	Rozsos István		2 Cases	Results
27	Late Diabetes Complications	Miléder Margit		2 Cases	Results
29	Peripheral Arterial Disease	Bernát Sándor Iván	2009	30	Study
35	**Ophthalmology**				
35	Diabetic Macular Edema	Tomáš Sosna	2010	7 Cases	Study
38	General Ophthalmology	Dr. Garai Borbála		3 Cases	Results
40	**Surgery**				
40	Neurosurgery	Németi Zoltán		232 + 3 Cases	Lecture
45	Triple and Fatigue Fracture	Rolf Oesterle	2005	1 Case	Lecture
46	Oral Surgery	Cséplő Krisztina		1 Case	Results
48	**Dermatology**				
48	Necrotic Ulcers	Horváth Ilona		4 Cases	Results
51	Visible Cosmetic Effects	R Klopp	2008		Study
54	Psoriasis Auricularis, Ulcus Cruris	Elisabeth Olszewsky	2000	3 Cases	Report
57	**Oncology**				
57	T-cell Lymphomia	Blanka Rihovah	2011		Study
67	Cancer Cell Radioresistance	Katja Storch	2016		Study
84	**Gynaecology**				
84	Chick Embryo Study: Teratogenesis	Jelinek Richard	2002		Study
90	Chick Embryo Study: Teratogenesis	Jelinek Richard	2002		Lecture
95	**Otorhinolaryngology**				
95	Tinnitus	Imre Szilágyi	2010	214	Study
107	Tinnitus, Balance Disorders	Habil Géza József		67	Study
108	Hyperacusis	Mikael Bäckman	2004	39	Study
125	Tinnitus	Imre Szilágyi	2010	214	Lecture

Page	Category / Specialty	Doctor / Researcher	Year	Subjects	Type
127	**Endocrinology**				
127	Hypothyroidism, PPD, GB, EOP, etc.	Balogh Imre			Report
131	**Internal Medicine**				
131	Cystic Fibrosis	Kesserü P, Kiss	2011		Study
139	**Pain Therapy**				
139	Rheumatology	Gomez Roberto	2011		Lecture
140	Pain Therapy	Eva Csecsei	2011	165	Lecture
142	Pain Therapy in Neurosurgery	Zoltän Nemeti	2011	232	Lecture
144	Fatigue in Multiple Sclerosis	Piatkowski J	2009	37	Study
152	Fatigue in Multiple Sclerosis	Piatkowski J	2009	37	Study
159	Multiple Sclerosis Tensor Fascia Lata	Duray Péter		20	Study
160	Musculoskeletal Physiotherapy	Franciska Gyulai	2015	100	Study
170	**Neurology**				
170	Strokes and Motor Neurone Disease	Terezia Szemerszki		3 Cases	Results
171	Delayed Speech Development	Szabolcs M. Horváth	2007		Summary
172	**Orthopedics**				
172	Osteoporosis	Kafka W	2005		Study
177	Various Orthopaedic Diseases	Hans Härtling			Study
179	Fibromyalgia	Freitag-Perez K	2002	150	Study
182	Knee Osteoarthritis	Sabsabi Y	2005	100	Study
189	**Physiology**				
189	Microcirculation	Klopp R			Study
218	Microcirculation and Vasomotion	Klopp R	2009	48	Study
219	Organ Blood Flow	Wolfgang Bohn	2011		Lecture
220	Mitochondrial ATP	Klopp R	2011		Lecture
221	Hemoglobin Oxygen Affinity	Wolf A Kafka	2003		Study
229	Autorhythmic Arteriolar Wall Movement	Klopp R	2010	28	Study
231	Pseudomonas Aeruginosa	Kesserü Péter			Study
232	Embyotoxic Cyclophosphamide	Jelinek Richard			Study
240	Erythrocytes	Krzysztof Spodaryk		32	Study
247	Quality of Life	György Seress	2011		Lecture
248	**Rehabilitation**				
248	Rehabilitatoin	Kovács Matild		110	Study
251	Physical Vasomotion	Klopp R	2013		Abstract
252	Rehabilitation and Orthopaedics	Stryla W	2004	497	Study

Page	Category / Specialty	Doctor / Researcher	Year	Subjects	Type
258	**Sports Medicine**				
258	CK Elimination Curve	Möbes K	2003	17	Study
262	Performance Capacity	J. Malomsoki	2006	12	Study
270	Sports Medicine	Klaus Jung	2010		Lecture
272	Sports Competition	Armin Dirschauer	2001		Lectuer
273	Musculoskeletal Sports Injuries	L. Weisskopf	2011		Abstract
274	Muscle Soreness	Krzysztof Spodaryk	2002	36	Study
281	**Dentistry**				
281	Odontogenic Disease	Zehner P	2007	35	Study
281	Dental Anxiety	Michels-Wakili S	2003		Study
282	**Veterinary Medicine**				
282	General Veterinary	Mezősi László		117 + 3 Cases	Report
284	Bovine Fertility	Preissinger M	2001	14	Study
291	**History**				
291	Technological History of Bemer	Wolfgang Bohn	1013		Editorial

BEMER Therapy Applied in General Medical Practice

Schönfeld, Rolf; MR Dr. med.; Berlin

SUMMARY: The BEMER therapy is outstanding for treatment of acute symptoms. Approx. 90% of patients had no symptoms or experienced improvements within a short period of time.
Rolf Scaahönfeld

ABSTRACT: *The BEMER therapy is an excellent tool. Following ad hoc applications, 90% of acute complaints were improved or resolved within short periods of time.*

The BEMER therapy is outstanding for treatment of acute symptoms. Approx. 90% of patients had no symptoms or experienced improvements within a short period of time.

To want to praise the benefits of the BEMER therapy at this congress would be to carry coals to Newcastle. But if, nonetheless, I present the benefits of the BEMER therapy as a result of my case studies in general medical practice, it is not to carry coals to Newcastle, but to provide answers to the following questions.

1. Is the BEMER therapy used more for acute or chronic illnesses in general medical practice?
2. For what illnesses or symptoms is the BEMER therapy particularly appropriate?
3. Are certain age groups preferred regarding the use of the BEMER therapy?
4. Are their gender-specific differences when using the BEMER therapy?
5. Can the BEMER therapy also be used effectively for short treatment periods?
6. Is the BEMER therapy a suitable treatment method at all for a general practice?

The answers to these questions will provide us with further clues as to how the BEMER therapy can be used even more effectively and will also supply us with arguments to convince other colleagues of the benefit of the BEMER therapy in general practice.

At this point, without anticipating my results, I would like to point to the need for the BEMER therapy to be widely used in general practice. The general practitioner – the family doctor – is in most cases the first point of contact for patients and is the most important source of advice for further diagnosis and therapy. The GP is also the doctor who sees the largest variety of patients, the greatest diversity of illnesses and symptoms to be treated and therefore also with the most diverse treatment spectrum. The GP can therefore exploit the most common possible applications of the BEMER therapy.

However, this depends on bringing this excellent, painless therapy with virtually no side-effects, which has as good as no contraindications to the attention of as many general practitioners as possible. This is the aim of my investigation.

At this point, I will show you a statement that I actually planned for the end of my lecture:

We are not only responsible for what we do, but also for what we do not do!

Let us turn now to the concrete results of my investigations of the BEMER therapy as applied in general medical practice.

A total of 201 patients were included in the investigation from April 1999 to July 2000.

The investigation only took into account those patients who received the BEMER therapy in practice or took a therapy device back home for treatment over a limited period of time. The investigation did not look at all those patients, who have purchased a therapy device and use it independently following a recommendation by their doctor. As the overview indicates, the number of female and male patients was almost the same. However, there are significant differences in terms of application for acute or chronic illnesses and symptoms and in terms of whether the therapy sessions were in practice or at home. More than 60% of sessions took place for acute illnesses/symptoms or in practice.

The patients universe

	Number of patients	In %
Total	201	100.0
Female	103	51.2
Male	98	48.8
Acute	123	61.2
Chronic	78	38.8
Practice	136	67.7
At home	65	32.3

The following overview shows that the BEMER therapy was used in all age categories, although it is also clear that the therapy was used in approx. 80% of cases between the ages of 31 and 60 for acute illnesses and symptoms and in approx. 70% of cases between the ages of 41 and 70 for chronic illnesses and symptoms.

BEMER – Application – Overview

| Age | Acute | Chronic | Application | | Male | Female |
			Practice	At home		
-10		2		2		2
-20	4		3	1	4	
-30	6	2	8		6	2
-40	31	7	28	10	22	16
-50	39	15	42	12	26	38
-60	27	14	26	15	19	22
-70	10	26	23	13	14	22
-80	3	7	5	5	4	6
>80	3	5	1	7	3	5
	123	78	136	65	98	103

Before entering into a closer analysis of acute and chronic illnesses and symptoms, I will show you how the patients evaluated the success of therapy by symptom-free and improved.

Therapy – Successes

	No.	Symptom free	in %	Improvement	in %
Male	98	58	59.2	30	30.6
Female	103	35	34.0	53	54.1
	201	93	46.3	83	41.3

This evaluation shows that 87.6% of the patients treated with the BEMER therapy device experienced no symptoms or an improvement in symptoms after completing the treatment. That statement overall applies almost identically to men and women. However, in terms of freedom from symptoms, there is a significant difference between the genders.

I shall start with a few short comments on the following analyses regarding acute and chronic illnesses and symptoms. The investigation only recorded the illnesses and symptoms specified by the patients at the start of treatment. It turned out during treatment and thereafter that many patients reported an improvement in symptoms that they had not specified or not really noticed. This was the case in particular for insomnia, agitation, general feelings of weakness and functional abdominal symptoms, to mention but a few. However, high blood pressures were reduced and the metabolic control in insulin-dependent diabetics was improved so that daily insulin doses could be reduced. Most frequently, patients reported improved sleeping patterns and associated improved general activity.

Among those suffering from acute illnesses/symptoms, a total of 63.5% experienced freedom from symptoms and a total of 30% reported improvement in their symptoms. Overall, therefore, the therapy had a positive outcome for more than 90% of those treated.

Acute Illnesses / Symptoms

Diagnoses	Number	in %	Symptom free	Improvement	Unchanged
Lumbar/back pain syndrome	29	21.2	11	15	3
Shoulder pain	27	19.7	20	5	2
Myogelosis Shoulder/neck	19	13.9	16	2	1
Bruising	12	8.8	11		1
Distortions	9	6.6	8	1	
Epicondylitis	9	6.6	3	4	2
Cephalgia/migranes	5	3.6	3	2	
Sleep disorders	4	2.9	2	2	
General physical performance	4	2.9		4	
Fractures (detumescent)	4	2.9	3	1	
Vegetative symptoms	4	2.9	2	2	1
Joint pain	3	2.2	1	2	
Teeth after tooth extraction	3	2.2	3		

Whiplash/Cervical spine	2	1.5	1	1	
Forearm tendonitis	2	1.5	2		
Burns 1+2°	1	0.7	1		
Totals	**137**		**87**	**41**	**9**

The discrepancy in the number of patients is due to multiple symptoms.

By contrast, only 18% of those treated with chronic illnesses/symptoms (see the following table) described freedom from symptoms at the end of treatment. This significant different in treatment outcome compared to acute illnesses/symptoms confirms the finding that longer therapy periods may be required for chronic illnesses/symptoms, including periods of significantly more than 4 weeks.

Nonetheless, a total of 69% of those treated in this group reported a significant improvement in symptoms, even if they did not report freedom from symptoms. So even under chronic illnesses/symptoms, the treatment had a positive outcome in approx. 83% of cases.

At this point, I would like to make a few short comments about using the BEMER therapy device. The therapy mat and the applicator are used both as individual therapy devices and in combination one after the other. The therapy programs for specific illnesses/symptoms are outside the scope of this lecture, as they would take some time to describe. I can, however, confirm that I have followed the therapy recommendations of the Academy for Bioenergetics (AFB) as far as possible. When using the applicator in combination with the mat, I found that it was more effective to start with the applicator and finish with the mat. Programs P3 or P4 with the mat proved to be most effective for treatment of lumbar symptoms.

Chronic Illnesses / Symptoms

The discrepancy in the number of patients is due to multiple symptoms.

Diagnoses	Number	in %	Symptom free	Improvement	Unchanged
Poor performance	16	11.7	3	12	1
Lumbar/back pain syndrome	12	8.8	1	9	2
Knee joint symptoms	10	7.3	3	6	2
Sleep disorders	10	7.3	4	6	
Cervical pain	9	6.6	1	6	2
Shoulder pain	9	6.6	3	4	2
Psychological symptoms	8	5.8	3	5	
Hip joint pain	5	3.6		4	1
Hypertension	4	2.8		3	1
Myogelosis Shoulder/neck	3	2.2		1	2
Arthralgia/Finger joints	3	2.2		3	
Cephalgia/migranes	3	2.2		2	1
Osteoporosis pain	2	1.5		2	

Abdominal pain post operation	2	1.5	1		1
Bronchial/asthma	2	1.5		2	
Other	8	5.8		4	3
Totals	106		19	69	18
			17.9	65.1	17.0

I have analyzed the duration of treatment by days to answer the question whether the BEMER therapy is also suitable for short treatment periods:

Treatment Period in Days

Days	Number of patients	In %
-3	10	5.0
-7	46	22.9
-10	55	27.4
-14	21	10.4
-21	28	13.9
-28	30	14.9
>28	11	5.5

This analysis show that a treatment period of up to 10 days was sufficient for approx. 50% and a period of 14 days was sufficient for a further 10% (so for a total of approx. 60%).

Therapy – Successes for Acute Illnesses

	Number	In %
Symptom free	82	66.7
Improvement	32	26.0
Unchanged	9	7.3
	123	

	Number	1st week	in %	2nd week	in %	After 2nd week	in %
Male	69	26	37.7	23	33.3	49	71.0
Female	54	17	31.5	9	16.7	26	48.1
	123	43	35.0	32	26.0	75	61.0

This overview shows that approx. 93% of patients reported a positive treatment outcome after treatment for acute illnesses/symptoms.

Taking into account the duration of treatment, it can be seen that approx. 35% reported freedom from symptoms or improvement after just one week of treatment and a total of 61% reported freedom from symptoms or improvement after the second week of treatment.

The overview of acute illnesses/symptoms you have already seen includes 16 different types of illness and symptom. Categorizing the illnesses and symptoms reveals that approx. 60% of acute illnesses/symptoms are musculoskeletal and approx. 20% are the result of accidents.

Separate evaluation of successful therapy outcomes shows that in fact more than 95% of patients suffering after accidents reported improvement. That is significant evidence of the special therapeutic effectiveness of the BEMER therapy device for treatment of injuries from accidents, in particular when treating distortions and bruising associated in conjunction with swelling.

Acute Illnesses / Symptoms

Total: 137, of which:	Number	In %
Musculoskeletal	87	63.5
Injuries after accidents	28	20.4
	115	83.9

Therapy – Successes

	Musculoskeletal		Injuries after accidents	
	Number	in %	Number	in %
Symptom free	51	58.6	24	85.7
Improvement	28	32.2	3	10.7
Total	79	90.8	27	96.4

Successful therapy outcomes for chronic illnesses/symptoms demonstrated significant deviations compared to acute illnesses/symptoms over the period of investigation.

Chronic Illnesses/Symptoms

	Total 106, of which:	Number	In %
1.	Musculoskeletal	53	50
2.	Psychological symptoms	18	16.98
3.	Poor performance, Various causes	16	15.1
		87	82.1

Therapy Successes

	For 1.		For 2.		For 3.	
Symptom free	8	15.1	7	38.9	3	18.8
Improvement	35	66.0	11	61.1	12	75.0
Total	43	81.1	18	100.0	15	93.8

The proportion of successes in the musculoskeletal category in acute illnesses/symptoms was 63.5%, but only 50% in chronic illnesses/symptoms. Psychological symptoms and general poor performance from various causes, including poor performance in malignant illnesses, are very prominent at approx. 15% in each case.

It is extremely interesting that all patients with psychological symptoms and approx. 90% of those with poor performance reported improvement.

These results show very clearly further specific possible uses of the BEMER therapy.

As a result of these investigations, my answers to the questions we began with are as follows:

1. In general practice, the BEMER therapy device is primarily used for acute illnesses/symptoms.
2. The BEMER therapy is particularly useful for acute illnesses/symptoms of musculoskeletal origin or following accidents. It is particularly suited to treating swelling after bruising and distortions, as well as to reducing pain.

In chronic illnesses/symptoms, musculoskeletal complaints are also relevant, but so are psychological symptoms such as sleep disorders, agitation and general poor performance from various causes.

3. Preferred age groups arise solely from the frequency of the specific illnesses at the different stages of life. The BEMER therapy is suitable for all age groups.
4. Gender-specific differences were not generally to be found. Patients who underwent treatment with the BEMER therapy device were approx. 50% female and male and each gender reported approx. 90% positive treatment outcomes. However, it was found that significantly more men were treated for injuries after accidents. There was also a significant difference alone in terms of perceived freedom from symptoms at the end of treatment. A total of 60% of men confirmed freedom from symptoms, but only approx. 35% of women. This difference may be explained by the different proportions of men and women treated for injuries after accidents and the particularly good therapy outcomes identified in that category.
5. The BEMER therapy is also very suited to short treatment periods. More than 60% of patients reported significant alleviation of their symptoms or freedom from symptoms after just 2 weeks. For specific illnesses/symptoms, application for just a few days is also an option, e.g. for bruising, burns or after tooth extraction.
6. In my opinion, the answer to the last question, whether the BEMER therapy is a suitable treatment method for a general practice, is an unambiguous "YES". The BEMER therapy device is a medical treatment device with a broad spectrum of application that we cannot – in my opinion – withhold from our patients... because all our patients are VIPs!

In the original meaning of the word, trust in the doctor or in the practice. Image of a practice or innovations product or practice specialisms such as BEMER therapy. Let us walk this path together to success.

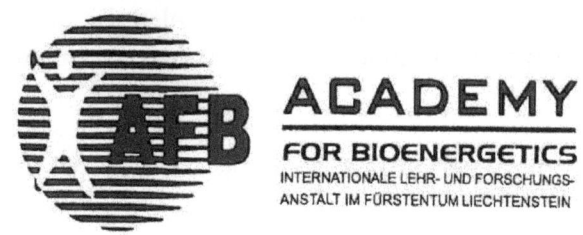

Academy for Bioenergetics

Schliessa 12FL-9495 Triesen
Tel. 00423 399 38 28
Fax. 00423 399 38 29
Email: afb@afb.li

May 1999 to December 2002

Michaelis Horst, Director of the Academy for Bioenergetics (AFB), Liechtenstein

SUMMARY: A total of 1,116 patients were treated using the BEMER therapy and documented over 6 weeks in 220 medical facilities (clinics, practices etc.).

A total of 851 (76%) of the patients reported freedom from symptoms or significant improvement in at least one symptom; a total of 196 (18%) reported improvements; and just 69 (6%) experienced no change in their state of health during the treatment period of 6 weeks.

Commissioned to perform the study: Academy for Bioenergetics, International Teaching and Research Institute, Triesen, Michaelis, H.

Objective: Identification of the therapeutic effects of the BEMER signal in a multi-center medical user study.

A total of 220 medical facilities participated in the study. Participation was voluntary and was not compensated; only the study devices were made available on loan.

Materials and methods: Patient selection and treatment was done independently of the AFB by the treating physicians. As the therapists wanted to test the effect of the BEMER 3000 critically, they predominantly selected cases untreatable by conventional medicine (patients treated using conservative therapies based on conventional medicine but without therapeutic progress over a prolonged period). Diagnoses were made using conventional medical standards. In polymorbid patients the different symptoms were assessed individually. The specific symptom status or the degree severity of the illness was classified on a five level evaluation scale.

The BEMER 3000 was generally used as a monotherapy in accordance with general therapeutic indications. Patients who were taking medication to treat their specific symptoms continued their medication in scope and dosage. The study protocol documented previous therapeutic methods and the therapeutic parameters with respect to the BEMER therapy, as well as the subjective and objective assessment of the course of therapy.

All treatments lasting at least four weeks and the cases in which satisfactory therapeutic outcomes were achieved in the past were included in the assessment. The five level evaluation scale was reduced to the categories "symptom-free/good", "better" and "unchanged" for greater clarity.

A total of 1,116 protocols satisfied the evaluation criteria. As a number of participating patients were suffering from several symptoms, there were a total of 2,031 cases. A total of 42 different main illness groups with at least ten cases are listed. The average period of therapy was six weeks.

Results:
- Patient-based evaluation
    - 851 patients (76%) are symptom-free/good in at least one symptom
    - 196 patients (18%) demonstrated improvement in at least one symptom
    - 69 patients (6%) showed no imporvement in health within the treatment period.

- Illness-based evaluation:
    - 65% of illnesses treated were evaluated as "symptom-free/good"
    - 23% of the illnesses showed improvement
    - 12% did not experience any change in the treatment period.

The AFB wishes to thank the many participants who made this study possible, especially the medical practitioners, the medical device consultants and BEMER Medizintechnik GmbH (Germany and Hungary). All participants demonstrated tremendous commitment and co-operation in collating the many protocols.

Horst Michaelis
Director of the AFB

AFB 11.19.2003

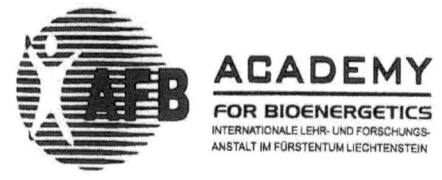

Multi-center medical user study with the BEMER 3000 System©AFB 24.10.2003 1116 Patient protocols // Therapy period > 4 weeks or freedom from symptoms 2031 cases (frequency) // in short period // 42 main illness groups // Average therapy period: 6 weeks

Total Cases: 2031

Symptoms	Freq	Number of Patients			Percent			Therapy period (weeks)
		Good / sympt free	better	Unchd.	Good / sympt free	Better	Unchd.	
General wellbeing	223	165	42	16	74	19	7	6
General pain	32	23	8	1	72	25	3	5
Allergies	23	16	4	3	70	17	13	5
Arthrosis / arthritis	236	112	83	41	48	35	17	6
Bronchial asthma	21	11	5	5	52	24	24	6
Spinal disc complaints	33	13	7	13	39	22	39	6
Depression	42	27	11	4	64	26	10	6
Diabetes mellitus	28	15	6	7	54	21	25	7
Circulatory disorders	67	46	16	5	69	24	7	6
Endoprosthesis	15	4	7	4	27	46	27	8
Inflammatory	46	38	4	4	82	9	9	4
Fibromyalgia	12	3	3	6	25	25	50	7
Fractures	22	22	/	/	100	/	/	5
Joint pain / arthralgia	47	37	6	4	79	13	8	4
Heart diseases	22	11	3	8	50	14	36	7
Hypertension	54	32	13	9	59	24	17	6
Weak immune system	16	12	4	/	75	25	/	5
Incontinence / Urination disorders	10	6	3	1	60	30	10	5
Sciatica / lumbago	46	38	4	4	82	9	9	4
Headaches	50	37	9	4	74	18	8	5
Stomach complaints	16	14	1	1	88	6	6	4
Meniscus complaints	11	8	3	/	73	27	/	4
Migranes	49	30	14	5	61	29	10	6

Bekhterev's disease	11	6	2	3	55	18	27	7
Fatigue / fatigue sydr.	63	45	14	4	72	22	6	6
Multiple sclerosis	14	4	6	4	28	44	28	8
Muscle tension	48	32	13	3	87	27	6	5
Edemata	17	13	3	1	76	18	6	5
Osteoporosis	30	18	9	3	60	30	10	6
Psycho-vegetative disorders	21	11	9	1	52	43	5	5
Rheumatic symptoms	48	34	11	3	71	23	6	6
Sleep disorders	176	115	42	19	65	24	11	6
Shoulder impingement syndrome	46	35	8	3	76	17	7	6
Dizziness	14	5	5	4	36	36	28	6
Metabolic disorder	16	7	5	4	44	31	25	7
Tennis elbow	20	16	3	1	80	15	5	6
Tinnitus	33	8	17	8	24	52	24	6
Conseq's of trauma	48	48	/	/	100	/	/	2
Ulcers	22	18	3	1	82	14	4	7
Spine syndrome	243	162	54	27	67	22	11	6
Wound disorders	29	26	1	2	90	3	7	4
Condition after stroke	11	4	4	3	36	36	28	5

Successful medical outcomes BEMER 3000

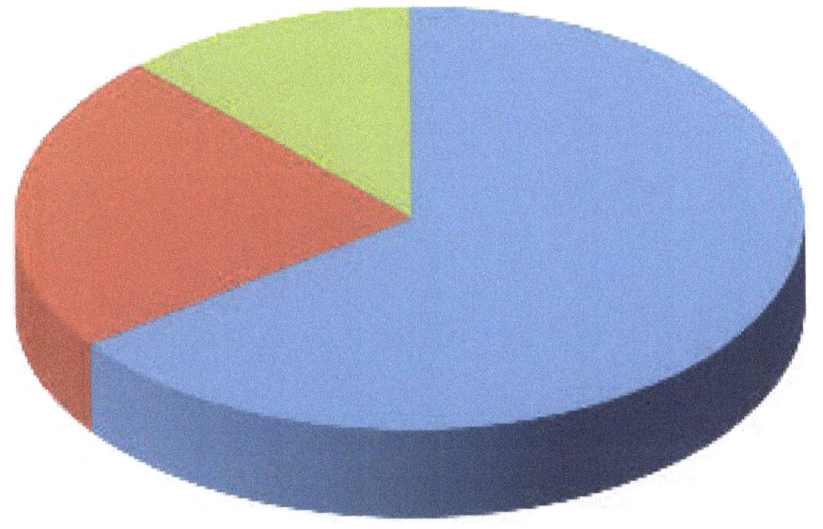

Good/symptom-free	Improved	Unchanged
65%	**23%**	**12%**

The effects of the "physical BEMER® vascular therapy", a method for the physical stimulation of the vasomotion of precapillary microvessels in case of impaired microcirculation, on sleep, pain and quality of life of patients with different clinical pictures on the basis of three scientifically validated scales

Wolfgang Bohn/ Lorenzo Hess/ Ralph Burger

ABSTRACT: As part of the statutory market monitoring of certified medical devices, 658 valid patient questionnaires were evaluated between April 2011 and March 2013. The questions consisted mainly of three scientifically recognized scales for assessing the changes of sleep, pain and quality of life in patients who had used the "physical BEMER® vascular therapy" for different diseases over 6 weeks. The result clearly shows that there are significant improvements in all areas surveyed through the application of this complementary treatment option, regardless of the underlying disease.

WOUNDCARE

Independent evaluation of BEMER© PHYSICAL VASCULAR REGULATION THERAPY

Liezl Naudé
Advanced nurse specialist: wound management
Advanced lower limb and wound management centre, Pretoria

**Heart 4 the Wounded
5-7 July
Pretoria**

Introduction
Lower limb wounds have always been a challenge not only due to the complexity of the trauma, but also because of the nature of chronic ulceration. In wound management we can utilise the best possible first world dressings we can get our hands on, but if we do not treat the cause of chronic ulceration, we will not be able to heal the wounds completely.

The pivotal point within wound management remains wound bed preparation (WBD) and we still regard moist wound healing techniques as the cornerstone of modern wound healing.[1,2] WBD was first proposed in 2000[3,4,5] and is now regarded as the prerequisite for a successful outcome in wound management globally.[6]

The difference with this module is that we have to treat the cause first before we even try to deal with the wound bed.[6] Macro-circulation is essential for life but without adequate micro-circulation we will not be able to facilitate the exchange of nutrients and waste products between the blood and surrounding tissue.[7] Circulatory disorders and the resulting oxygen deprivation leads to a serious shortage of adenosinetriphosphate (ATP), the universal biological energy generated at cellular level.

Improved circulation, especially an improved micro-circulation, increases the manufacture of sufficient biological energy in the form of ATP, improves cellular metabolism, provides a better supply of nutrients and removal of toxins in tissue and organs and hence results in a better functioning of the self-regulating mechanisms. This also ensures the organism's ability to adapt and to optimise all biological processes.

It is the protein bio-synthesis which is of paramount importance for human life and health. As a reproducing process, it is highly dependent on sufficiency of oxygen supply in the oxygen-driven ATP energy production process.

As a wound management specialist working in an advanced wound management centre, our patient profile consists of patients having several pathologies such as venous insufficiency, arterial insufficiency, lymphoedema, diabetes, malignancy, immune deficiency, arthritis, pain syndrome and many others.

Aim
The purpose of this independent evaluation is to document the impact of physical vascular BEMER therapy as a patented broad-spectrum low-intensity pulsed electromagnetic field therapy on these patients' wound healing, overall well-being and specifically their micro-vascular status.

By increasing cellular energy, BEMER treatment has been shown to improve cellular performance which facilitates the body's inherent ability to self-regulate its important physiological parameters and heal itself by:
- Improving blood circulation (micro and macro circulation)
- Strengthening the immune system through increased t-cell release
- Increase in oxygen partial pressure
- Improving blood viscosity
- Improving cell metabolism and ion pumping.

Method
In 2012 and 2013 a series of case studies were conducted on a range of different chronic wounds including foot ulcers and mixed lower leg ulcers. In this evaluation several cases will be discussed where BEMER formed part of the treatment regime. The cornerstone of this treatment was also the application of the wound bed preparation guideline enabling moist wound healing.[6]

Cases had varying medical pre-conditions, which included prior sharp debridement of devitalised tissue and different levels of bacterial load. A range of wound dressings were used according to the phase of wound healing.

Independent evaluation of BEMER© physical vascular regulation therapy utilisation

Standard BEMER protocol for all advanced lower limb and wound management centre patients

1. Patient was started on initial treatment on the body mat (BM), intensity 3 (10.5 µT), which is thereafter increased at one level for the first four treatments up until a level six intensity (21µT), which is then maintained when using the BM.
2. After the BM session (eight minutes) mini-mat (MM *Large intense applicator*) is applied directly on affected area at level 10 intensity (35 µT) for eight minutes.
   After MM session (eight minutes) the special light applicator (SLA *Small LED light applicator*) is applied directly on the wound surface at level 10 intensity (35 µT) for eight minutes.

Patient SHO001: diabetic arterial foot ulcer right maleoli		
Patient history	**Photo 1**	**Photo 2**
Mr S is a 59-year old male with a history of arterial insufficiency and diabetes. Patient had angioplasty and bypass surgery, small ulceration still remained for longer than one year. BEMER therapy was started with moist wound healing.		
Evaluation		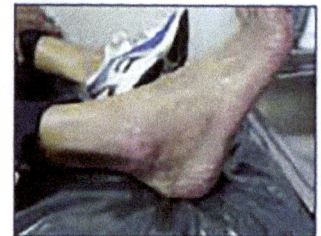
Patient intially experienced severe claudication, he had no quality of life and could not even go shopping with his wife. Within two weeks of using the BEMER, the wound healed and the patient was able to walk without pain. He was also able to start swimming again without experiencing calf cramps halfway through his exercises. His saturation rate improved significantly to a constant 93%. After six months the wound was still healed. Patient now has his own BEMER at home and his overall health has improved significantly. He is able to exercise and have an active lifestyle for the first time in more than a year. He also got a clean bill of health from the vascular surgeon and no further vascular interventions were indicated at this point in time.		

Patient CRO005: arterial foot ulcer		
Patient history	**Photo 1**	**Photo 2**
A 25-year old male patient with a history of ulceration for more than three months. Patient has a history of intermittent claudication over the past two years. Capillary refill count five. Poor pulse quality with severe pain 9/10.		

Evaluation

Patient's wound improved significantly even though basic wound dressings were used. Within the first four BEMER sessions capillary refil changed to three and stayed at three for the last month. Pulses are now bounding and overall condition of the foot improved. No oedema present. Patient had a computer topograph angiogram and the vascular surgeon decided not to do any surgery due to the significant improvement without any intervention at this stage. BEMER therapy is the main focus of treatment and wound dressings are used to facilitate autolytic debridement. Patient is able to sleep better and mobility has improved. Pain now 6/10. This patient benefited significantly from the BEMER units at the centre as part of the evaluation. He is undergoing as many sessions of BEMER as possible.

Independent evaluation of BEMER© physical vascular regulation therapy utilisation

Patient DEA001: chronic venous leg ulcer

Patient history	Photo 1	Photo 2
Patient is a 70-year old male with a history of chronic venous ulceration. He also had localised infection and severe arthritis. At the start of his treatment the ulcer was very painful 8/10.	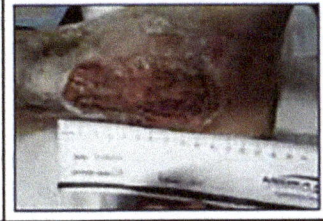	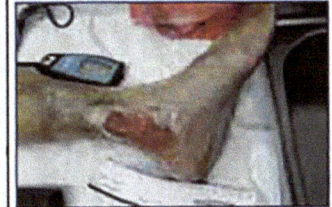

Evaluation

BEMER therapy is combined with compression therapy and advanced wound care products. A significant increase in vascular flow and oxygen levels are seen after each BEMER session.

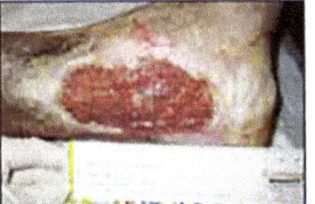 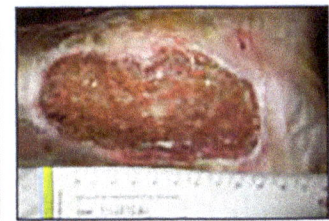

Patient BRI002: Reynaud's syndrome and connective tissue disorder

Patient history	Photo 1	Photo 2
A 57-year old female patient with auto-immune disorder, Reynaud's syndrome, arterial insufficiency, arthrosclerosis and connective tissue disorder. Pain 9/10 at start of treatment.	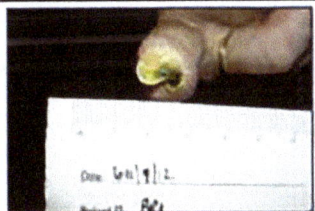	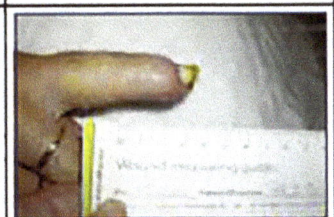

Evaluation

Improved circulation within two weeks of using the BEMER. All digit wounds healed with no new ulcerations for the first time in one year. Patient has had no new wounds for the past five months since using the BEMER three times per week as maintenance treatment. Saturation improved from 85% to 92% after BEMER sessions. Patient experienced better mobility as well. Whilst using the BEMER once a week patient had no recurrence of ulceration. Patient stopped coming to the centre for three months. Pain started flaring up again and small ulceration occurred. Patient is now using the BEMER once a week in a maintenance programme and for the last two months and had no recurrence.

Patient KHA001: diabetes, severe oedema, pain and heart failure

Patient history	Photo 1	Photo 2
A 76-year old female diabetic patient with a history of pressure sores after hospitalisation for heart failure. Patient could not mobilise at all and had severe pitting oedema bilateral. Wound slow to heal and pain 8/10. Biphasic pulses with doppler evaluation.	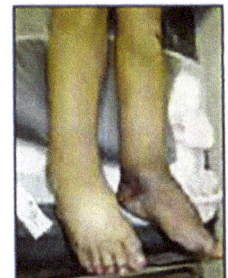	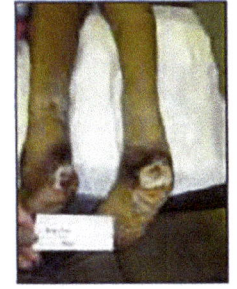

Evaluation

Decrease in oedema within one week of BEMER therapy three times per week. Only very light crepe bandages were applied below the knees to assist with managing the oedema in between BEMER sessions. Both the ulcers demarcated well and overall condition improved significantly. Pain decreased to 4/10 and patient is now able to stand on her own with minimal assistance.

Independent evaluation of BEMER© physical vascular regulation therapy utilisation

Patient POT003: venous ulceration

Patient history

A 72-year old female diabetic patient with a history of ulceration after falling and creating a degloving injury one month ago. Wound slow to heal and pain 8/10. ABPI = 0.9

Photo 1 | **Photo 2**

Evaluation

Wound healing improved significantly with better perfusion after application of BEMER therapy. Patient's pain decreased and oedema also decreased. Wound healed in less than two months with good epithelial skin requiring weekly dressings with light compression and weekly BEMER sessions.

Patient DEB003: burn wound diabetic patient

Patient history

A 44-year old type 1 diabetic patient with a history of a nonhealing deep partial thickness burn wound. Pain 8/10. Bounding pulses. Wound present for two months. Patient was not able to walk on the foot at all.

Photo 1 | **Photo 2**

Evaluation

Patient had an immediate decrease in pain with the first BEMER session. After one week pain levels were experienced as 2/10 and after two weeks the patient was able to go back to work. He was also able to walk normally without crutches. To his delight some pigmentation also returned as can be seen in the photographs.

Patient BEY002: spider bite left hand

Patient history

A 32-year old male patient bitten by a spider on his hand resulting in severe oedema and discomfort. Pain 8/10. Patient immediately started with antibiotics and BEMER standard protocol.

Photo 1 | **Photo 2**

Evaluation

Initial swelling was severe, but decreased within 30 minutes after the first session. Patient was able to utilise the BEMER initially for three times per day. By day three he had no discomfort and swelling was gone. Two weeks after the incident he had no pain and no complications.

Independent evaluation of BEMER© physical vascular regulation therapy utilisation

Comparison photographs before and after BEMER therapy sessions

Standard protocol for all wound management patients:
Patient starts on initial treatment on the Body Mat (BM) intensity three (10.5 µT), which is thereafter increased at one level for the first four treatments up until a level six intensity (21 µT), which is then maintained when using the Body Mat.
After the BM session (eight minutes) Mini-mat (MM large intense applicator) is applied directly on affected area at level 10 intensity (35 µT) for eight minutes. After MM session (eight minutes) the small LED light applicator is applied directly on the wound surface at level 10 intensity (35 µT) for eight minutes.

Before treatment session	After treatment session	Wound photograph before BEMER therapy	Wound photograph before BEMER therapy
SpO2 = 87% Pulse = 84 BP = 142/88mmHg Pain = 7/10	SpO2 = 92% Pulse = 78 BP = 135/78mmHg Pain = 6/10 *Improvement in tissue colour and perfusion*		
SpO2 = 92% Pulse = 85 BP = 130/85mmHg Pain = 5/10	SpO2 = 94% Pulse = 78 BP = 125/80mmHg Pain = 4/10 *Long term improvement in oedema and suppleness of the skin*		
SpO2 = 85% Pulse = 80 BP = 137/82mmHg Pain = 8/10	SpO2 = 92% Pulse = 76 BP = 125/78mmHg Pain = 7/10 *Drastic improvement in wound bed colour and perfusion*		
SpO2 = 90% Pulse = 70 BP = mmHg Pain = 0/10	SpO2 = 96% Pulse = 68 BP = mmHg Pain = 0/10 *Increased sensation, patient experiencing heat sensation at wound site*		
	Showed in these photograhs is the immediate effect of using the BEMER therapy. Keeping in mind the effects of the pulsating physical vascular regulation therapy on all the cells in the body, we can see an improved perfusion which also means increased oxygenation. This resulted in every patient having an improvement in their oxygen saturation percentage.		

Results

At the Advanced Lower Limb and Wound Management Centre in Pretoria, treatment is based on the standard BEMER protocol described on the previous page. We have seen significant results with regards to improved vascularisation, improved granulation tissue as well as tissue oxygenation (as can be seen from the before and after comparison photographs).

Overall improvement in patient well-being was significant especially with mobilisation and reduced pain levels. We have also been using the therapy in treating patients with sleep disorders and 60% of patients reported an improvement in their sleep patterns, which resulted in an overall better quality of life.

Conclusion

The cases seen in this evaluation showed a significant improvement with the use of BEMER therapy. This technology is invaluable in patients with microvascular disorders or insufficiency and has been shown to assist in saving limbs.

This technology enables me to provide the best possible care for the compromised patients that we treat. Significant to our centre is also the improvement in sensation that some of our diabetic patients experience with regards to their neuropathy, this is still very early in the studies that we do and more data need to be collected in this regard.

Overall the decrease in pain is the most significant result when dealing with patients that have wounds. We also see a remarkable difference in athletes with muscle injuries as well as bruising. Athletes recover faster from injury and have less swelling and bruising after therapy.

Improved vascular flow cannot be ignored and the value of this treatment modality is hugely underestimated in the medical fraternity. I am excited about the results so far and can't wait to improve more patient's quality of life, allowing them to take their rightfull place in society.

References available on request

BEMER Therapy Applied in Cardiology and Hematology

Mikrozirkulation im Fokus der Forschung; ISBN 978-3-033-01464-0; P510-517

KLOPP R (2008); effective support of established treatment concepts by using a specific electromagnetic AC field with additional vasomotoric stimulation in patients with diabetic polyneuropathy over 60 days.

SUMMARY: *In illnesses associated with major disruption of the microcirculation, such as diabetic polyangioneuropathy, complementary treatment using the BEMER plus system is promising.*

Chronic complications in diabetes mellitus include diabetic polyangioneuropathy and its consequences ("diabetic foot"). The so-called diabetic foot is the consequence of diabetic polyneuropathy in conjunction with diabetic microangiopathy and weakened resistance to infection. "Diabetic foot" and arterial occlusive disease often occur together, which poses a therapeutic dilemma.

A glance at the pathogenesis of chronic complications in diabetes mellitus shows clearly that the rate of success can be increased by employing other therapy options (in addition to established clinical therapy), which are aimed at influencing the functional status of the microcirculation and improving the microhemodynamic general conditions so that the first steps in immunologic reactions are not inhibited. The results of clinical observation demonstrate clearly that application of specific electromagnetic AC fields in conjunction with vasomotoric stimulation may be considered in this regard.

Figures 335 and 336.

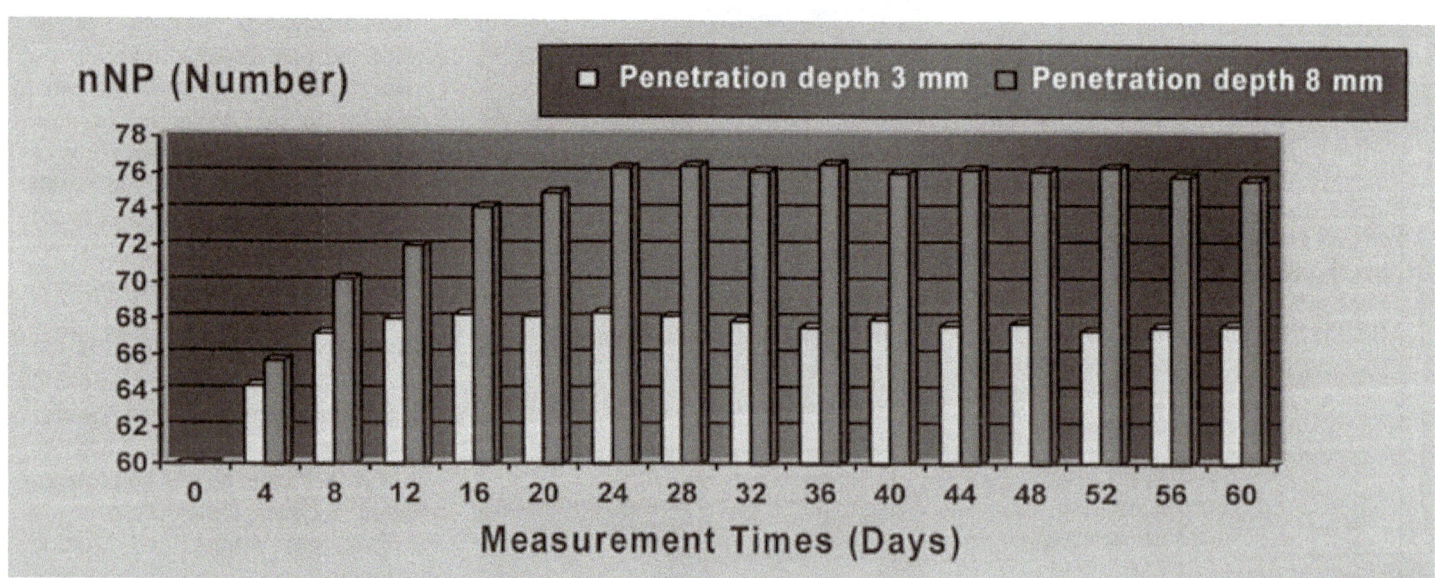

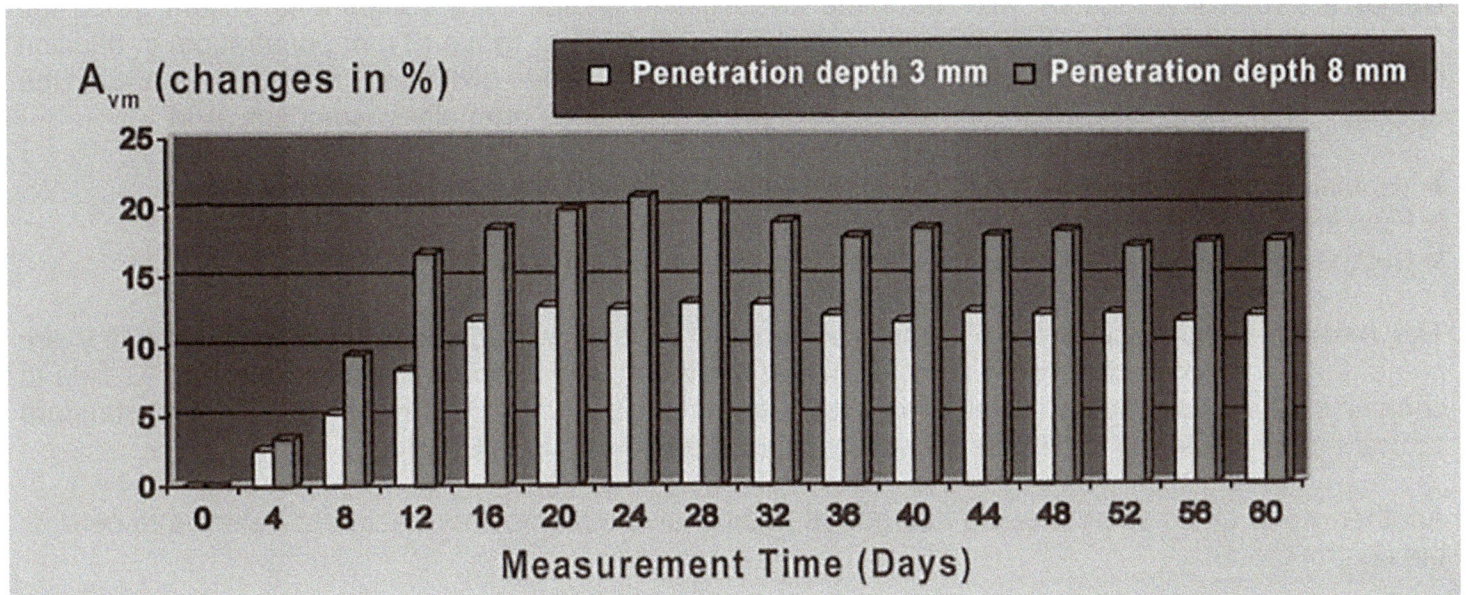

The data from the control group, which experienced worsening in the function of subcutaneous microcirculation over the 60-day period of observation, is not provided here.

In Figure 337, a selected vitalmicroscopic example exemplifies the effects of the complementary application of an electromagnetic AC field in conjunction with vasomotoric stimulation.

Figure 337

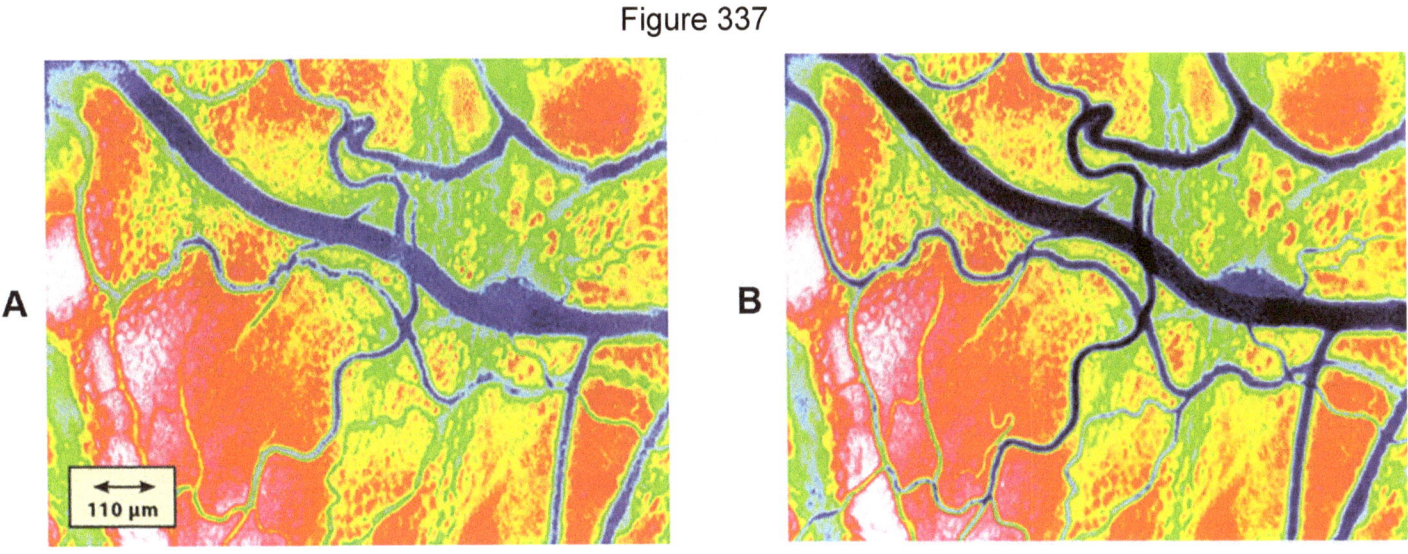

A: before additional treatment
B: after a 60-day treatment period.

Change of distribution of the plasm-blood cell mix in subcutaneous microvessels (3 mm penetration) in a male patient with diabetic polyangioneuropathy before and after 60-day treatment with a specific electromagnetic AC field.

Vitalmicroscopic finding, 1/250 sec.; pseudo-color transformation of the primary image: the blood cell perfused microvessels are indicated in blue.

During a further investigation with the same investigation design on a comparable patient group the following characteristics were recorded in the subcutaneous target tissue (3 mm penetration) in addition to the above characteristics ("Number of blood-cell perfused nodes nNP" and "Surface area under the envelope of the amplitude-frequency spectrum of the spontaneous arteriolar vasomotion AVM"):

► Venular flow stream Qven.
► Flow stream of the initial lymph QL.
► Number of adhering white blood cells at a defined venular wall area A = 18,000 µm², nWBC/A.

The measurement results from a sample of geriatric patients with diabetic polyangioneuropathy are presented. One group underwent complementary treatment with a specific electromagnetic AC field in conjunction with vasomotoric stimulation over a treatment period of 60 days in additional to standard clinical therapy (referred to here as the verum group, treated with BEMER plus).

Another group of the same size did not receive additional complementary treatment (referred to here as the control group).

Data on the characteristic "**Number of blood-cell perfused nodes nNP**" (average values) in the subcutaneous and infracutaneous target tissue of geriatric diabetics with polyangioneuropathy over a 60-day treatment period (complementary application of a specific electromagnetic AC field with additional vasomotoric stimulation). Data obtained simultaneously at two tissue depths: 3 mm and 8 mm.

Figure 338

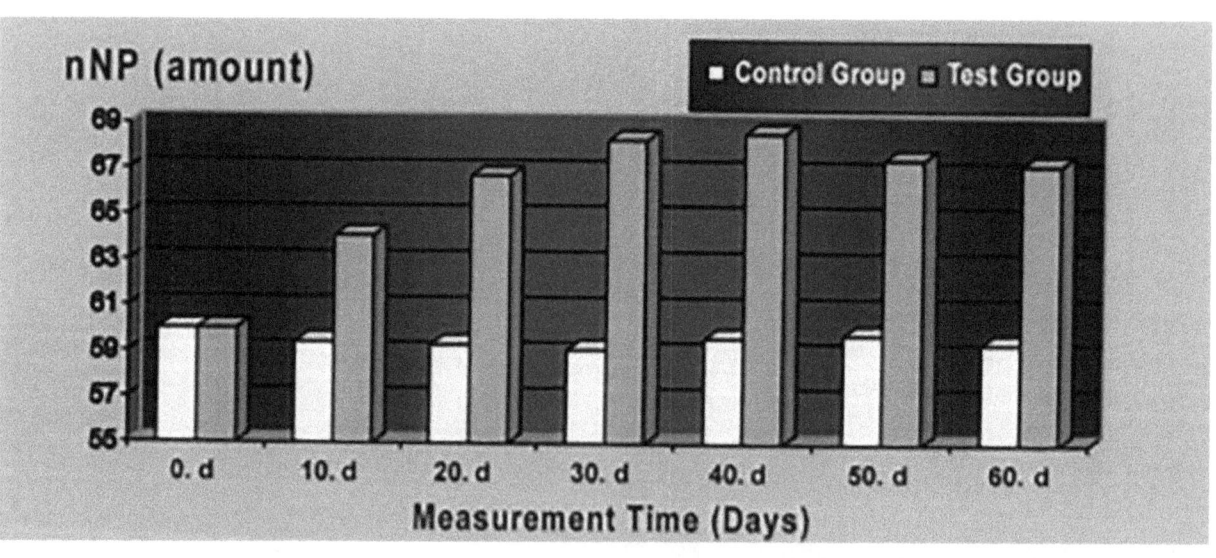

Significant characteristic differences between the data of a control group and the data of the verum group treated additionally with a specific electromagnetic AC field occurred from day 8.

Data on the characteristic "**Surface area under the envelope of the amplitude- frequency spectrum of the spontaneous arteriolar vasomotion AVM**" (average values) in the subcutaneous and infracutaneous target tissue of geriatric diabetics with polyangioneuropathy over a 60-day treatment period (complementary application of a specific electromagnetic AC field with additional vasomotoric stimulation). Data obtained simultaneously at two tissue depths: 3 mm and 8 mm.

Figure 339

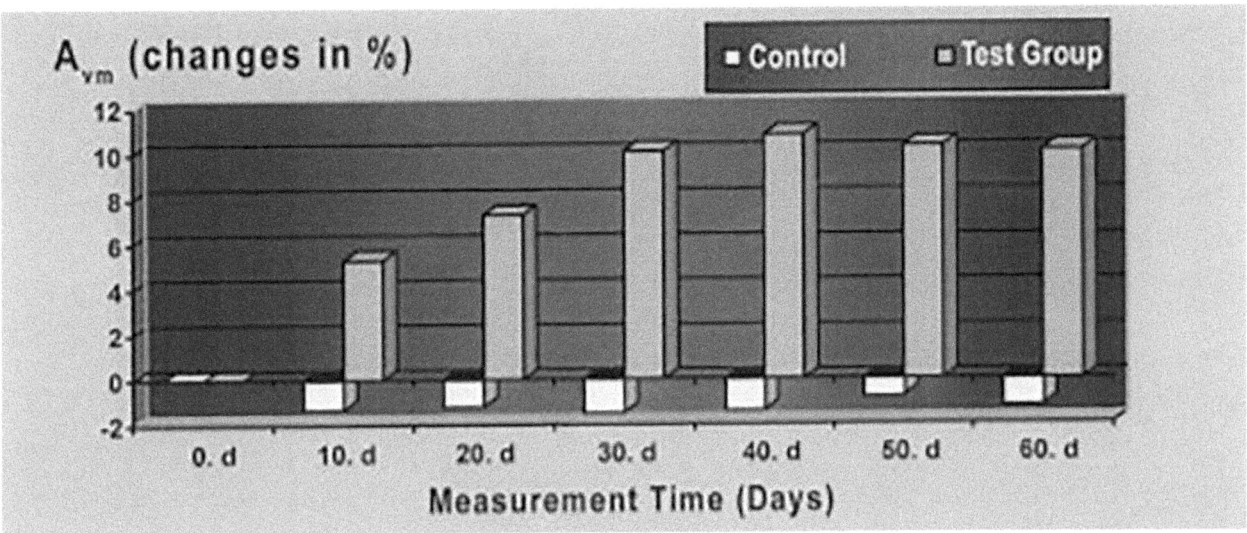

Significant characteristic differences between the data of a control group and the data of the verum group treated additionally with a specific electromagnetic AC field occurred from day 8.

Data on the characteristic "**Venular flow stream Qven**" (average values) in the subcutaneous target tissue over a 60-day treatment period in a sample of geriatric diabetics with polyangioneuropathy undergoing complementary treatment with a specific electromagnetic AC field in conjunction with vasomotion stimulation in addition to standard clinical therapy (verum group) compared to a sample that did not undergo complementary treatment (control).

Figure 340

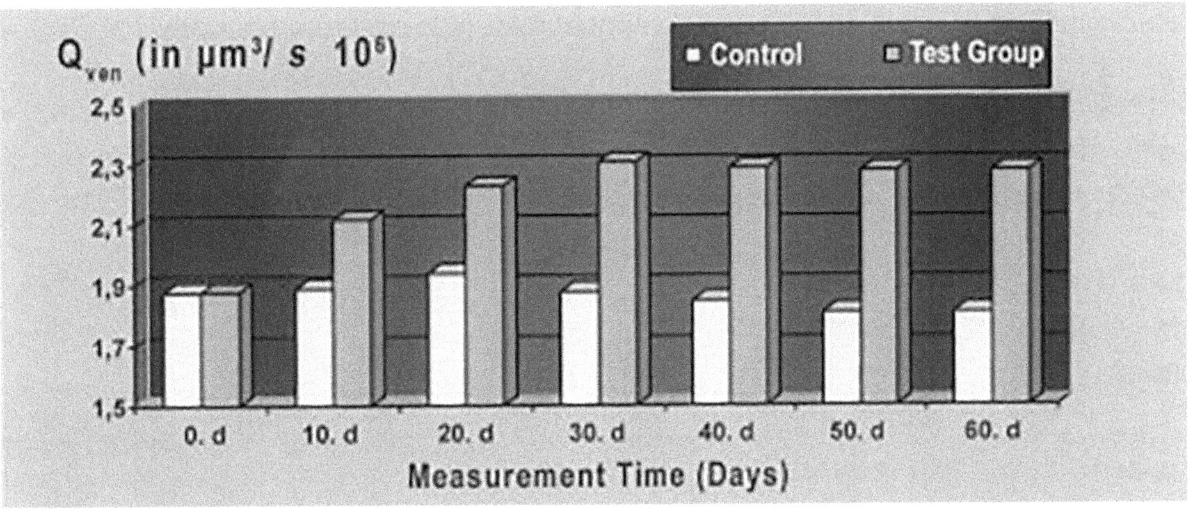

Significant characteristic differences between the data of a control group and the data of the verum group treated additionally with a specific electromagnetic AC field occurred from day 10.

Data on the characteristic "**Flow stream of the initial lymph QL**" (average values) in the subcutaneous target tissue over a 60-day treatment period in a sample of geriatric diabetics with polyangioneuropathy undergoing complementary treatment with a specific electromagnetic AC field in conjunction with vasomotion stimulation in addition to standard clinical therapy (verum group) compared to a sample that did not undergo complementary treatment (control).

Figure 341

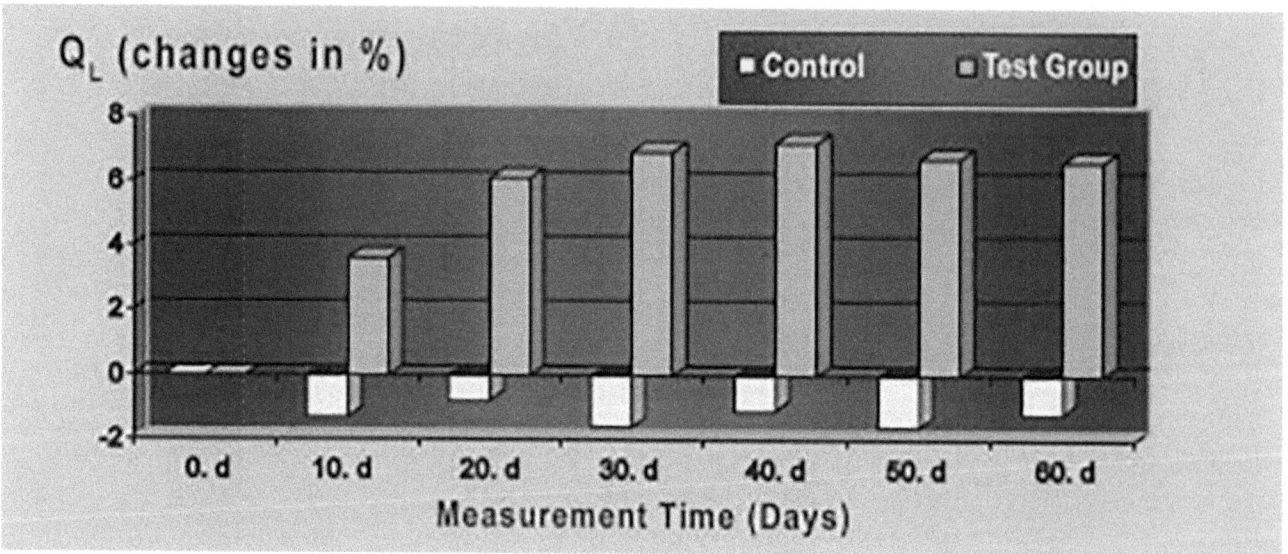

Significant characteristic differences between the data of a control group and the data of the verum group treated additionally with a specific electromagnetic AC field occurred from day 10.

Data on the characteristic "**Number of adhering white blood cells at a defined venular wall area nWBC/A**" (average values) in the subcutaneous target tissue over a 60-day treatment period in a sample of geriatric diabetics with polyangioneuropathy undergoing complementary treatment with a specific electromagnetic AC field in conjunction with vasomotion stimulation in addition to standard clinical therap y (verum group) compared to a sample that did not undergo complementary treatment (control).

Significant characteristic differences between the data of a control group and the data of the verum group treated additionally with a specific electromagnetic AC field occurred from day 10.

Figure 342

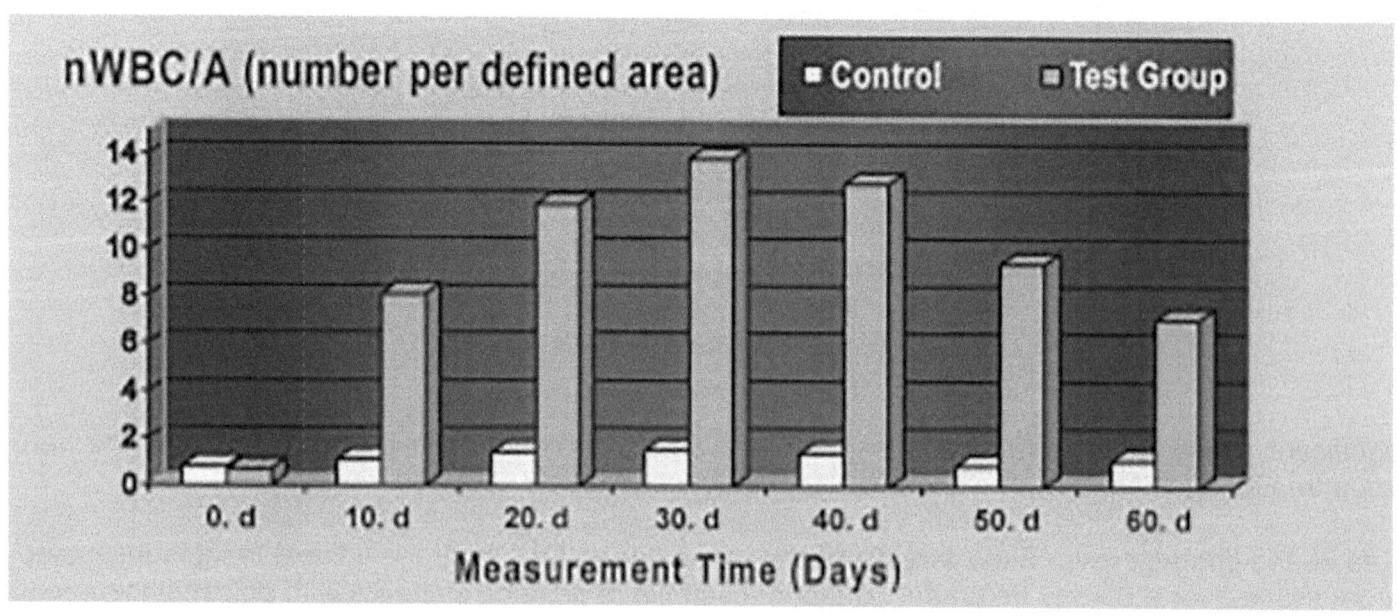

Change of distribution of the plasm-blood cell mix in subcutaneous microvessels (3 mm penetration) in a male patient with diabetic polyangioneuropathy before and after 60-day treatment with a specific electromagnetic AC field (vitalmicroscopic finding, 1/200 sec.).

Figure 343

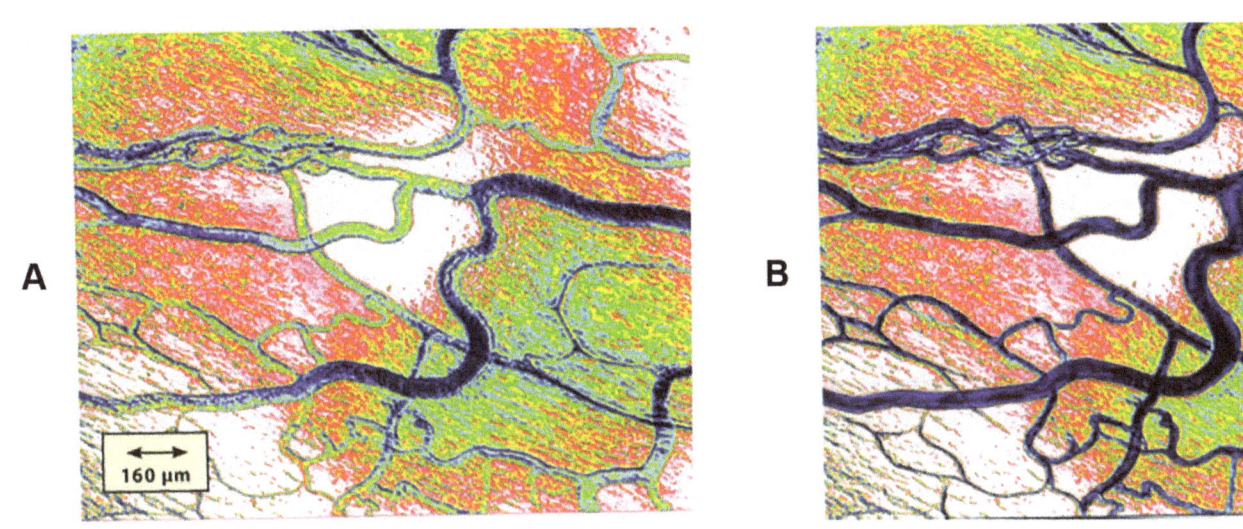

A: Before additional treatment
B: After a 60-day treatment period.

Immunologic behavioral characteristics (formation and adhesions) of white blood cells in a subcutaneous venule in a patient with diabetic polyangioneuropathy before and fater 60-day treatment with a specific electromagnetic AC field (vitalmicroscopic finding, 1/100 sec.).

Figure 344

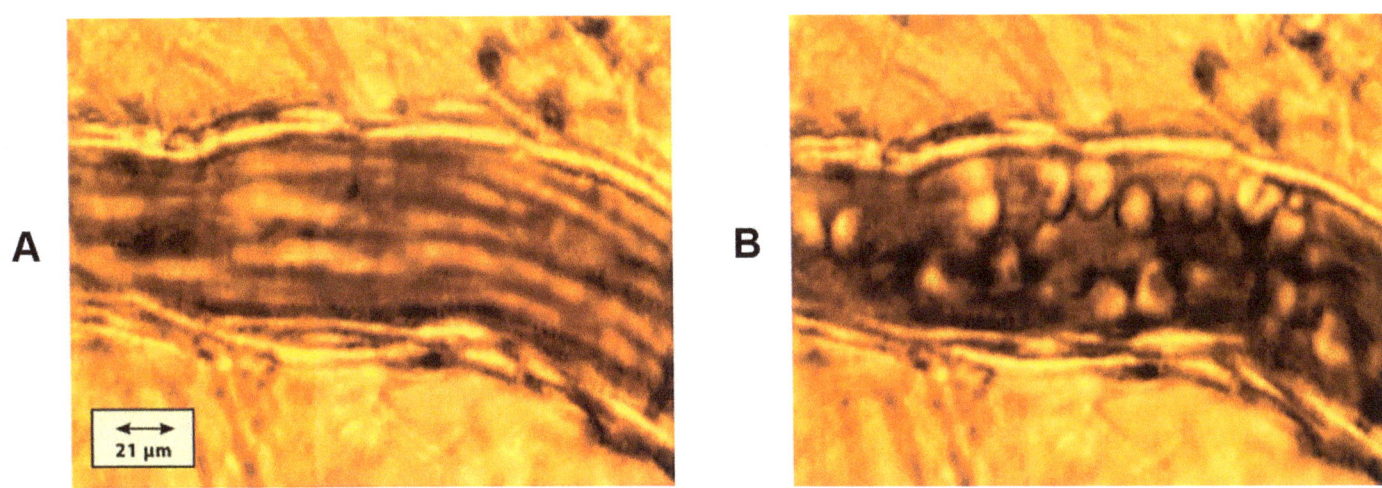

Immunologic behavioral characteristics (formation and adhesions) of white blood cells in a subcutaneous venule in a patient with diabetic polyangioneuropathy before and fater 60-day treatment with a specific electromagnetic AC field (vitalmicroscopic finding, 1/100 sec.).
A: venule section before additional treatment.
B: same venule section after 60-day treatment period.

The results of the investigation may be summarized as follows:

Complementary use of specific electromagnetic AC fields in conjunction with vasomotoric stimulation to increase the therapeutic success of established therapy concepts is promising for illnesses associated with significant disruption of the microcirculation and the cause of which cannot be treated, such as diabetic polyangioneuropathy.

BEMER Therapy in Complementary Treatment of Necrotizing Fasciitis Patients
Lecture at the BEMER Budapest Conference 2007

Zsófia Borbély; Physical Therapist

SUMMARY: *The BEMER treatment is an effective complement to causal therapy. Tissue necrosis, ischemia and edema induced by infection significantly reduce oxygenation of the tissue. Regular and adequate BEMER treatment, however, can reduce the disruption of microcirculation and the deficiency of oxygen in the tissue significantly – and increase the strength of the body's protection system. The saved extremities heal with a satisfactory level of function.*

In recent years a significant change occurred in the increase in the number of invasive infections. Globally, more and more infections caused by streptococcus pyogenes have been diagnosed. Among such infections, particular attention should be paid to necrotizing fasciitis and its serious complication, streptococcal toxic shock syndrome (STSS). In the traumatology department of our hospital, we have treated five patients in the last year with illness caused by this infection. The seriousness of infection was variable. In three cases we were able to save the extremity. In one case we were forced to amputate the extremity to save life and we lost an elderly patient, who died for another reason after remission of the underlying illness.

METHOD: The pathogenesis of the process caused by necrotizing fasciitis is not entirely unknown. The bacterial toxin and the damage to vessels play the main role in the development of the inflammation. The lethality of infection is 30%, so the therapy primarily involves adequate and regular surgical excavation, empirical therapy with antibiotics and, in the case of STSS, intensive therapeutic care.
AIM: Prevention of the continued progression of the illness, general prevention, reduction of the loss of function caused by loss of tissue.

RESULT: The BEMER treatment is an effective complement to causal therapy. Tissue necrosis, ischemia and edema induced by infection significantly reduce oxygenation of the tissue. Regular and adequate BEMER treatment, however, can reduce the disruption of microcirculation and the deficiency of oxygen in the tissue significantly – and increase the strength of the body's protection system.

The saved extremities heal with a satisfactory level of function. Despite long hospitalization for a number of months, the patients were able to return to their families and their former ways of life.

Lower Limb Curculatory Disorders and Efficient Supplemental Therapy
BEMER Therapy – 5 Years of Experience

Dr. Rozsos István Ph.D. MBA Theta Center, Pécs

Surgical techniques tend to develop towards minimally and optimally invasive methods. In addition, standardized conservative methods provide a well-set base for these treatments.

The pathological processes are based on circulation defects, so any improvement of the circulation leads to reappearance of the conditions required. This, of course, is not sufficient in many pathological events, but it is part of the whole in any case. Angiologists have an easy task since they have to deal not only indirectly, but also directly with circulation insufficiency cases. In everyday practice, efficacy is largely influenced by patient compliance. In addition, the harmful effects of improper healing factors are also permanently present. In this confusing mixture of therapies, there is a stable bastion, a real team player, that is, the BEMER therapy. Taking into account that the device currently used it is not a simple magnetic therapeutic unit, but a device that can address several challenges of a sick body. It is clearly a device for conservative treatments, to be used together with the other components of traditional healing such as training, exercises, fluid therapy and drug therapies. The steal effect may be harmful in case of many therapies if we cannot establish the necessity of local treatments. A condition following multistage lower limb amputation with difficult healing. [Results can be observed only after a long treatment period.]

A good circulation is essential in the healing of ulcus cruris as well. Ulcus cruris – PTS is almost an epidemic which affects not only an individual but the entire family. It is in the border zone of several specialties, i.e. in "no man's land". Its treatment is expensive and is made even more costly by loss of work. Due to the defined circulatory depletion, the efficiency of the BEMER therapy is indisputable.

Extreme angiospasm may lead to limb amputation that requires prompt and intensive treatment. Inflammatory processes are also problematic in case of inappropriate circulation. The area of the elbow also presents difficulties.

Multiple explorations had no effect since these do not necessarily improve circulation. Diabetic limb complications are caused by microangiopathies and macroangiopathies, but we are the ones who bear the responsibility of treating these conditions.

ASO and diabetic neuropathy

A 79 years old male patient was released home at his own risk; otherwise the limb would have been amputated at the Surgical Department of a municipal hospital.

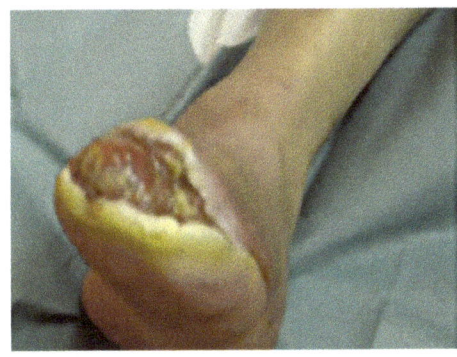 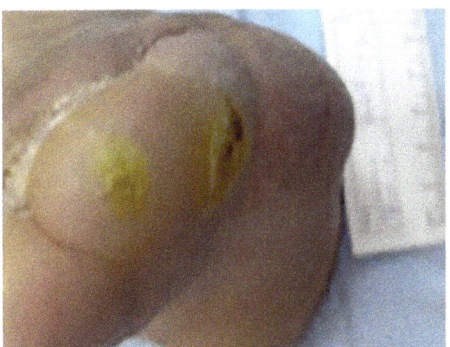

An almost dramatic story with a happy end.

A story that happened over two years ago (54 years old male patient).

In comparison: nothing special happened, we only wanted to save this leg from amputation!

How?

In our practice, we always combine BEMER therapy with fluid and oxygen therapy in addition to classic drug treatments and local wound care methods. Never alone and never conventionally.

What for?

In addition to the success stories, the lack of adverse effects and other risk- free therapeutic options, it should be emphasized that results can be obtained based on the appropriate indication and well-chosen programs; if the BEMER therapy is used as a "supplement", we lose the efficiency provided by targeted treatments and we jeopardize its validity. Diagnostics, treatment plan, intermediate control, confirmation or correction, and follow-up.

Why?

To illustrate this problem: we can use a screwdriver to hammer a nail into a wall, but it is laborious and the result is doubtful because, although the screwdriver is a really great tool, it was made for a different purpose.

Possible Application of the BEMER Therapy in Late Diabetes Complications

Dr. Miléder Margit

"Csolnoky Ferenc" Hospital of Veszprém County. Center of Internal Medicine, Diabetes and Metabolic Conditions

According to the data published by IDF in 2003, a significant increase in the incidence of diabetes is expected worldwide. Diabetes constitutes a significant burden both for the society and the individual. When analyzing the economic aspect of this social burden, based on a survey in 2009, the health costs related to patients with diabetes account for 13% and 0.65% of the National Health Fund (NHF) and the GDP, respectively.

As regards diabetic patients, their disease leads to a significant decrease in quality of life, the factors of which include the disease and its complications, the diagnostic and therapeutic interventions, the psychological and social problems and the financial burden. These burdens are further increased when subsequently the late diabetic complications occur.

50% of the type 2 diabetes cases are already associated with microvascular and macrovascular complications and risk factors at diagnosis. The cardiovascular and cerebrovascular mortality rates in patients with diabetes also increase despite the fact that social efforts have been made for decades in both healing and prevention. In 1989, the Statement of Saint Vincent established that the incidence of blindness, renal insufficiency and limb amputation caused by diabetes should be decreased by 30% to 50%.

Nevertheless, 1 in every 4 patients with T2DM has his or her leg amputated, 1 in every every 5 patients has myocardial infarction and every 6th patient suffers from end-stage renal insufficiency.

From a pathophysiological point of view, the diabetic leg is an autonomous peripheral neuropathy and a condition that develops as a result of lower limb vasoconstriction of different severity and progresses in most cases.

It is the main risk factor of non-traumatic lower limb amputations.

Diabetic leg ulcer has a poor prognosis for healing and even if it heals, in 30% to 100% of the cases the wound recurs within one year, which results in 3000- 4000 amputations annually in Hungary.

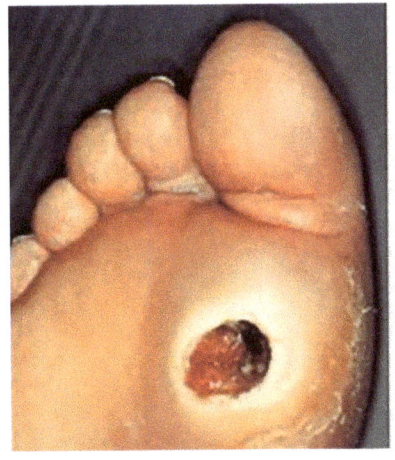
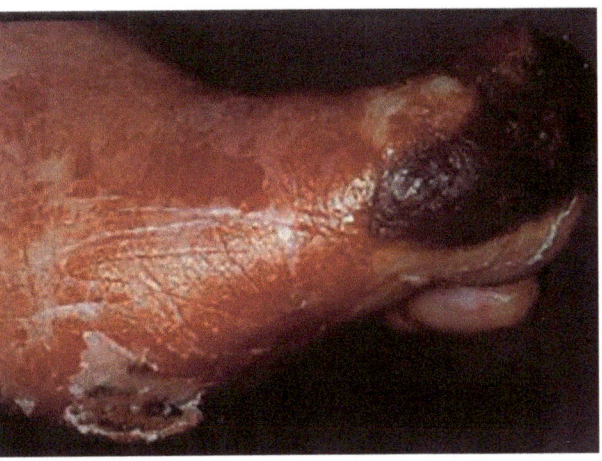

[Lower extremity amputation is a huge trauma for the patient and involves great expenses for the society. No groundbreaking results have been achieved in the prevention and treatment of diabetes. Subsequently we present the results of BEMER therapy as an alternative method, which has proven to improve microcirculation.]

Data were collected retrospectively on the manner BEMER 3000 treatment influences carbohydrate metabolism, the ankle/arm index and the calibrated tuning fork values, the pain based on the VAS scale and the rate of wound healing. HbA1c values decreased from 7.71% to 7.325% (p=0.053), without being statistically significant, but a tendency can be observed in the changes. The ankle/arm index (right side: p=0.037, left side: p=0.048) significantly improved. Although the values measured using a calibrated tuning fork also showed an improvement, the change was not significant. The level of pain determined using the VAS scale was reduced.

We also achieved spectacular results in the treatment of diabetic ulcers and stump wounds and none of the patients required further surgical interventions. The BEMER therapy, proven to improve microcirculation, may be used in the primary, secondary and tertiary prevention of late diabetic complications as well.

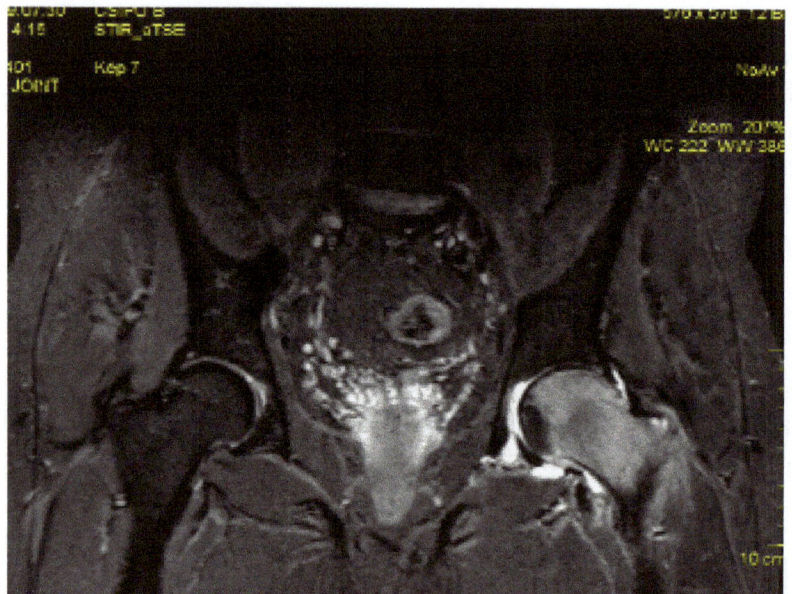
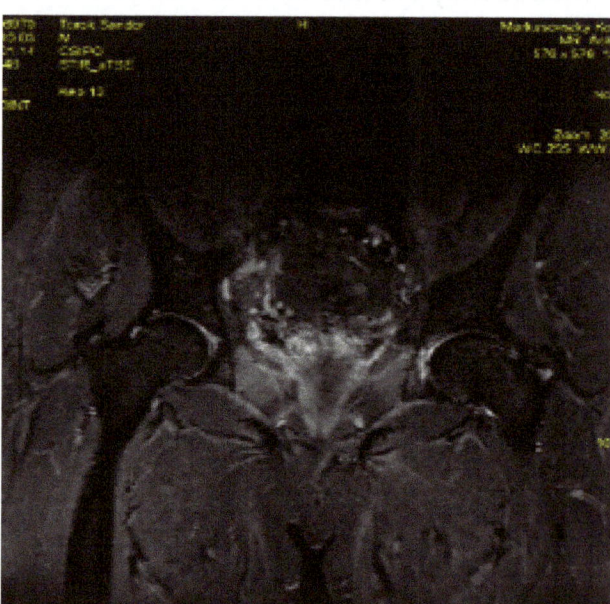

A 57 year old male patient was referred to us by the Rheumatology Department where aseptic necrosis of femoral head was confirmed using MRI. After 6 weeks of BEMER therapy, the pain was relieved and no abnormality was detected on the femoral head during the control MRI.

Effects of pentoxifylline and BIO-ELECTRO-MAGNETIC-ENERGY- REGULATION Therapy in obliterative arterial disease of the lower extremity

Bernát Sándor Iván, Ph.D.1 and Pongrácz Endre Ph.D.2
1State Health Center, 1st Dept. Internal Medicine – Angiology, Budapest, Hungary County Hospital, Department Neurology and Laboratory for Clinical Hemorheology

SUMMARY: In conclusion it can be stated, that in our study series BEMER therapy was efficient and highly efficient in 43% of patients, during combination treatment 71% of the patients experienced efficient and highly efficient results.

Background

The number of conservative therapeutic options is limited in peripheral arterial disease (PAOD) of the lower extremity. In clinical practice vasodilators, including prostaglandin E1, and haemorheologics such as pentoxifylline and naftidrofuryl are used. Isovolumic haemodilution is also a haemorheological treatment, which decreases the viscosity of blood and plasma. In addition, platelet inhibiting drugs (aspirin, clopidogrel) are also used for thrombosis prophylaxis (6,12,18,22).

Limited number of therapeutic options is available to improve microcirculation. Therefore when we had learnt about microcirculation improving effect of Bio- Electro-Magnetic-Energy-Regulation (BEMER) the question has emerged, whether it can be used in PAOD patients in combination with pentoxifylline to improve therapeutic effect. In his book Klopp R. published the results of several studies on the effects of BEMER therapy (8). The studies have shown that the microcirculation can be improved by BEMER therapy. It causes significant increase in vasomotion of microvasculature (AVM envelope curves of arteriolar and venular frequency spectra), in the difference in arterio-venous pO2, in the number of opened capillaries, in the number of junctions of capillaries (nNP), in the number of Kirchoff's junctions perfusing red blood cells of the given time, in arteriolar and venular flow (Qart and Qven) and in flow rate of the red blood cells at the specific microcirculation area (8). The above findings were supported by other studies (13, 14). After 2 minutes of BEMER therapy, significant improvement of the gingival microcirculation was shown (9). Pentoxifylline – despite common misbeliefs– is not a vasodilator, but it too improves microcircular blood flow (haemorheological effect). It significantly improves the deformability of red blood cells and decreases the aggregability of red blood cells and platelets (3, 4, 11, 15, 16, 23, 24). Although there are studies that could not show beneficial haemorheological effects for pentoxifylline (2).

Theoretically the effects of BEMER and pentoxifylline are additive, as the former increases the patency of microcircular blood vessels, and the number of opened capillaries in the microcirculation, while the latter improves the blood flow in the microcirculation through improving the rheological properties of blood. To put it simply BEMER acts on microvasculature, while pentoxifylline acts on the microvascular blood flow.

The effects of BEMER in obliterative vascular disease of the lower extremity have not been studied so far. While making the clinical study plan, our aim was to find out whether BEMER technique has any effect at all. If we can find a clinical efficacy, it would be worth to study the extent of efficacy comparing it with treatment options that have been used to date.

Patients
The mean age of the patients (21 male and 9 female) was 69.3 years. The youngest patient was 57, the oldest was 85 years old. 26 patients had hypertensive disease, 11 patients had diabetes mellitus and 13 patients were smokers at the time. We did not change the patients' current medications.

Throughout the study period patients received their treatment with antihypertensive and cardial drugs, beta-blockers, Ca-antagonists, platelet inhibitors, diuretics and antilipemics in an unchanged dosing regimen. No lifestyle changes were made.

Inclusion criteria

Diagnostic conditions of PAOD were the following: typical intermittent claudication, physical examination (inspection, palpation of the temperature of the extremity, palpation of the vessels – bilateral femoral artery, popliteal artery, dorsalis pedis artery, posterior tibial artery), during ankle/arm index examination – ratio of systolic pressure measured above the ankle (in mmHg) and systolic pressure measured on the arm (mmHg) – diagnostic criteria was that the value should be lower than 0.9.

Doppler examination: above arteries of the lower extremity abnormal curve can be detected or arterial flow cannot be detected. By means of the above examinations patients (N=54) could be assigned to Fontaine stages IIa and IIb (no pain at rest, pain-free walking distance >200m /stage IIa/ or <200m /stage IIb/, limb pain ceases after a few minutes).

Exclusion Criteria:

Patients with severe ischaemic heart disease, effort or rest angina pectoris, evidence of circulatory insufficiency (dyspnea, physical and radiological signs of pulmonary congestion, anasarca), symptoms of respiratory insufficiency (dyspnea, spastic rales above the lungs on auscultation, respiratory function test suggesting moderate to severe obstruction),complaints affecting the locomotive organs which affect or prevent the examination of walking distance: coxarthrosis, gonarthrosis, lumbar spondylosis, lumbar discopathy, lumbago-ischias syndrome etc.

Fontaine stage III–IV (limb pain at rest, or gangraena) which would have made the measuring of the pain-free walking distance impossible.

After 54 consecutive patients' enrolment, 24 patients were excluded from further studies as a result of applying the above exclusion criteria.

Subsequently 30 patients signed the series of treatments and study information leaflet and the informed consent form. There were no other patients withdrawn from the study; therefore after completion of the study series, the results of all 30 patients were processed.

It was a randomised, open-label, self controlled study series which was conducted between October 2008 and December 2009.

Study design

After the enrolment, patients' pain-free walking distance (PFWD) and maximal walking distance (MWD) were measured by a Schiller (made in Switzerland) MTM 1500 med - CS 200 No 030.02431 type treadmill equipment. The settings of the equipment were the following: 3.6km/h (60m/min, 1m/sec) constant speed and 0% slope.The time elapsed until the occurrence of the first pain, and the maximal time period during which a patient could walk with the increasing pain was measured. With the rate (m/min) and the time elapsed (min) available, the walking distance (m) could be calculated. In the first case we got PFWD, in the second case we got MWD values.

Following a one week placebo period, PFWD and MWD values were again measured. Then, in the analysis of the results the placebo period PFWD and MWD values were deducted, and thus change of "net" walking distance during therapy was measured.

In the second part of the study series patients received 2x8 minutes of BEMER therapy 8 times. BEMER, Bio-Electro-Magnetic-Energy-Regulation technique is application of a special changing magnetic field with gradually decreasing amplitude, which, as previous studies indicated, has beneficial effects on the microcirculation (1, 7, 19, 17). The manufacturer of the equipment is: BEMER International (Lichtenstein). Patients received 8 minutes of BEMER 3000 plus therapy every time (daily), with P1 type program of the equipment, by a mattress applicator. In the second part of the treatment a 20 minute long therapy took place with the use of an applicator pad around the right and left legs.

After the total 16 BEMER therapies PFWD and MWD values were measured again. Before and after each BEMER radiation patients' blood pressure and pulse rate were measured in supine position.

In the third part of the study series patients received 8 times, 2x2 ampoules (400 mg/day in total) pentoxifylline every time infunded in 2x250ml of normal saline solution. After the 16 infusion therapies PFWD and MWD values were measured again.

For the assessment of the therapy, the following quartiles were defined: if the increase in walking distance was less than 15%, the therapy was declared ineffective, identical to placebo. If the walking distance increased by 16–50%, 51–100 % or more than 100% the therapy was assessed subsequently weakly effective, effective, and highly effective.

Results

At the end of placebo period the mean increase in PFWD was 8.7%, and in MWD was 11.6%. The maximal decrease in walking distance was 9% and 3%, the maximal increase was 16% and 22% subsequently.

The baseline PFWD and MWD values were the ones measured at the end of the placebo period. Compared to these values, after 16 BEMER therapies the mean increase of net painfree walking distance was 57.4% (P=0.005), and of net maximal walking distance was 36.6% (P=0.0042).

After 16 infusion therapies with 200mg pentoxifylline further increase in PFWD and in MWD could be observed. There was further 15.5% (P=0.047) increase in pain-free walking distance compared to the time between BEMER and infusion therapy, and maximum walking distance increased by further 20.5% (P=0.137).

As a result of combination of the two types of therapies the total mean increase in PFWD and in MWD was subsequently 81.9% and 84.0%. Both values increased significantly: P value of the PFWD was 0.000373, and of MWD was 0.00741.

Summarizing the results, there were no examples of measuring decrease in walking distance after therapies. In 7 patients of 30 BEMER therapy was ineffective, i.e. walking distance did not decrease but its increase did not exceed 15%. BEMER therapy had moderate effect in the case of 10 patients. In 5 and 8 patients the therapy was subsequently effective and highly effective.

Combination (BEMER and infusion) therapy had further therapeutic benefit. After combination therapy there were 5 patients in total who experienced ineffectivity of the therapeutic interventions. In 4 patients the combination therapy had moderate effect, in 7 and in 14 patients was subsequently effective and highly effective.

Patients' blood pressure was measured before and after BEMER therapy. Both measurements took place in supine position. At the first measurement the patient had been lying for 3–5 minutes, the second one was taken place after further 40 minutes in supine position. In 8 out of 30 patients the decrease in blood pressure was more than 10%, and in 22 patients, the change (decrease of increase) was less than 10%. During BEMER therapy the pulse rate did not change in 27 patients, it decreased in 3 patients by more than 10%.

In conclusion it can be stated, that in our study series BEMER therapy was efficient and highly efficient in 43% of patients, during combination treatment 71% of the patients experienced efficient and highly efficient results.

Discussion

Pentoxifylline is a widely used treatment to alleviate the complaints of dysbasia in peripheral, obliterative vascular disease. Previous studies have demonstrated that pentoxifylline increases the deformability of red blood cells, and decreases the aggregability of red blood cells and platelets, thus improving the microcirculation. The Bio-Electro-Magnetic-Energy-Regulation (BEMER) therapy too improves the microcirculation by increasing vasomotion, opening capillaries, increasing flow rate of red blood cells and difference between arterial and venous pO2. On the basis of the aforementioned data, we assumed that concurrent effect of pentoxifylline and BEMER therapy will result in significant increase in pain-free and maximal walking distance, improving the quality of life of patients with PAOD.

After reviewing relevant professional literature, it could be stated that no such type of clinical study has ever been conducted to date.

The enrolment of patients proved to be a difficult task. Approximately half of the patients eligible for the inclusion criteria (Fontaine stage IIa and IIb) were not eligible for the study because of other cardiovascular, locomotive organ, and respiratory diseases. The mean age of the patients enrolled was high; most of the patients had advanced PAOD.

Patients had Fontaine IIb stage disease. Many PAOD patients were suffering from hypertension and diabetes as well. During the study period no change of previous medication treatment, lifestyle and smoking habit has been implemented.

In order to prevent placebo effect well-known from professional literature, a therapy-free period was implemented before the therapeutic period. Placebo effect is due to the fact that during repeated treadmill tests the patients are no more afraid; they have a better technique, and can walk on the treadmill equipment more economically.

Although the number of patients taking part in the study was low (pilot study) both pain-free and maximal walking distance was significantly increased due to BEMER and to pentoxifylline therapy as well.

Combination of the two treatments had further therapeutic benefits. There were in total 5 out of 30 patients who experienced an increase in PFWD less than 15%. Walking distance did not decrease in any patient, and the therapy was effective or highly effective in 21 patients. Side effects or complications did not occur. Maximum daily dose of parenteral pentoxifylline is 0.6mg/bodyweight kg/hour, in a 70kg patient this is 1008mg/day (20). In this study patients received 400mg pentoxifylline daily, i.e. a medium daily dose was applied.

Conclusion from tables presenting the results would be that BEMER is more effective in increasing PFWD and MWD than pentoxifylline. However this fact is only apparent. In the background of this is the fact that the therapy applied first has greater efficacy than the second one. Based on this finding it is worth to conduct a study series in the future where patients will be treated first with pentoxifylline and then BEMER.

It is very difficult to compare the efficacy of the different pentoxifylline therapies, because in certain studies the compound was given parenterally and in others orally, pain-free walking distance was measured with different methods and different therapeutic dose and time was applied.

During their study Triebe G et al. found that in the pentoxifylline treated patient group PFWD increased from 155m to 191m compared to the controls, which is equivalent to an increase by 23%, and P value was less than 0.01. (21).

In a meta-analysis published by Girolami B et al. they found that in the 6 reviewed clinical studies the mean increase in PFWD was 21.0m (from 0.7m to 41.3m) and in MWD was 43.8m (from 14.1m to 73.6m) with pentoxifylline (5). Moher D et al reviewed fifty-two clinical studies including the data of 5088 patients in total. During pentoxifylline therapy the mean increase in PFWD was approximately 30m while in MWD was 60m (10).

No previous studies on the effects of BEMER in PAOD have been conducted before our present publication. As this was the first study, and because of the low number of patients taking part in the study, no far-reaching conclusion can be drawn from our results. However it can be stated, that it seems worth conducting further – maybe cross over – studies to evaluate the efficacy of BEMER, pentoxifylline and combined conservative therapy.

References

1. J. Beck and I. Horváth: Bio-elektromágneses energia reguláció (BEMER). Érbetegségek 2004; 11: 135-140. D.L. Dawson, Q. Zheng, S.A. Worthy, B. Charles, D.V. Jr. Bradley DV: Failure of pentoxifylline or cylostasol to improve blood and plasma viscosity, fibrinogen, and erythrocyte deformability in claudication. Angiology, 2002; 53: 509-520.
2. M.T. DeSanctis, M.R. Cesarone, G. Belcaro: Treatment of intermittent claudication with pentoxifylline: a 12-month, randomized trial-walking distance and microcirculation. Angiology, 2002; 53: S7-12
3. W. Drozdz, J. Panek, W. Lejman: Red cell deformability in patients with chronic atheromatous ischemia of the legs. Med.Sci.Monit. 2001; 5: 933-939
4. B. Girolami, E. Bernardi, M.H. Prins et al.: Treatment of intermittent claudication with
5. physical training, smoking cessation, pentoxifylline, or nafronyl: a meta- analysis. Arch.Intern.Med. 1999; 159: 337-345.
6. Guide of Angiological Practice (Angiológiai Útmutató – Klinkai Irányelvek
7. Kézikönyve), 2007. Medition Press Budapest.
8. W.A. Kaffka: The physical and phisiological basis of the BEMER 3000 signal 2. Int. World Congress of Bio-Electro-Magnetic-Energy- Regulation. Emphyspace, 2001; 2: 9-14. R. Klopp: Mikrozirkulation – Im Fokus der Forschung. Mediquant Verlag AG in Schliessa, 2008
9. R.C. Klopp: Elektromágneses terápia (BEMER) mikrocirkulációra kifejtett hatásának placebo kontrollált, dupla vak vizsgálata. Érbetegségek 2005; 12: 27-30.
10. D. Moher, B. Pham, M. Ausejo, A. Saenz, S. Hood, G.G. Barber: Pharmacological management of intermittent claudication: a meta- analysis of randimized trials. Drugs. 2000;59(5):1057-1070.

11. A.V. Muravyov, I.A. Tikhomirova, A.A. Maimistova et al.: Extra- and intracellular signaling pathways under red blood cell aggregation and deformability changes.
12. Clin.Hemorheol. Microcirc. 2009; 43: 223-232. L. Norgren, W.R. Hiatt, J.A. Dormandy et al.: Inter-Society Consensus for the Management of Peripheral Arterial Disease (TASC II). J.Vasc.Surg 2007; 45: 5-67Ch. Ohkuba, H. Okano: Static magnetic fields and microcirculation, In: Rosch P.J., Markov M (Eds.): Bioelectromagnetic Medicine. Taylor & Fracis, Boca Raton 2004; 563-591. Ch. Ohkuba, S. Xu: Acute effects of static magnetic fields on cutaneous microcirculation in rabbits. Invivo 1997; 3: 221-226 Pentoxifyllin – www.wikipedia.org.de/pentoxifyllin
13. V. Perhoniemi, K. Salmenkivi, S. Sundberg: Effects of flunarizine and pentoxifyllin on walking distance and blood rheology in claudication. Angiology, 1984; 35: 366-372 M. Quittan, O. Schuhfried, G.F. Wiesinger, V.
14. Fialka-Moser: Klinische Wirksamkeiten der Magnetfeldtherapie – eine Literaturübersicht. Acta Medica Austriaca. 2000; 3: 61-68.
15. P. Scheffler, D. de la Hamette, J. Gross, H. Mueller, H. Schieffer: Intensive vascular training in stage IIb in peripheral arterial occlusive disease: the additiv effects of intravenous prostaglandin E1 or intravenous pentoxifylline during training. Circulation 1994; 90: 818-822
16. K. Spodaryk, W.A. Kaffka: Oxidant stress clearence in human erythrocytes by non-invasive stimultion with extremly weak (BEMER type) pulsed electromagnetic fields: A blinded, randomised, plecebo- controlled study. Arch. Biochem-Biophys. 2003. Suppl. Summary of therapeutical product characteristic (Trental – Sanofi Aventis)(Gyógyszer alkalmazási előírat)
17. G. Triebe, U. Münnich, F. Liebold: A therapieutic comparison between hemodilution and pentoxifylline in arterial obstructive disease. An objective assessment by quantitative Doppler sonography. Dtsch. Med. Wochenschr. 1992;117(14):523-530.
18. K.J. Waters, A.D. Craxford, J. Chamberlain: The effect of naftidrofuryl (Praxilene) on intermittent claudication. Br. J. Surg. 1980; 67: 349-351
19. D.J. Weiss, R.J. Georg, K. Burher: Effects of pentoxifylline on hemorheologic alterations induced by incremental treadmill exercise in thoroughbreds. Am.J.Vet.Res. 1996; 57: 1364-1368.
20. *C.C. Wu, M.H. Liao, S.J. Chen, M.H. Yen: Pentoxifylline improves circulatory failure and survival in murine models of endotoxaemia. Eur.J.Pharmacol. 1999; 28: 41-49.*

BEMER Therapy Applied in Ophthalmology

Experience with the Use of the BEMER Device in the Treatment of Diabetic Macular Edema

Pilot study abstract of the Konsensus Konferenz Freudenstadt
[Freudenstadt Consensus Conference] from 10/02/2010

Doc. MU Dr. Tomáš Sosna, CSc. Eye Clinic - Thomayer University Hospital, Charles University in Prague, Diabetes Centre at the Institute for Clinical and Experimental Medicine, Prague

SUMMARY: As a focus of the clinical application of the BEMER 3000 device, I envision short-term intensive application prior to treatment of clinically significant macular edema, which would simplify laser treatment by reducing edema in patients with focal and diffusion maculopathy. Subject to the requirement of regular daily use, in other words in patients with high compliance, and indeed all forms of diabetic retinopathy – from the initial to moderately advanced – as well as initial but not clinically significant macular edema. The third indication would be clinically significant macular edema of the previous types that do not respond adequately to laser treatment.

During the pilot study, whose aim was to evaluate the efficacy, harmlessness and compatibility of the treatment of patients with diabetic macular edema with concomitant diabetic retinopathy conducted using the BEMER 3000 device, I was able to observe the electromagnetic effect of the device on diabetic macular edema in five patients.

Theoretical conditions for the effect of the device
Diabetic retinopathy is characterized by a number of disorders, and with regard to the effect of the device, I find the following the most important:

Hyperglycemia and oxidative stress
The increase in hexose concentration in the blood of a diabetic supports the biochemical theory of hyperglycemia as a basic element for the development of diabetic retinopathy.

The cell membrane is practically impervious to sorbitol, which leads to its tissue accumulation as well as pathological changes in oncotic pressure. The excessive accumulation of advanced saccharification products (AGE - advanced glycation endproducts) also supports microvascular changes in the retinal vessels. Through direct action, these products can not only change vascular rigidity but also damage the connective tissue. The oxidative stress accompanying hyperglycemia is the cause of the imbalance between free radicals and the antioxidant cell protection mechanism. The resulting pseudohypoxia can damage cell membranes - by protein denaturation or the arising DNA damage as a result of the conversion of glucose into toxic peroxide and oxoaldehyde. The reduced amount of glucose transporter 1 resulting from long-lasting hyperglycemia leads to a paradoxically occurring reduced supply of glucose to the cells and subsequent apoptosis.

Diacylglycerols (DG) and Ca^{2+} together with other substances form a protein kinase C (PKC) activating complex. In the process, DG represents a precursor to prostaglandin synthesis. Particularly with diabetics, the enzyme activity of PKC and DG is significantly higher. It has been determined that PKC significantly affects not only vascular permeability, but also contractility, blood flow and the angiogenesis. It also has an effect on the cell adhesion molecules and cytosine as a transforming growth factor-beta (transforming growth factor- PKC-beta). The vascular endothelial growth factor (vascular endothelial growth factor-VEGF) is also activated by PKC in severe hypoxia.

Hemorheological changes

Long-term hyperglycemia leads to microcirculation disorder via different mechanisms. This is accompanied by capillary hyperpermeability.

Hyperglycemia increases blood viscosity and changes the concentration of plasmatic proteins. Thrombocyte aggregation is simultaneously increased.

Changes in the rigidity and flexibility of erythrocytes lead to microtraumatisation of the capillary endothelium, where at the same time the amount of the exposed von Willebrand factor, which has a direct influence on the aggregation, is increased. The mechanical damage is evidently more distinctive at an accelerated blood flow through the capillaries, which accompanies hyperglycemia. At the same time, however, oxygenation decreases significantly. The reducedoxygen transport function of erythrocytes in diabetics also has a negative effect on the development of diabetic retinopathy. Leukocytes also play an important role in the pathogenesis of diabetic retinopathy. The size of the leukocytes almost reaches the diameter of a capillary. Thanks to its remarkable deformability, they fit through the capillaries in a healthy human. In diabetics, its adherence to the endothelium is increased and the proteolytic enzymes can therefore be released. With the increase of blood flow resistance, oxygen radicals are released simultaneously. These changes can also result in a capillary occlusion. The glycated Golgi enzyme obviously has an impact on increased adhesiveness.

Hemodynamic changes

At the start of uncontrolled diabetes, changes appear in the blood flow through the capillaries. For example, this is significantly increased by experimentally induced glycemia of about 25 mmol/l. A similar phenomenon, of little importance, however, was also observed in hypoglycemia. The blood flow changes lead directly to the reduction of vascular reactivity. In animal models, it was proven that these changes also damage the vascular endothelium.

Certainly blood elements are also involved in this damage, specifically on a mechanical basis, by changing its rigidity. As already mentioned, microtraumatization of the capillary endothelium is expected. Paradoxically, laminar flow changes with increased blood flow through the capillaries into turbulent flow. At the time of emergence of diabetic retinopathy, blood flow decreases in the middle periphery of the retina. This is a protective mechanism by which normal blood flow through the retina is maintained in a functionally more important central region. Only as a result of further reduction of blood flow through the retina and by the emergence of extensive ischemic zones, the perifoveolar area, where blood flow decreases dramatically, is damaged.

Retinal pigment epithelium (RPE)

With the emergence of the DR, the retinal pigment epithelium (RPE) plays a very important role. In diabetics, there is an increase of sorbitol concentration in RPE, and as a result there are primary changes in the osmotic gradient and the Na+- K+- ATP activity. With this mechanism, the disorder of the nerve cell metabolism, the ganglion cell layer and the granular layer of the retina are explained primarily. Hyperglycemia, but also hypoglycemia cause intraocular pressure to drop in diabetics. With this relative hypotension, the structure of RPE can be changed both morphologically and functionally. This is termed a "emargination" (infolding) of the cell membrane on the Bruch's membrane of the RPE cells that sit closely to the lamina chorioidocapillaris. The functional alteration of the RPE may be one of the causes for the collapse of the inner and outer blood-retinal barrier. The abnormal transport through the RPE therefore allows some proliferative factors to slightly penetrate into the vitreous body and increase the proliferative potential of the eye. The perfusion pressure of the retinal vessels is defined by the difference between intravascular and intraocular pressure. The lowering of intraocular tension leads to a relative increase in the perfusion pressure, however, this then also leads to the progression of venous dilation until a later collapse of the auto- regulation mechanisms. The relative increase in perfusion pressure also leads to more prominent exudation as well as to the weakening of the capillary walls and participates in the formation of microaneurysms – frequent signs of diabetic retinopathy. This mechanism would eventually provide an explanation for why the fragile pericytes in the retina perish more frequently than those in other organs (except the heart), where different perfusion pressures also have an effect.

Based on these pathogenetic mechanisms, we have assumed a possible effect on diabetic retinopathy and/or diabetic macular edema.

Evaluation type and results
Highly specialized methods were used for evaluating treatment results such as fluorescent angiography, 7-field fundus photography according to a ETDRS study (Early Treatment Diabetic Retinopathy Study), optical coherence tomography, non-contact tonometry and more.

A total of 7 patients were observed in the study. 2 patients refused the treatment immediately after delivery of the device: a younger patient due to difficuties maintaining the treatment regimen (often traveling); an older patient refused treatment because of her concern that the device could harm her. 5 patients completed the study. 3 patients continue the treatment in a follow-up study. In the course of the study, neither negative effects of treatment nor cataract genesis were observed. In two patients, there was progression of the findings during observation - for poor compliance. Grid laser photocoagulation had to be carried out; the need for laser treatment could therefore not be avoided. In one of the patients who showed excellent compliance, there was clinically significant improvement of the eye findings. The biochemical parameters as well as cognitive intrusion also improved insignificantly, whereby this also includes this improvement and among others the more regular regime, which he kept. In two other [female] patients, an accelerated resorption of macular edema after treatment with grid laser photocoagulation was observed. This is obviously due to improved hemodynamics and haemorheology of blood and blood elements, including retinal capillaries. In patients with high compliance, changes in the hemodynamic and haemorheologic conditions in the eye were the probable result with a high probability in the overall application of the device. This is also confirmed by QOL - decrease of neuropathic difficulties. Other effects (ATP, etc.) can currently only be speculated. A direct effect on the capillary network can not really be required in relation to the location of the local application - the bony structure of the eye socket.

Application possibilities
As a focus of the clinical application of the BEMER 3000 device, I envision short-term intensive application prior to treatment of clinically significant macular edema, which would simplify laser treatment by reducing edema in patients with focal and diffusion maculopathy. Subject to the requirement of regular daily use, in other words in patients with high compliance, and indeed all forms of diabetic retinopathy - from the initial to moderately advanced - as well as initial but not clinically significant macular edema.

The third indication would be clinically significant macular edema of the previous types that do not respond adequately to laser treatment.

Follow-up study. Thanks to the kindness of BEMER, I have an opportunity to observe three patients whose conditions after the pilot phase of the study have improved. In two patients with a very high compliance, their condition gradually improves or their edema reduction stabilizes and the disintegration of hard focuses is apparent in the photographic documentation. Subjectively, they tolerate the method very well, neuropathic symptoms have been significantly reduced. The most interesting is the third patient, who initially had the highest compliances. Because of an acute lower back pain, he has ceased using the device entirely. The findings on the retina deteriorated quite dramatically within 4 months but so far not to the stage where laser intervention would be necessary. The patient was informed of this deterioration and has subsequently started using the device again. The question remains as to whether or not his condition will improve and if so, how quickly. All patients are observed according to the protocol of the previous study.

Dr. Garai Borbála Ophthalmologist, private practice

The vast majority of the information from the environment is perceived by vision.

In a study, the following theoretical question was asked: what would one rather choose for his or her old age – vision impairment or limited movement capacity? A substantial proportion of the respondents preferred to preserve their vision.

According to the WHO, there are approx. 314 million visually impaired persons worldwide with about 45 million blind persons. In welfare societies 3 persons in 1000 go blind. In Africa this value is 10 persons in 1000. The two most common causes of blindness (in welfare societies) are the ophthalmological complications of DM (diabetic retinopathy) and the age-related macular degeneration (Degeneratio maculae luteae).

The anatomical unit responsible for central vision is extremely small. It has a diameter of approx. 2 mm with a mean thickness of 185 microns in the region of the fovea and 250 microns on average in an area of 2 mm.

In many cases we do not know the primary reason of the diseases affecting the macula lutea, but it is sure that the second factor is oxygen deprivation, which can be influenced by improving the circulation.
I will present three cases to illustrate the therapeutic effect of the BEMER therapy as physical agent.

Case 1. Ms. B. Gy. 66 years old woman

The vision of the patient was 0.7 in the right eye, while on left side she could count the fingers right before her eye. The patient feels that her vision deteriorates every day, especially in the left eye. Vision correction did not help. Peaceful bulbs and clear refractory media. Fundus: pale pupils with clear delimitation; arteries narrower than average and moderately filled veins; the retina is tightened on both sides in the region of the central vision; uneven regions and drusens at the level of the pigment epithelium. Exudation was not found. Following basic mat therapy and daily use of the intensive applicator in the temporal region, after three months the patient's vision improved to 0.9 and 0.15 on the right and left, respectively. The OCT (Optical Coherence Tomography) revealed that the thickness of the retina remained the same. The functions improved. A secondary result was that the patient was able to interrupt a part of the medications used to improve her circulation. Her condition remained unchanged for 8 months.

Case 2. Ms. Sz. G. 79 years old woman

The vision of the patient was 0.4 in the right eye with correction, while on left side she could count the fingers right before her eye. Peaceful bulbs, mild phacosclerosis in the lens on both sides. Fundus: pale pupils with clear delimitation on both sides; arteries narrower than average; drusens on the right side in and around the macula and scattered at the periphery; an unevenly pigmented athrophic scar on the left side in the region of the macula with a couple of choroideal artery below this; the periphery seems to be intact.

The patient's most important complaint was that reading is becoming increasingly difficult. Following basic mat therapy and daily use of the intensive applicator in the temporal region, after six weeks the patient's vision improved to 0.6 and 2 m o.u. on the right and left, respectively, with correction. During this period, the fundus seemed to remain unchanged. The functions improved and the patient feels that she reads more easily and her spatial sense of security is improved. A secondary result was that her prior obstipation complaints resolved.

Case 3. B. M. 50 years old man

The vision of the patient was 0.4 in the right eye with correction, while on left side it was uncertain 1.0. His complaint was that he is almost unable to see colors in his right eye and feels that his vision started to deteriorate in his left eye, as well, and the weak right eye bothers him in binocular sight. According to him, this condition appeared during the last six months. During the two weeks after the first examination, his vision in the right eye further deteriorated to 4 m finger counting. Peaceful bulbs and clear refractory media. Fundus: intact pupils with clear delimitation; phys. arteries. On the right side, uneven pigmentation in the macula and plate neuroretinal detachment was found. On the left side, a small detachment can be seen under the fovea. Following basic mat therapy and the use of the intensive applicator in the temporal region three times a week, after three months the patient's vision improved to 0.4 and 0 on the right and left, respectively. To his great joy, he can see colors again. Fundus: the uneven pigmentation on the right side remained unchanged and no detachment could be observed. On the left side, the biomicroscopy showed no PE unevenness. A secondary result was that her arrhythmia resolved. His condition has not deteriorated since March 2009.

In the first two cases the diagnosis was macular degeneration l.u. AREDS Stage 3 in the better eye and AREDS Stage 4 in the weaker eye. In the third case the diagnosis was diffuse pigment epitheliopathy l.u. (Central serous chorioretinopathy?). None of the patients showed neovascularization (formation of new arteries).

Summary

The precise cause of the vision impairment described in these case studies is not clarified.
The functions improved (visual acuity, color vision and peripheral vision) as a result of the circulation improving effect of the BEMER therapy.

BEMER Therapy Applied in Surgery

Dr. Németi Zoltán Neurosurgeon

Kenézy Hospital, Department of Trauma and Arm Surgery, Neurosurgery Ward, Debrecen

The majority of the central nervous system syndromes are basically non-surgical conditions. Generally speaking, surgery is required only in well circumscribed focal diseases which, by their very nature, destroy, injure or hinder the functioning of the normal neural tissue, and due to their volume, they can displace normal tissue elements (brain tissue, blood or brain fluid), otherwise in a closed space, which sooner or later will cause local symptoms and, subsequently, can create life-threatening overpressure in the skull. The same applies to spine diseases, as well.

These syndromes require surgical intervention depending on their type, place and rate of progression, the timing of which also differs within a wide range.

For example, 70-80% of disc herniation cases do not require surgery or can be postponed for years, while traumatic intracranial bleeding, acute hydrocephalia or tumors that cause herniation must be immediately operated.

Regardless of the algorithm used to establish or project the indication of surgery, the fact of a surgery is not the same as healing, because the latter is often just T0 time point of that process, where the actual regeneration begins. It is not uncommon that this process is hindered by serious factors, and the more efficient circulation and metabolism induced by the BEMER therapy can eliminate several of these factors.

Neurosurgery showed a huge development in the last years. The diagnostic equipment gathering image and functional data (through rapid leaps in the development of IT and precision instruments) provide the treating physicians with detailed information never seen before.

The current performance of computers allows for the integration and simultaneous and spectacular presentation of data in real time and in several dimensions. All these data can be precisely adapted to a specific patient. The same improvement renders the surgical interventions and instruments more precise. Based on these improvements, a neurosurgeon can remove possibly the entire pathological process using the best approach and with as less destruction as possible. Although the scale of development is huge, we are still only able to "take", and the things we can "give" are very limited. This is explained by the very limited regeneration capacity of the highly differentiated neural tissue, as well as the complexity and uniqueness of the functional connection system.

The abovementioned options are all aimed at removing the pathological process WHILE DAMAGING AS LITTLE HEALTHY TISSUE AS POSSIBLE AND PRESERVING AS MUCH INJURED BUT FUNCTIONAL TISSUE AS POSSIBLE IN FUNCTIONAL STATE.

After the surgeon has done his or her job, the brain is "left alone" during healing. The battle for the penumbra starts, that is, the healthy tissue surrounding the areas permanently lost, and the reorganization of the useful neural connection system.

One of the key steps in this process is to ensure the appropriate metabolism and efficient circulation. The rest is the job of the brain. In this process, it is relevant whether it is a disease requiring surgery or not. Non-surgical healing methods before and after or instead of the intervention, as well as complex rehabilitation is and will always be maximally justified. However, we can use the amazing effects of the professionally created pulsating magnetic field to improve microcirculation which plays a key role in healing.

Nonetheless, the spine is not only the "home" of the spinal marrow, but also one of the most important locomotor organ and therefore all changes typical to this disease category can frequently occur: arthritis, inflammation, herniation, swelling, fracture, other injuries, osteoporosis, instability or stenosis.

A neurosurgeon spends much of his or her time with patients who have these complaints.

According to the professional guidelines, surgical cases are identified from this considerable patient group. The proportion of surgical cases does not exceed 30% at international level, as well, which means that 2/3 of the patients has to solve their spine pain using non-surgical means. Therefore, it is not irrelevant which methods can be used to relieve pain without surgical solutions, to achieve the most optimal healing, to prevent complaints and to slow down progression.

During my 15 years of work, I have met a great number of patients for whom I was not able to recommend any neurosurgical intervention, or for whom there was no appropriate efficient medicine or method for the problems before and after surgeries, and the extent of residual symptoms and complaints did not allow for normalizing the patient's lifestyle. I started to use the BEMER magnetotherapy based on these cases to extend and supplement the existing neurosurgical treatment options.

It is important to note that diseases affecting the central nervous system, the head and the spine frequently have a serious impact on the entire body and therefore should not be considered taken out from this context. For example, a brain disease or injury associated with severe impairment of consciousness, immobility and modified hormonal status can have so many complications that these cause permanent damages or we lose the patient because of them, although the underlying disease alone would have healed. We can provide qualitative support in the recovery of the patient by using the beneficial effect of a pulsating magnetic field to reduce the risk and severity of these complications.

And now, let's see the numbers!
In 3 years, more than 200 patients (232) received BEMER therapy. 50% of them suffered from cervical and lumbar spine disease; 10% of these patients underwent surgery in the first step or later due to unsuccessful conservative treatment. A large proportion of patients (14%) were injured in accidents; another large group of patients (12%) suffered from neural complications related to other diseases. Some patients have completely lost their faith in classic medical care because they have not experienced improvement for a long period of time and believed that their case is hopeless. The following section describes a couple of instructive examples. However, there were cases where no substantial results were obtained (8%).

Case		Number of Patients		Percentage distribution	
Spine disease (10% surgeries)	Lumbar	82	115	71	50
	Cervical	33		29	
Trauma	Spine injury	21	32	65	14
	Head injury	11		35	
Nervous system complications		28		12	

Other diseases	85	24
Total	232	100

Competent medical examination and the necessary care were provided for all patients. The recommended magnetotherapy was administered alone or as part of a complex treatment. In addition to monitoring the objective symptoms, the extent of the change in the symptoms and complaints was evaluated based on the patients' opinion and experiences, and documented using the popular Visual Analog Scale (VAS) which measures the initial pain, the symptoms and the improvement obtained using a ten-grade scale.

Based on practical considerations, 4 classes of efficiency were established. At the beginning, the VAS value exceeded 7 in all cases (1 indicates the best state, free of pain, while 10 is the worst state with intolerable symptoms).

- 40% of the patients became complaint-free or recovered.
- 36% of the patients reported significant improvement with residual complaints that only minimally hindered their further life.
- 16% of the patients reported that their complaints were reduced to more than half, which included, among others, reduced need for drugs, better manageability, longer resistance and less sick pay for our patients.
- 10 cases (8%) showed no improvement mainly because of sacroiliac arthritis or repeatedly operated severe spine disease where the serious mechanical harm could not be eliminated not even after the administration of therapy.
- Negative effects were observed in 2 cases. After myocarditis, tachycardia occurred that caused complaints as a result of the therapy. In the case of another patient, itching skin rash appeared all over the body, as a result of which the otherwise efficient treatment had to be discontinued.

Case studies

Let me begin by saying that I could describe the case of almost any of my patients as regards the successes obtained in degenerative spine diseases. Sometimes statistics can be more eloquent than concrete examples. However, the following cases tell a more special story. Notwithstanding this, they have in common that they are not unique cases in my practice and the BEMER therapy showed the same efficiency in other cases, as well.

Case 1

46 years old male patient: negative history without known cervical injuries. He felt from his bike, fractured his nasal bone and sprained his neck. After a couple of hours, numbness in all four limbs started to appear, followed by tetraparesis; he was paralyzed with limited movement in his hands. The emergency CT scan was negative, only the cervical vertebrae IV and V showed a calcified beak. However, the MRI showed that there was a disc hernia that did not caused symptoms, but during the accident it hit the spinal marrow and caused the symptoms.

Subsequently, steroid therapy and surgical decompression was applied, followed by acute rehabilitation. He was discharged from our department with spastic-ataxic gait and clumsy hands, but in improving condition; 2 weeks later he started the BEMER therapy. The patient showed an exceptionally rapid improvement and was able to start working again after 6 weeks, in symptom-free condition, although in such cases the healing process can last for months with uncertain final outcome.

Case 2

64 years old male patient: after a couple of days of physical fatigue observed that his right arm is weaker which rapidly resulted in severe paralysis and muscle loss. He was not able to lift his shoulder, bend or partially stretch his elbow. In 10 months the upper limb became contracted, which further reduced its function. The ENG showed the lesion of the upper brachial plexus that remained unchanged after several months of treatment and physical therapy. At this point, the patient started the BEMER therapy and continued the physical therapy. After two weeks a subjective and objective improvement was observed, the numbness ceased, the movement range improved and the circumference of the arm increased by 2 cm in 5 weeks due to the increase in the muscle mass.

Case 3

The 44 years old male patient was taken by surprise by a storm in August in a forested area was hit by a broken branch. He suffered an impression skull fracture and multiple cheekbone fractures associated with severe open brain injury and leakage of cerebrospinal fluid.

He was not able to either open his mouth or talk. He was at risk of vision impairment, meningitis and permanent brain damage. Together with an oral surgeon we performed a surgery. The skull bone was raised, the brain damage was treated, plastic surgery of dura mater, and reconstruction of the cheekbone was performed.

After the surgery, the leakage of cerebrospinal fluid and the brain contusion temporarily worsened, and edema occurred, the patient's thinking slowed down associated with irritability and symptoms of memory disorders. His mouth movement was resolved, but he had serious pain during chewing. The leakage of cerebrospinal fluid was stopped and meningitis did not develop. He was discharged home.

During convalescence the patient experienced headache, painful chewing, permanent and disturbing memory impairment, depression, vertigo and weakness. As his wife put it, "he was a half-zombie".

The patient started the BEMER therapy with little hope. However, after 6 weeks of treatment, gradually ALL COMPLAINTS were resolved. First the headache and the vertigo disappeared; the last complaint was the pain during chewing. At the present, the patient is able to work, solves crosswords and has no pain. So, the "zombie is gone".

In all three cases, the BEMER therapy efficiently broke the impasse in the healing process and resulted in clinically and subjectively significant qualitative improvement and recovery within a fraction of the average healing time.

Summary and evaluation
Beyond these figures, based on my experiences so far, I have reached some relevant practical conclusions.

As regards the spine as a locomotor organ, it can be established that for the BEMER therapy it is almost irrelevant which region is affected. What is more important is the nature of the disease, its duration, the extent of the degeneration and progression, and the proportion of the primary mechanical and secondary symptoms. If this is taken into account during the administration of the treatment, it can be very efficient and efficacy and the patient can be prepared for the changes expected, the improvement and the time required.

In my opinion, in case of diseases or injuries that affect the brain and the spine, the greatest advantage of the BEMER is that it reaches even the most vulnerable areas without complications or adverse effects and eliminates the auto-destructive vicious circles that hinder recovery, which increases the efficiency of other medical treatments and auto-healing processes.

Today, I use the BEMER therapy in my everyday work and it became part of my thinking. Based on my increasing experiences and with full confidence I recommend this therapy to both surgical and non-surgical patients to their and my greatest satisfaction.

Lecture at the 7th BEMER Therapy World Congress, Bad Windsheim, 10.1.05

Successful BEMER 3000 magnetic field therapy in an extremely rare and complicated cluster of symptoms: H fracture (triple fracture) of the sacrum as fatigue fracture in manifest osteoporosis

Dr. med. Rolf Oesterle; Practice of Holistic Prevention and Promotion of Health

SUMMARY: After only 7 weeks of BEMER 3000 therapy: "Healed sacral H fatigue fracture on both sides with signs of spongiose reconstruction with diffusely increased sclerosing. Almost complete osseous consolidation is evident in the fracture with a pitch in ventral direction."

Traumatology Example Case: Female patient, I. L., 73 years old. 2003: Long-term high-dose cortisone therapy for seronegative rheumatoid arthritis of the large joints and the finger joints.

Further diagnoses: Condition after bladder cancer 1992. Arterial hypertension. Wet macular degeneration of both eyes.

Since June 2004, increasing pain in the area of the left buttock and deep-seated sacroiliac pain. Alleviation only when standing and lying, whereas sitting is almost impossible because of strong pains. 07/11. – 07/15/2004 inpatient at the Neurosurgical University Clinic.

Diagnosis: Sciatica of uncertain origin in the form of a pseudo-radicular pain syndrome. Neurosurgical indication excluded. CT lower lumbar spine with negative result, X-ray of pelvis and left hip joint also with negative result 07/28 – 08/06/2004 in-patient in orthopedic specialty clinic:

07/29/2004: Magnetic resonance imaging of the os sacrum: "Two-sided fatigue fracture of the massa lateralis of the os sacrum with pronounced edema and root canals S1 and S2 affected on both sides. In addition, transverse fracture line with slight buckling between first and second sacral segment in the form of a H fracture of the sacrum." Incomplete weak foot dorsiflexion. Manifest osteoporosis.

Conservative symptomatic therapy and physiotherapy as well as monthly Aredia infusions (biphosphonate) to treat the osteoporosis.

02/04/2005: Magnetic resonance imaging of the pelvis to monitor progress: "Fracture lines still visible in the massa lateralis on both sides of the sacrum with persisting fluid containment. The fractures are still not consolidated."

02/25/2005: Start of BEMER 3000 magnetic field therapy: Coil mat 3x daily on P4. An additional application of the intensive applicator was not tolerated by the patient.

04/13/2005: The head physician of the Orthopedic Clinic intends to transfer the patient to a specialist for surgical treatment, as the cluster of symptoms was extremely rare and very complicated. Multislice spiral computed tomography brings about a turning point: "There is diffuse osteosclerotic reconstruction of the massa lateralis of the os sacrum on both sides. In the distortion of the ventral cortex of the os sacrum ..... the bone is almost completely healed ..... There is inhomogeneous increased sclerosis in the second sacral segment in the area of the transverse fracture."

Conclusion:
After only 7 weeks of BEMER 3000 therapy: "Healed sacral H fatigue fracture on both sides with signs of spongiose reconstruction with diffusely increased sclerosing. Almost complete osseous consolidation is evident in the fracture with a pitch in ventral direction."

Using the BEMER Therapy in Oral Surgery
New Option in the Treatment of the Osteonecrosis of the Jaw Caused by Bisphosphonates

Dr. Cséplő Krisztina

Military Hospital, Oral Surgery Ambulance

A hardly treatable and commonly therapy-resistant defect in the oral cavity membrane is the osteonecrosis of the jaw caused by medicines containing bisphosphonates (ONJ). The pathomechanisms of this disease, known since 2003, is still not charted in detail and several factors may be involved.

Bisphosphonate therapy is widely used in patients with bone metastases from a primary tumor, osteoporosis, myeloma multiplex, or other diseases with loss of bone. Medicines may be intravenous or tablets. In patients with myeloma multiplex and tumor metastasis, intravenous medicine is part of the treatment protocol.

Osteonecrosis of the jaw is observed in patients who received long-term oral or intravenous bisphosphonate therapy, and afterwards they suffered some bone trauma in the oral cavity, or underwent a dental intervention or eventually oral surgery.

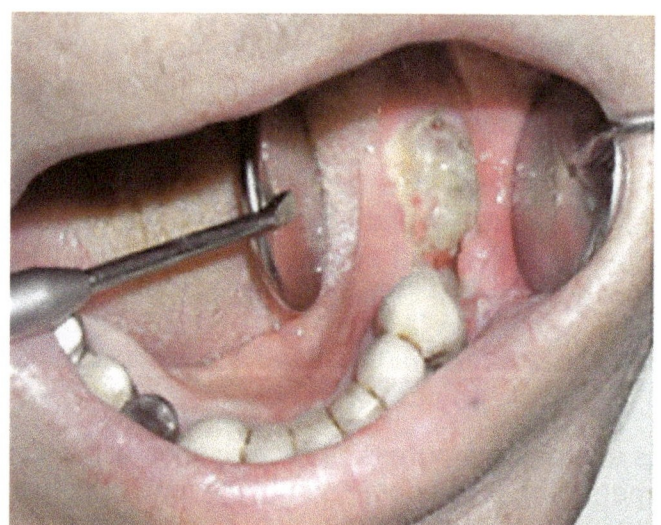 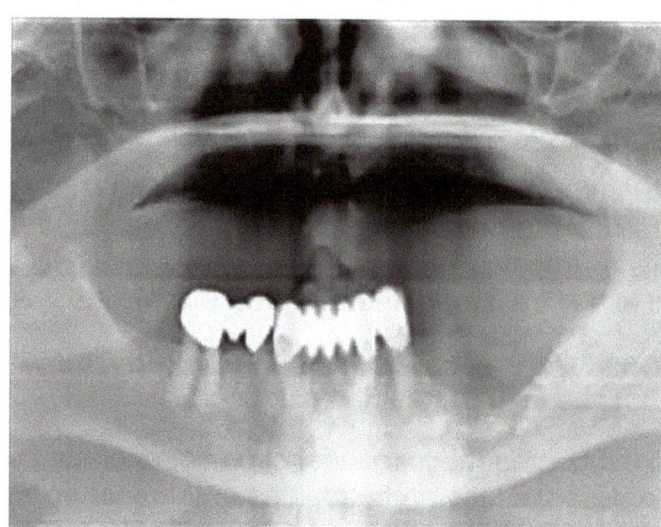

Osteonecrosis of the jaw in Stage 3.
A great portion of the lower jaw bone is clearly necrotic and exposed
The panoramic X-ay shows the necrotic portion on the lower left jaw

One of the leading symptoms of the bisphosphonate-induced osteonecrosis of the jaw is the development of a defect of the mucous membrane, the exposed jaw bone and the necrosis of the jaw bone. After dental interventions, the disease starts to develop at the place of the tooth extraction with a small and painless wound of the mucous membrane.

The exposed bone (without epithelium) may be a further source of infection that can lead to the extension of the necrosis.

Thus, with the progression of the disease, osteonecrosis may affect an increasing area of the jaw. At this stage, symptoms may include pain, swelling of the face, purulent fistula and pathological fracture.

In early stages of the disease, conservative treatment with antibiotics is recommended based on the recommendations and classification of the American Association of Oral and Maxillofacial Surgeons (AAOMS); however, in more advanced stages surgery is unavoidable. After removing the bone sequester or sometimes a larger portion of the necrotic jaw bone, slower healing of the mucous membrane, wound breakdown or dehiscence during healing may frequently occur, eventually associated with a relapse of bone necrosis.

The disease is likely to develop as a result of the fact that the jaw bones are separated from the environment by a very thin mucosa (unlike the other bones in the body) and that the oral cavity, by default, contains a large volume of diverse bacteria.

Any intervention affecting the mucous membrane may directly injure the bone, and therefore the protection of the jaw against bacteria becomes an important task. Bisphosphonates remain in the bone for 5 to 10 years, and although they aim at strengthening the bones (with great success) by inhibiting the functioning of the osteoclasts, they interfere with the dynamics of the bones and make them more prone to infections.

BEMER therapy is successfully used in several medical areas in the treatment of chronic inflammation. Its mechanism is based on a special pulsating magnetic field through which a physical agent, administered to the body, improves microcirculation which consequently also leads to an improvement in the artery metabolism.

One of the characteristics of necrotic tissues is that the blood flow is stopped. It is well known that microcirculation is of key importance in wound healing as well. Healing of a tissue with impaired blood supply is very doubtful, often completely beyond hope.

It was proposed that if the necrotic bone is surgically removed, post-operative magnetic resonance therapy may play a role in the prevention of the recurrence of jaw osteonecrosis by improving the blood circulation in the remaining healthy bone.

Improper healing of the mucous membrane observed in the osteonecrosis of the jaw (ONJ) is likely to improve as a result of the microcirculation enhancing effect of BEMER therapy.

The efficacy of BEMER therapy was studied after surgical interventions due to bisphosphonate-induced ONJ showing a very poor healing tendency and in patients with ONJ and mucosa defect to be treated with conservative therapy based on the relevant recommendations. Our study showed that BEMER therapy may be efficiently used during post-operative recovery to improve healing and to prevent relapse of the bone necrosis. Further studies are ongoing in initial stage, that is, in patients who do not yet require surgical care, assuming that BEMER therapy may also be useful in their case in the reduction of the progression of the disease.

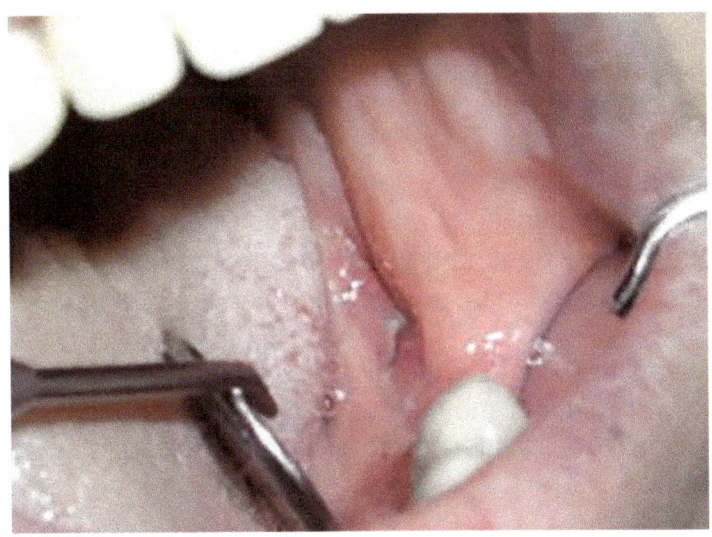

A symptom-free area after multiple surgical interventions necessitated by relapses and treated with the BEMER therapy following the last surgery.

BEMER Therapy Applied in Dermatology

Experience with the BEMER Therapy in the Treatment of Chronic Wounds and Other Dermatologic Syndromes

Dr. Horváth Ilona
Dermatologist, BIO-MED private practice, Gödöllő

BEMER therapy improves microcirculation and modulates the immune activity and positively influences the self-regulatory mechanisms of the body that provides a supplementary therapeutic option in the treatment of several skin diseases. One of the most important effects of this therapy is helping the healing of acute and chronic wounds.

The efficient treatment of chronic wounds with different etiologies has an exceptionally important role in terms of epidemiology since these wounds occur in 2-3% of the population. When complications appear, these can lead to life-threatening conditions (thrombosis, sepsis or limb amputation). The medical care of these complications constitute an exceptionally heavy burden for both the health care system and the patient.

75% of the chronic leg wounds are caused by chronic venous circulatory insufficiency. Other etiological factors: diabetes mellitus, vasoconstriction, chronic lymph edema, neuropathy, vasculitis and so on. These causes can be present simultaneously in many patients. A correct diagnosis and an adequate complex treatment are essential for the faith of the patient. In patients not eligible for angiosurgical reconstruction, improving the circulation is usually an extremely difficult task. An efficient therapy is typically hindered by the metabolic condition of the patients (diabetes mellitus), impaired movement (age, overweight or eventually previous amputation) and the lack of patient compliance (resistance to the use of a compression bandage in patients with chronic venous insufficiency).

Regardless of the etiology, the development of the wound is ultimately caused by the circulation problems in the affected region and the deficiencies in tissue metabolism and immune response.

The effects of the BEMER therapy confirmed by clinical studies (unique vasomotion effect, improving microcirculation and tissue oxygenation, increasing the quantity of bioavailable energy and stimulating protein synthesis) play a beneficial role in every stage of wound healing.

We have been using the BEMER therapy in our practice as supplementary therapy in the treatment of various dermatological syndromes for 5 years. The main fields of application:

- treatment of chronic leg wounds, diabetes feet ulcers, pressure sores and amputation stubs,
- facilitating the healing of acute traumas that affect the skin and the soft parts,
- supplementary treatment of post-herpetic neuralgia,
- reducing skin redness, swelling and itching in allergies.

Our patients received the BEMER therapy 2-3 times a week on average for 60 minutes in outpatient care. Our patients with limited movement or bedridden patients (due to their general condition) were treated by our specialized assistant in their home. If requested, we also provide BEMER devices for long- term home use.

Summing up the experiences of these 5 years, it can be stated that the systematic use of the BEMER magnetotherapy as supplementary therapy had a positive influence on the healing and quality of life of our patients with ulcers in all cases. We illustrate our therapeutic results with the following clinical images.

Patients with chronic ulcers typically "wait for a miracle" and try for years to find a "miracle doctor", "magic ointment" or "miracle treatment".

Of course, the BEMER therapy is not a miracle treatment in itself. However, it is efficacy, it can be used without pain or adverse effects, it is suitable for use at home, and may be an efficient supplementary therapy to the complex health care of these patients.

Case study 1 (82 years old woman)

The patient had a leg ulcer that appeared 6 months (after erysipelas developed in relation with chronic venous circulatory insufficiency) earlier above the external side of the right ankle and continued to deepen and extend despite adequate dermatological treatment.

Accompanying diseases: treated type 2 diabetes mellitus, treated hypertension, severe degenerative musculoskeletal complaints.

Due to the largely limited movement capacity, the patient was treated at home twice a week (basic therapy + intensive application on the leg and lower back + SLA phototherapy applied on the ulcer). After 30 sessions of treatment the leg ulcer was resolved, the musculoskeletal status significantly improved and the patient is able to walk on the street with an attendant though she was confined to her higher-floor apartment up until that moment.

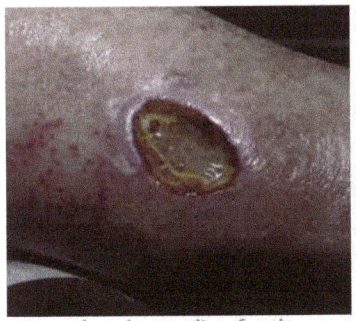
Leg ulcer (extending for the last 6 months) above the external side of the right ankle

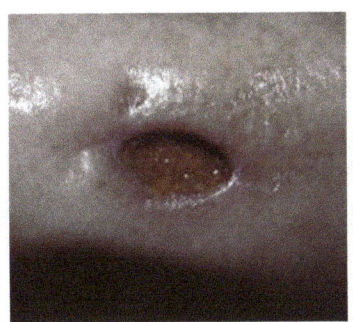
After 10 sessions of treatment

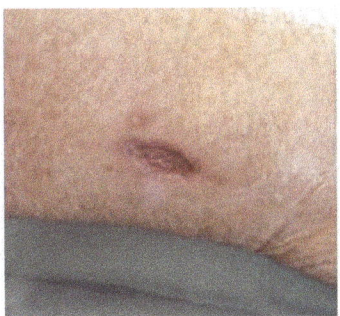
After 20 sessions of treatment

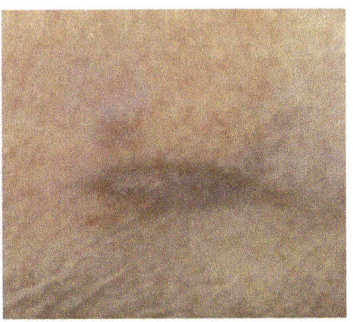
Healed after 30 sessions of treatment

1 Leg ulcer (extending for the last 6 months) above the external side of the right ankle
2 After 10 sessions of treatment
3 After 20 sessions of treatment
4 Healed after 30 sessions of treatment

Case study 2 (58 years old woman)

After an appendectomy at 40, deep vein thrombosis and a small ulcer developed on the left leg.
After a couple of years, the thrombosis recurred on the same leg.

This leg ulcer recurred 1.5 year after the BEMER therapy. The wound on the external side of the left ankle did not heal despite hospital care and periodic dermatological care; moreover, after 18 months it grew to several inches.

Accompanying diseases: hypertension treated 5 years earlier.

After 9 months of treatment (at the beginning 3 times, then 2 times a week) with the BEMER therapy, her ulcers completely healed. At the present, the patient is symptom and complaint free with only 1 session a week and with the use compression stocking.

Case study 3 (72 years old woman)

A couple of months before the BEMER therapy, multiple (in total 9) deep, coated and necrotic ulcers appeared on both legs.

Accompanying diseases: largely limited movement of both hip joints, hardly controlled hypertension for 30 years, type 2 DM for 8 years, deep vein thrombosis in the left leg for 5 years, ischaemic heart disease (IHD) and vasoconstriction in both legs.

The BEMER therapy was administered twice a week at her home. As a result of the accompanying diseases, the epithelization of the ulcers took almost 3 years because of their extremely low healing potential. Despite the ulcers recurring repeatedly over these years, the patient's quality of life significantly improved, is self-sufficient in her home and has a chance to eventually undergo a hip replacement surgery.

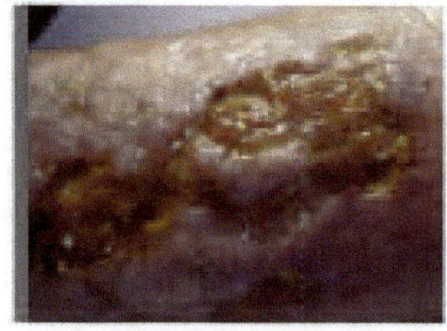 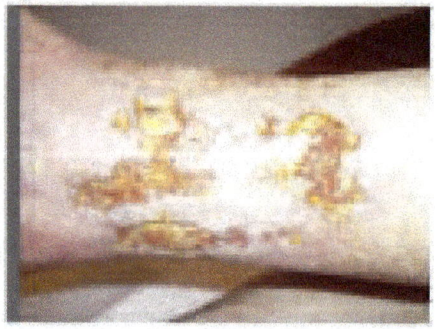 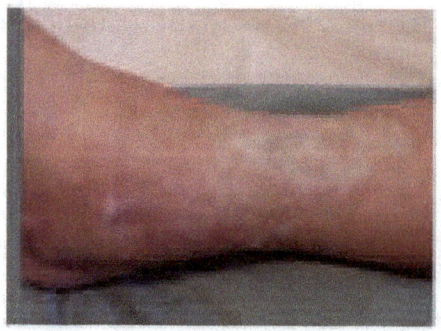

The lateral side of the left leg at the beginning of the BEMER therapy.

After the 30 BEMER therapy

Current state with two maintenance sessions a week.

Case study 4 (16 years old boy)

The BEMER therapy was administered for seven days immediately after a corrective surgery for the traumatic cheek injuries associated with nasal bone fracture.

As a result of the intensive treatment with a B.PAD applicator once a day, the average 2-3 weeks healing time significantly decreased, his hematomas completely absorbed by Day 7 and the pain ceased.

Complementary Application of the BEMER Plus System in Combination with Light Therapy of 'Visible Cosmetic Effects' on the Skin

KLOPP R (2008); Comparison of the immediate effect of a suitable electromagnetic AC field with additional vasomotoric stimulation (BEMER plus) and the effect of a suitable electromagnetic AC field with additional vasomotoric stimulation (BEMER plus) combined with soft laser-like light treatment on the surface microvessel networks of the subcutis (forehead).

SUMMARY: Complementary application of the BEMER plus system in combination with light therapy likewise promising to achieve "visible cosmetic effects" on the skin and to stimulate its function as an organ.

The main visible area of aging on the skin is the papillary dermis. The comparatively high tissue turgidity in early childhood is based on correspondingly high concentrations of hyaluronic acid in the conjunctive tissue basic substance, which gives this area a high level of viscosity and a large capacity to store water and electrolytes. After birth, retention of hyaluronic acid falls in stages and slows in the following years of life. The skin of an ageing person therefore appears flabbier and wrinkled. This effect may be amplified by UV-related degeneration of the elastic fibers and other influences.

These natural processes cannot be stopped and cannot be reversed at all. However, it is possible effectively to avoid ageing processes being accelerated (e.g. avoidance of damaging noxa, health-promoting measures and stimulation of microcirculation). It should be noted that the dermis is also a "waste site" and storage organ. Molecular and small corpuscular waste products (of endogenous and exogenous origin) are phagocytized and stored in almost limitless quantities. The reactions of the reticular dermis tend to be sluggish because of its functions as the mechanical base frame of the skin. Significant reaction patterns includes: scar formation, fibrosis, sclerosis and atrophy. The subcutaneous fatty tissue has a simple reaction. It reacts to the effect of mechanical, inflammatory or enzymatic noxa when fat cells die and fatty acids are released. These cause an increased inflammatory stimulus, which initiates a chain mechanism: Death of additional fat cells → Lipogranulomatosis → Sclerosis. From a general medical perspective, the significance of skin as the organ of homeostasis of the entire body is paramount. The dermis is representative of the circulation and, together with the intestine, is one of the most active organs of the body in terms of immunology.

From the perspective of microcirculation research, the combination of soft laser and electromagnetic AC field is seen as a form of stimulus modulation with the aim of increasing the effect of microcirculation. This stimulation effect - increased within certain boundaries – should not be overestimated, but also not denied, as the following examples from clinical investigations demonstrate.

The acquired data are presented in summary in Figures 350 and 351. Figures 352 and 353 present selected example findings.

The presented data show that more powerful effects (increased venule-side oxygen utilization and better surface quality of the skin) may be achieved by combined application of a specific electromagnetic AC field with vasomotoric stimulation (BEMER plus) and an adequately pulsed soft laser (SLT).

Data on the "venule-side oxygen utilization ΔpO_2" (average values) in subcutaneous target tissue over a 70-day treatment period in a sample of female patients ~ 50 years old treated with a specific electromagnetic AC field with vasomotoric stimulation (verum 1) or treated in combination with a specific electromagnetic AC field with vasomotoric stimulation and pulsed soft laser (verum 2) compared to a sample that underwent no treatment at all (control).

Figure 350

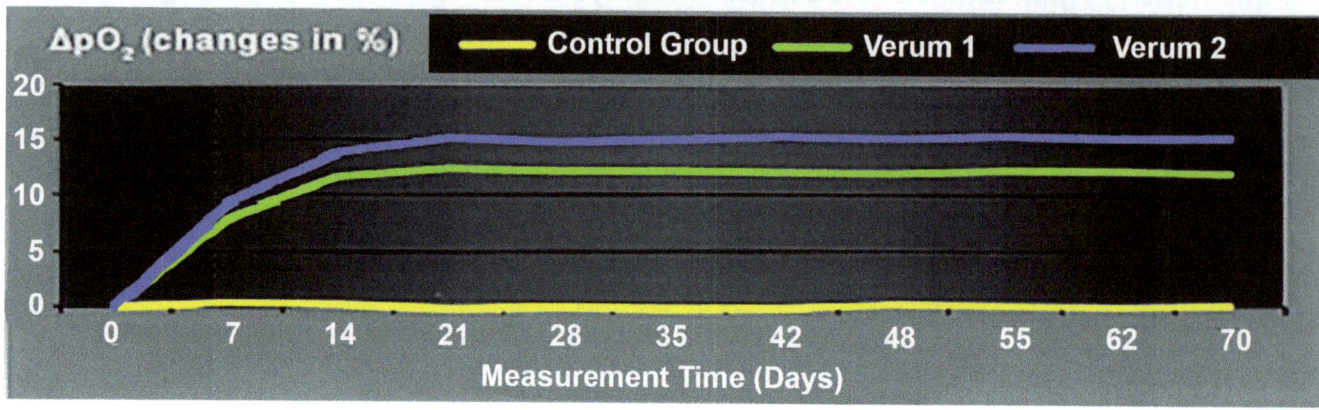

There were significant differences between the data of verum 1 group and the data of verum 2 group from day 14.

Figure 351

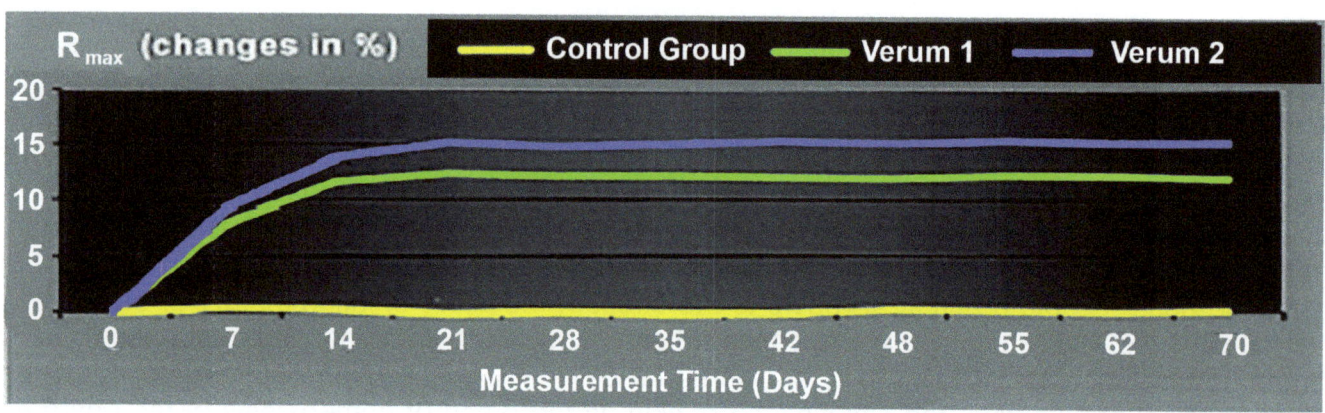

Data on the "maximum surface roughness Rmax" (average values) in subcutaneous target tissue over a 70-day treatment period in a sample of female patients ~ 50 years old treated with a specific electromagnetic AC field with vasomotoric stimulation (verum 1) or treated in combination with a specific electromagnetic AC field with vasomotoric stimulation and pulsed soft laser (verum 2) compared to a sample that underwent no treatment at all (control).

There were significant differences between the data of verum 1 group and the data of verum 2 group from day 14.

Figure 352

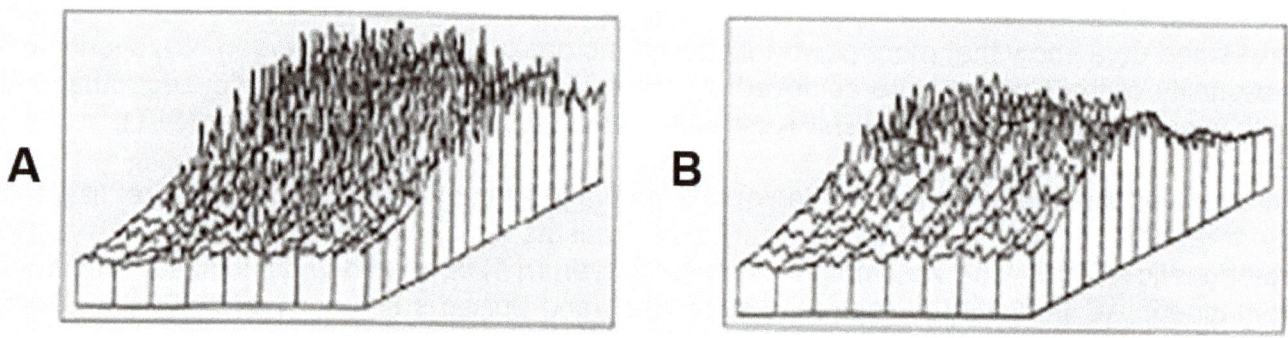

Surface condition of skin on the forehead before and after 70-day treatment with a specific electromagnetic AC field with vasomotoric stimulation in a 50- year-old patient (selected example finding).

A: Surface condition before treatment.
B: Surface condition after 70-day treatment.

Computer imaging of the measured surface quality: the roughness profiles along the defined measurement lines are combined to form a 3D image of the measured surface.

Figure 353

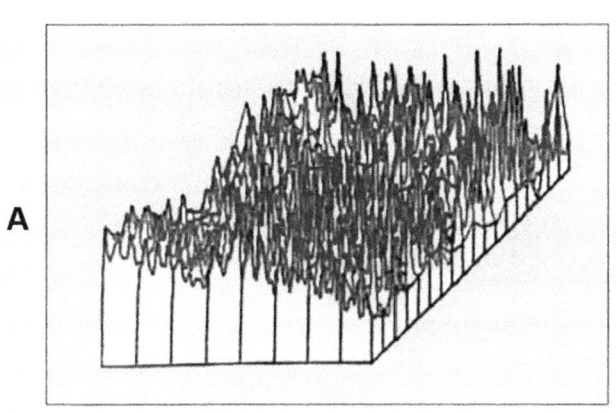
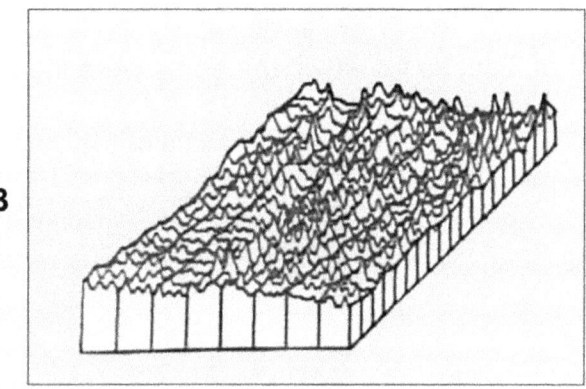

Surface condition of skin on the forehead before and after 70-day treatment with a specific electromagnetic AC field with vasomotoric stimulation and a soft laser (SLT) in a 50-year-old patient (selected example finding).

Computer imaging of the measured surface quality: the roughness profiles along the defined measurement lines are combined to form a 3D image of the measured surface.

It is notable that the surface area of the measurement fields to determine the surface quality of the target tissue after applying the electromagnetic AC field and the soft laser was 1,200 µm². The identified changes in maximum roughness surface roughnesses reflect the changed functional status of the microcirculation as a result of the applied treatments.

Even in the case of illness, the combined application of specific electromagnetic AC fields with vasomotoric stimulation and soft laser as a complementary treatment may be beneficial (examples include: diabetic polyangioneuropathy, various chronic inflammatory and degenerative processes, chronic venous insufficiency (CVI) with venous ulcers, etc.). When applying specific electromagnetic AC fields and the soft laser where disease is present, it must be noted that there are complementary treatment methods and precedence is given to established therapy concepts.

EMPHYSPACE REPORT
Emphyspace 2, 1-48(2000)

Maria-Elisabeth Olszewsky, Dr
Specialist in skin diseases, allergology and phlebology

On the symptoms of psoriasis auricularis; ulcus cruris ateriosum, and ulcus cruris neuropathicum.

In dermatology, there are a number of illnesses with a high resistance to therapy.

A total of 3 cases for which therapies were ineffective for years will be demonstrated in photographs:

Psoriasis of the auditory canal (Figures 1, 2 and 3)

I.

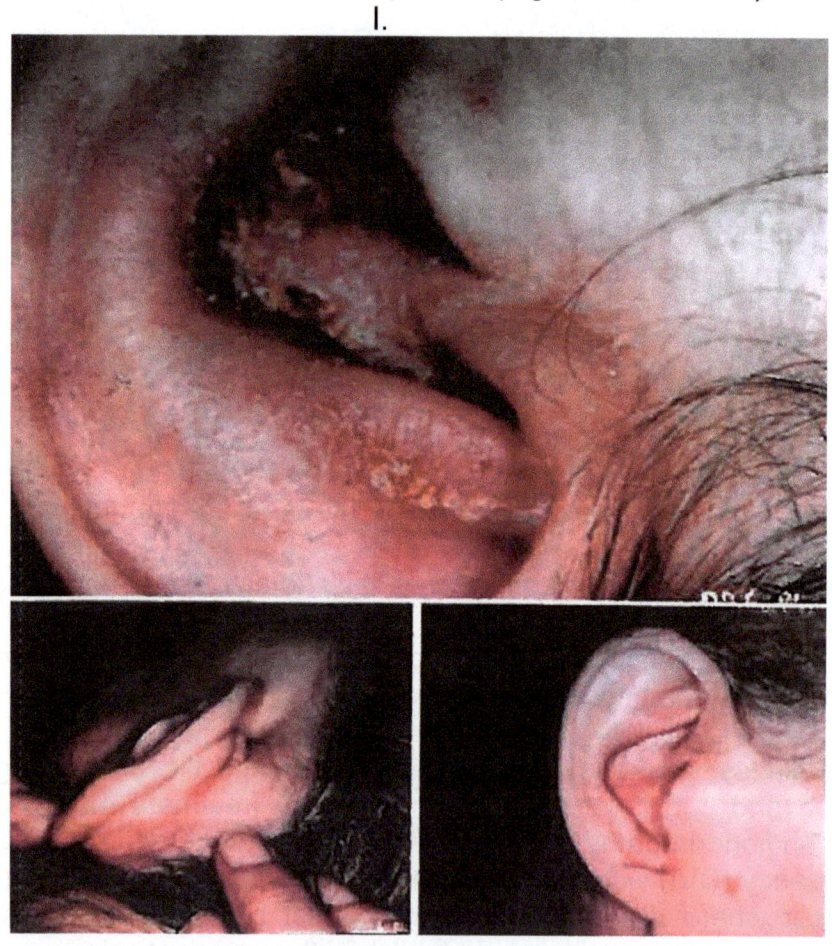

Definition: primary inflammatory dermatosis with acutely exanthematic or chronically stationary course on the basis of an inherited disposition. Example case: 53-year-old female patient with pruritic skin changes over approx. the last 4 years in auditory canal.

Treatments with dexpanthenol-based ointments and fat-based topical agents were ineffective.

Exclusive therapy with intensive applicator of the BEMER magnetic field device was applied for 2 weeks. Thereafter there was an increase in skin lesions.

A fungal culture identified a massive cutaneous candidiasis.

Therapy with antimycotic and cortisone-based topical treatments brought about healing within a few days.

Commentary: The virulence of the candida albicans fungus may have increased under the influence of the BEMER magnetic field therapy. The illness did not abate following anti-inflammatory, but not antimycotic therapy.

63-year-old female patient with arterial occlusive disease of the left leg, as well as chronic ulcus cruris with stasis dermatitis.

Previous therapy with aortocrural bypass operation in 1998, Prostavasin infusions daily over 3 weeks and femorocrural vein bypass operation in June 2000 did not heal the arteriovenous pretibial ulcer.
In August 2000, the BEMER magnetic field therapy was applied at strength P1* increasing to P3*, increasing to P4* 2x daily in September 2000 with intensive applicator over the ulcer.

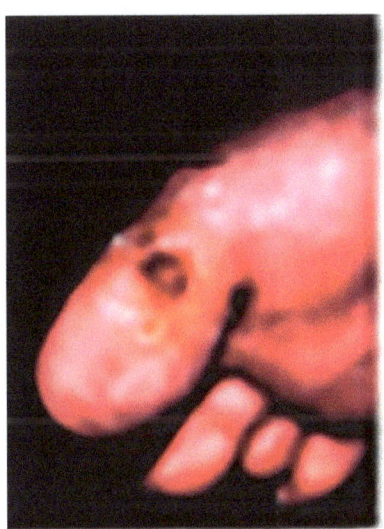
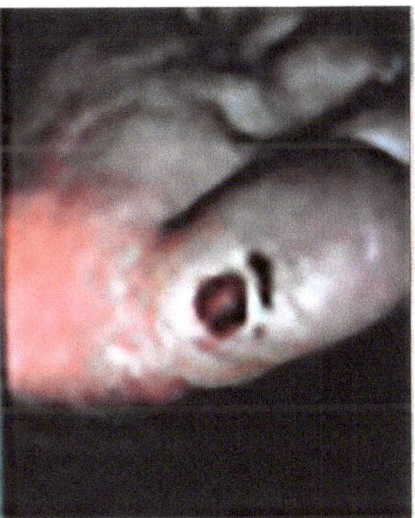
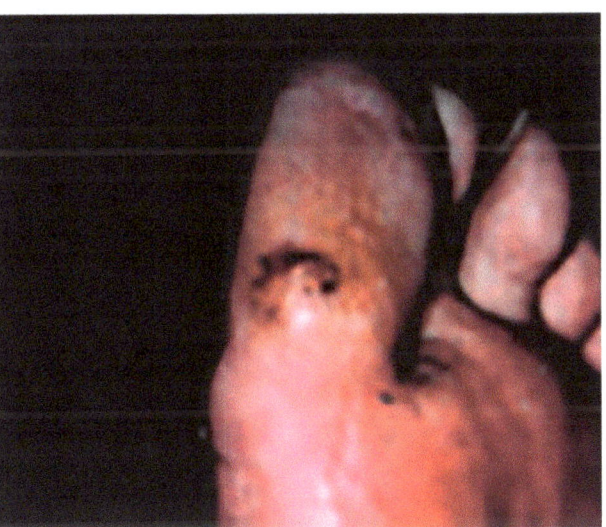

It was possible to reduce the dosage of analgesics at the end of October 2000. The patient was able to increase walking distance from 50 m to 400 m.

On a positive note, the zone of necrosis on the extensor tendons of the lower leg is becoming significantly smaller. The patient is also able to walk even longer distances without pain directly after applying the magnetic field.

3rd diagnosis: neuropathic ulcus with diabetes mellitus. Condition after deep leg vein thrombosis (Figures 4, 5 and 6)

Medical history: Pelvic and leg vein thrombosis on the right in 1975. Since then, Marcumar therapy I compression treatment of the legs. Diabetes mellitus since 1998. Since then, acro-osteopathia ulcero-mutilans with diabetic right plantar foot ulcer.

Therapies with complete relief of pressure on foot and optimum local treatment.

Intravenous vasopressin over 4 weeks showed no change in the depth and size of the ulcer. Treatment with BEMER magnetic field therapy, intensive applicator, intensity P4 since June 2000 3x per week 1x daily. No change in the findings up to the end of July 2000.

Following 2x daily therapy P4 with the intensive applicator, significant vascularization of the ulcer base and healing tendency observed in August 2000. Complete wound closure in September 2000. Stabilization of the callus in October 2000 following further therapy.

Commentary: In venous edema and diabetic vascular neuropathy, the magnetic field therapy with intensive oxygen supply had an optimum effect. The toe demonstrated significant detumescence, not achieved for the previous 2 years. Sensory stimuli, such as pain and sense of touch are slowly returning. This may open up a way to treat the diabetic neuropathy of the lower leg and feet.

BEMER Therapy Applied in Oncology

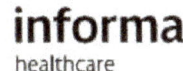

Synergistic effect of EMF–BEMER-type pulsed weak electromagnetic field and HPMA-bound doxorubicin on mouse EL4 T-cell lymphoma

Blanka Říhová[1], Tomáš Etrych[2], Milada Šírová[1], Jakub Tomala[1], Karel Ulbrich[2], and Marek Kovář[1]

[1]Department of Immunology and Gnotobiology, Institute of Microbiology, Academy of Sciences of the Czech Republic, V.V.I., Vídeňská Prague, Czech Republic and [2]Department of Biomedical Polymers, Institute of Macromolecular Chemistry, Academy of Sciences of the Czech Republic, V.V.I., Vídeňská Prague, Czech Republic

Abstract

We have investigated the effects of low-frequency pulsed electromagnetic field (LF-EMF) produced by BEMER device on experimental mouse T-cell lymphoma EL4 growing on conventional and/or athymic (nude) mice. Exposure to EMF–BEMER slowed down the growth of tumor mass and prolonged the survival of experimental animals. The effect was more pronounced in immuno-compromised nude mice compared to conventional ones. Acceleration of tumor growth was never observed. No measurable levels of Hsp 70 or increased levels of specific anti-EL4 antibodies were detected in the serum taken from experimental mice before and at different intervals during the experiment, i.e. before solid tumor appeared, at the time of its aggressive growth, and at the terminal stage of the disease. A significant synergizing antitumor effect was seen when EL4 tumor-bearing mice were simultaneously exposed to EMF–BEMER and treated with suboptimal dose of synthetic HPMA copolymer-based doxorubicin, DOX^{HYD}-HPMA. Such a combination may be especially useful for heavily treated patients suffering from advanced tumor and requiring additional aggressive chemotherapy which, however, at that time could represent almost life-threatening way of medication.

Keywords: EL4 T-cell lymphoma, athymic mice, DOX^{HYD}-HPMA, EMF, anticancer resistance, stimulation of the immune system

Introduction

Over the past three decades, potential health effects of exposure to electromagnetic fields (EMFs) have been extensively investigated in epidemiologic studies. This awareness has been triggered by the growing body of knowledge on how EMFs interact with cellular systems of living organisms. The EMF treatment is widely applied in clinical practice for prevention, diagnosis, and treatment of diseases with various etiologies. The mechanisms of biological and therapeutic effects of EMFs are still not entirely understood (Gapeyev et al., 2011). It was even suggested that low-frequency EMFs may be a risk for human health (Zheng et al., 2000; Erren, 2001; Porock & Gentry, 2002; Scott et al., 2002; Busljeta et al., 2004; Trosic et al., 2004; Chen et al., 2010; de Vocht, 2010).

Widespread concerns about whether EMFs could affect human health have been raised in epidemiologic studies trying to answer the question of their involvement in cancer appearance (Pollan et al., 2001; Weiderpass et al., 2003; Girgert et al., 2005). Low-frequency EMFs were suspected of being involved in carcinogenesis, acting as co-promoters during neoplastic transformation, modifying cell proliferation, and/or signal transduction pathways (Jin et al., 2000; Richard et al., 2002). Experimental findings also suggested that exposure to low-frequency EMFs may affect various cell functions via actions exerted on intracellular and membrane proteins, including ion channels, membrane receptors and enzymes, and cytoskeleton (Grassi et al., 2004; Lange et al., 2004). On the other hand, Scarfi et al. (2005) and Jian et al. (2009)

Address for Correspondence: Prof. Blanka Říhová, Department of Immunology and Gnotobiology, Institute of Microbiology AS CR, V.V.I., Videnska 1083, 142 20 Praha 4, Czech Republic. Tel: +420 2 4106 2345. Fax: +420 241 721 143. E-mail: rihova@biomed.cas.cz

(Received 13 July 2011; revised 26 August 2011; accepted 07 September 2011)

report that extremely low frequency (ELF) EMF induces apoptosis only in cancer cell lines which could be even enhanced by low doses of X-ray irradiation. Literature in the area of DNA strand breaks as a consequence of EMF exposure is also contradictory (Ruiz-Gómez & Martinéz-Morillo, 2009). Some investigators report on DNA damage (Vijayalaxmi & Prihoda, 2009), while others deny it (Phillips et al., 2009). So far, the findings gave no support to the hypothesis that EMF exposure increases the risk of cancer (Beniashvilli et al., 2005; Forssén et al., 2005; Sommer et al., 2007; Chen et al., 2010; de Vocht, 2010).

It is the reality that the data from scientific literature as well as from epidemiologic studies are still controversial. While some researches associate ELF-EMF exposure with carcinogenesis, other studies suggest that treatment with selected frequencies is feasible and well tolerated and may have biological efficacy in diseased patients (Lacy-Hubert et al., 1998; Lange et al., 2004; Ronchetto et al., 2004; Chen, 2010).

Here, we aim to study the biological effects of a low-frequency pulsed EMF produced by the BEMER device (EMF–BEMER) (Kafka, 1998) on an experimental cancer model, EL4 T-cell lymphoma (H-2b, Thy-1.2+) growing on normal immunocompetent mice of inbred strain C57BL/6 (B/6) and/or on immunodeficient athymic nu/nu CD-1 mice. It was demonstrated that EMF–BEMER influences microcirculation and the activity of antioxidant enzymes (Kafka & Spodrayk, 2003), especially after chemo- and radio-therapeutic cancer treatment (Gabrys, 2004) and wound healing (Kafka et al., 2005).

A new generation of polymeric anticancer drugs based on N-(2-hydroxypropyl)methacrylamide (HPMA) with improved therapeutic potential considerably decreased nonspecific side effects and the ability to stimulate anticancer immunity is already well documented (Kopecek & Kopeckova, 2010; Lammers & Ulbrich, 2010; Říhová & Kovář, 2010).

The main purpose of this study was to test (i) the effect of an exposure to EMF–BEMER on growth an experimental cancer model (EL4 T-cell lymphoma) and (ii) a possible synergizing effect of suboptimal treatment with HPMA copolymer-based doxorubicin (DOX^{HYD}-HPMA) as an anticancer agent and EMF–BEMER.

Materials and methods

Polymers conjugate DOX^{HYD}-HPMA

Polymers conjugate DOX^{HYD}-HPMA was prepared according to Etrych et al. (2008). It is a doxorubicin bound to N-(2-hydroxypropyl)methacrylamide (HPMA) copolymer carrier through a hydrazone bond with a MW ~34,000 (Figure 1).

EMF source and exposure

The BEMER device is a certified medical instrument. The control unit works with an operating voltage from 12 V to 15 V. In the connected coil mat the special multidimensional pulsating current generates a weak pulsating EMF. The basic BEMER impulse starts at a frequency of 0 Hz and constantly increases and within 30 ms reaches its maximum of 2 kHz. From there i falls back to 0 Hz and the impulse starts again. Paralle the magnetic flux intensity begins at 0 µT and pulse: upward until it reaches its maximum, according to the chosen level. From there, like the frequency, it falls back to 0 µT and the impulse starts again (Figure 2). For the experiment were chosen maximum levels of 3.5 µT, 10.5 µT, 21 µT, and 35 µT. The BEMER device neither offer: the choice of only one constant frequency nor only one constant intensity.

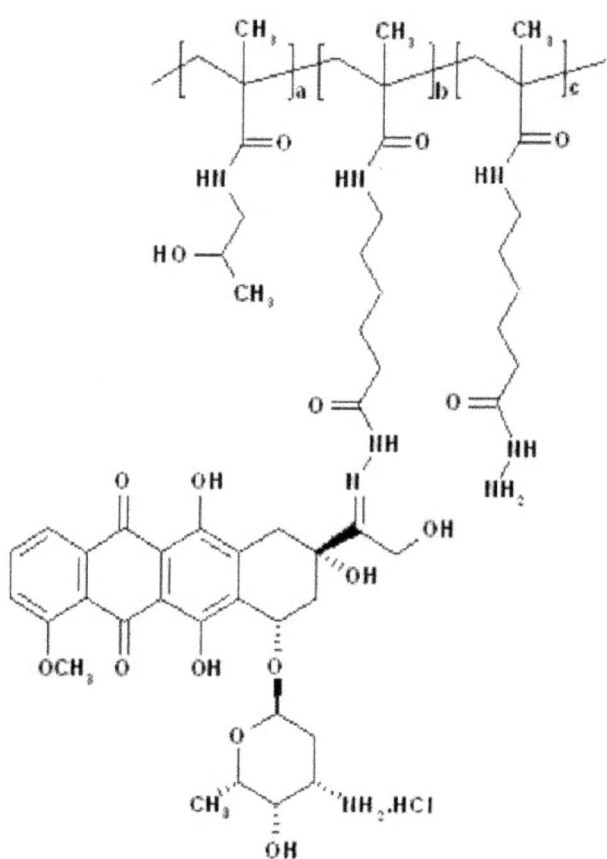

Figure 1. Structure of the DOX^{HYD}-HPMA conjugate.

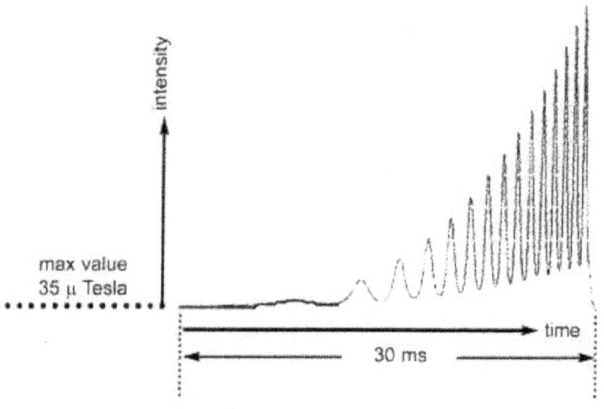

Figure 2. Typical form of electromagnetic impulse generated by the BEMER device.

Cancer cell line
Mouse T-cell lymphoma EL4 cells were obtained from American Type Culture Collection (ATTC).

Culture conditions
The EL4 cells were grown at 37°C with 5% CO_2 in RPMI 1640 medium (Gibco BRL) supplemented with heat-inactivated 10% v/v fetal calf serum (FCS) selected for low mitogenicity, 4 mM L-glutamine (Gibco BRL), 1 mM Na-pyruvate, 50 mM 2-mercaptoethanol, 4.5 g/L glucose, 100 U/mL penicillin, and 100 µg/mL streptomycin (Sigma).

Animals
All experiments were done either on conventional 8-week-old female mice of inbred strain C57BL/6 (H-2^b) purchased from the Animal Center of the Institute of Physiology, Academy of Sciences of the Czech Republic, V.V.I. or on 8-week-old female immunodeficient athymic nu/nu CD-1 mice obtained from AnLab Ltd., Prague. The mice were randomly assigned to either experimental or control groups and housed in accordance with approved guidelines. Food and water were given *ad libitum*. The animal room was maintained at 22°C. The experimental designs were in accordance with the Czech Republic Act for Experimental Work with Animals (Decrees No.311/97, 117/87, and Act No. 246/96), which is fully compatible with the corresponding European Community Acts.

In vivo tumor growth
Exposure to EMF only
On day 0, 1×10^5 EL4 T-cell lymphoma cells in 0.1 mL RPMI 1640 medium were injected subcutaneously (s.c.) on right back of C57BL/6 or nu/nu CD-1 mice. The experimental animals were exposed to low-energy EMF-BEMER. Controls were transplanted with cancer cells but were not exposed to EMF. At least 10 mice were used for each experimental group. The animals were observed daily for signs of tumor progression. The survival time, size of tumor, and the number of long-term survivors (LTS) were determined.

Exposure to EMF and DOX^{HYD}-HPMA conjugate
Mice were exposed to EMF-BEMER similarly as described above. The mice that developed palpable tumors reaching 5-8 mm^3 in diameter within 8 to 9 days after the implantation of cancer cells were intravenously treated with DOX^{HYD}-HPMA (15 mg of DOX eq./kg) diluted in PBS. Those surviving at least 60 days without any signs of a tumor were considered as LTS, and they were re-transplanted with a lethal dose (1×10^9) of the same tumor cells and left without treatment to determine the therapy-induced tumor resistance.

and quantitation of Hsp70 in serum according to the manufacturer's manual.

ELISA detection of anti-EL4 antibodies
Mice were bled from the tail veins and the separated serum was stored at −80°C until analyzed. The antibody level was estimated by an indirect ELISA method (double layer). Serum taken before the transplantation with cancer cells was used as a negative control. The sera of mice immunized five times with 5×10^5 dead EL4 cells incorporated in complete Freund's adjuvant (CFA) were taken as a positive control. Detection was carried out as reported previously (Říhová et al., 2002). Briefly, NUNC Immunoplate MaxiSorp F 96 microplates were coated either with EL4 cells (10^5 cells/well) or with EL4 cell lysate (25 µg of protein/well). Two plates were prepared simultaneously. After overnight incubation at 4°C, the plates were washed three times with PBS and PBS/0.2% Tween 20 and blocked with 1% BSA/PBS/0.02% gelatin at 37°C for 2 h. After five more washings with PBS, and PBS with 0.2% Tween 20, the microplate wells were filled with 100 µL of serial dilutions of tested sera and the plates were kept overnight at 4°C to allow quantitative antigen-antibody binding. The next day, the microplates were washed as described above and horse-radish peroxidase-conjugated, affinity-purified porcine anti-mouse Ig was diluted 1: 500 and added at 37°C for 1 h. The conjugate with the enzyme was removed, and the plates were developed with 0.015% H_2O_2-o-phenylenediamine for 10–20 min at 22°C in the dark. The reaction was stopped by the addition of 20 µL of 1M H_2SO_4 and the absorbance of the colored product was measured using an automatic ELISA reader (Tecan) at a wavelength of 492 nm against a series of wells treated only with substrate. The results were calculated as the arithmetic mean of the titer detected in three individual wells on each plate (altogether six individual wells/sample). Every assay included a negative control (serum tested alone, antigen without horse-radish peroxidase-conjugated anti-mouse Ig, or antigen without tested antisera) as well as a blank control of the specificity of the reaction.

Statistics
The statistical significance ($p < 0.05$) of the differences between volumes of tumors in the various groups was assessed by applying a two-sided Student's t-test. For each approach, three independent experiments were conducted and differences between exposed and control animals with an error probability of $p < 0.05$ were considered to be statistically significant.

Results and discussion

Figure 3A illustrates mean tumor volume change for each of the four treatment groups and Figure 3B documents survival of experimental animals. Both figures show significant retardation of tumor growth and prolongation of lifespan in mice exposed to EMF-BEMER with an intensity of 21 µT. The experiment was repeated three times with similar results.

The slight antitumor activity demonstrated in the experimental group exposed to EMF-BEMER of the intensity of 21 µT could be, among others, related to the activation of the immune system. To elucidate a tentative involvement of innate (natural or native) and/or adaptive (specific) immunity in the mechanism of action of EMF-BEMER on tumor growth, we used for further experiments immuno-compromised athymic nude (nu/nu) mice. Athymic mice suffered from an extremely limited number of T-cells, which is the reason why they have only marginal specific immunity and are routinely used to define the role of T/B lymphocytes in immunity and disease.

Similarly as in conventional mice, we have repeatedly observed in nude mice that EMF-BEMER to which the animals were exposed slowed down the growth of experimental EL4 T-cell lymphoma (Figure 4A) and significantly extended their average lifespan (Figure 4B). Interestingly enough, the exposure to EMF-BEMER gave a better result in terms of the tumor growth retardation and prolongation of survival time in immuno-compromised nude mice, where the effect was more pronounced than in conventional animals. This suggests that either innate immunity, that is strong in athymic mice, or absence of T-suppressive activity may contribute to the protective effect of EMF-BEMER.

Taken together, the results point to slight but clear-cut antitumor effects of low-frequency EMF-BEMER on EL4 mouse T-cell lymphoma or at least could be taken as a proof that exposure to EMF-BEMER is not a risk factor intensifying the development of experimental mouse T-cell lymphoma EL4.

There are numerous data confirming not only the safety but also certain antiproliferative effects of EMF

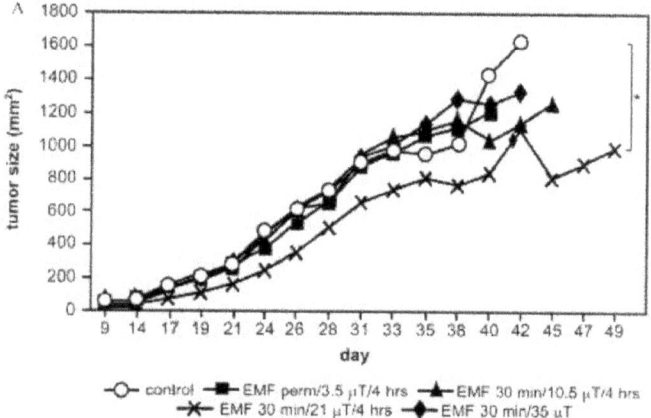

Figure 3A. Effect of pulsed EMF-BEMER on the growth of EL4 mouse T-cell lymphoma in conventional C57BL/6 mice exposed to EMF for 30 min every 4 h (intensity of 10.5 µT, 21 µT, or 35 µT) or permanently (intensity of 3.5 µT). The exposure to EMF started 4 days before cancer cell transplantation; *$p < 0.05$.

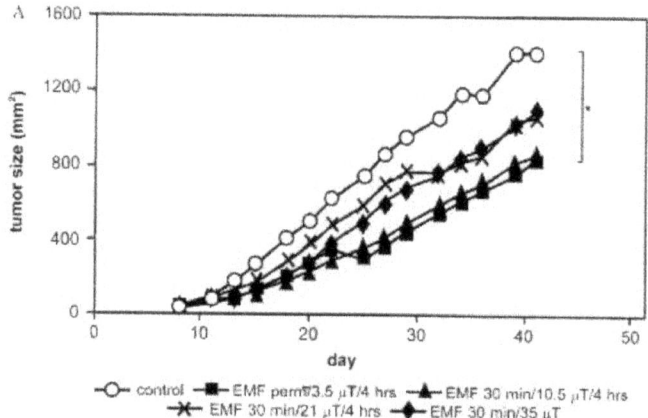

Figure 4A. Effect of pulsed EMF-BEMER on the growth of EL4 mouse T-cell lymphoma in nu/nu CD-1 mice exposed to EMF for 30 min every 4 h (intensity of 10.5 µT, 21 µT, or 35 µT) or permanently (intensity of 3.5 µT). The exposure to EMF started 4 days before cancer cell transplantation; *$p < 0.05$.

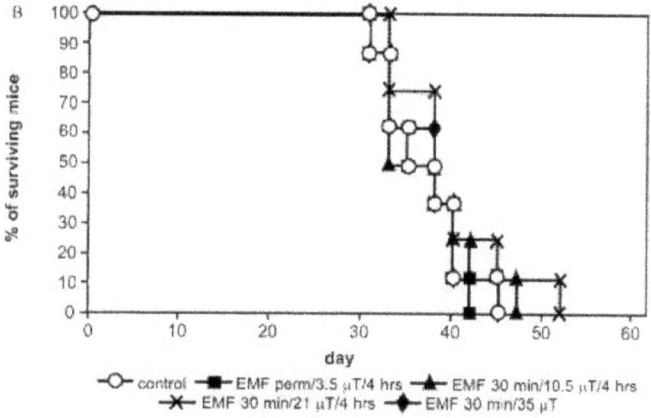

Figure 3B. Effect of pulsed EMF-BEMER on the survival of C57BL/6 mice bearing EL4 mouse T-cell lymphoma and exposed to EMF for 30 min every 4 h (intensity of 10.5 µT, 21 µT, or 35 µT) or permanently (intensity of 3.5 µT). The exposure to EMF started 4 days before cancer cell transplantation.

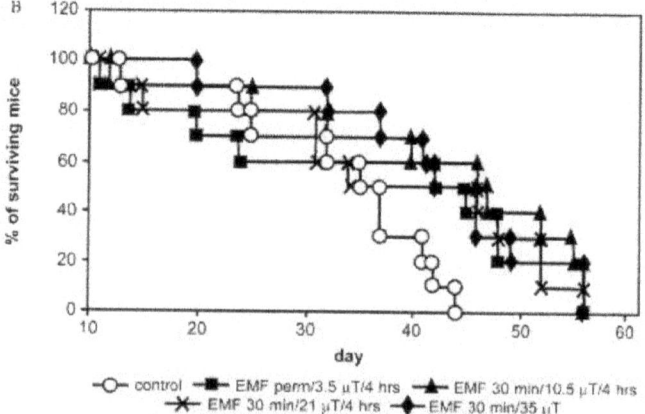

Figure 4B. Effect of pulsed EMF-BEMER on the survival of nu/nu CD-1 mice bearing EL4 mouse T-cell lymphoma and exposed to EMF for 30 min every 4 h (intensity of 10.5 µT, 21 µT, or 35 µT) or permanently (intensity of 3.5 µT). The exposure to EMF started 4 days before cancer cell transplantation.

treatment (Beneducci et al., 2005; Jiménez-García et al., 2010). Williams et al. (2001) were the first to report the reduction of tumor angiogenesis after exposure of mice with experimental cancer to pulsating EMFs. As a result, tumor growth was significantly reduced in female C57H/HeJ mice bearing mammary adenocarcinoma. Tofani et al. (2002) documented that the treatment of tumor-bearing nude mice with daily exposure to ELF-magnetic fields for 4 weeks caused significant tumor growth inhibition. Mice suffering from cancer xenograft had significantly fewer lung metastatic sites, slower tumor growth, and reduced vascularization, which together resulted in an increased survival time compared to untreated controls. Similar data were obtained with AKR/J mice suffering from spontaneous lymphoblastic lymphoma. The EMF exposure did not alter malignacy or the progression of the disease and lymphatic infiltration did not occur more often in EMF exposed than in control mice (Sommer et al., 2004; 2007). Cameron et al. (2005) report a decreased growth and reduced vascularization of human breast cancer xenografts in female athymic (nude) mice exposed to EMF either alone or in combination with gamma radiation. Similarly, a slight inhibition of the formation of chemically induced neoplastic foci in rat livers was observed when the animals were exposed to the EMF (Rannug et al., 1993).

The anticancer effects of EMF could result from inhibition of cell proliferation, targeted apoptosis induction, regulation of cellular homeostasis, affecting pathways associated with heat stress and/or activation of the immune system.

Tokalov & Gutzeit (2004) demonstrated the expression of heat-shock genes, in particular *Hsp70 (A, B, and C)* in human cells in response to ELF-EMFs alone and in combination with thermal stress. Since EMFs interact with moving charges, it is generally accepted that such treatment could stimulate the stress response by interacting directly with moving electrons in DNA (Blank & Goodman, 1999). The events mediating the EMF-stimulated stress response appear to be similar to those reported for other physiological stresses (e.g. hyperthermia, heavy metals, oxidative stress) and could well constitute the general mechanism of cell response to EMF (Lin et al., 1999). Detailed mechanisms of the processes of transduction of the electromagnetic signals into biological responses, especially changes in biosynthesis, are however still unknown. The full understanding of complicated mechanisms of action of LF-EMFs could take years. But meantime, the LF-EMF could be and has already been widely explored as a noninvasive way to treat cancers where a multimodality therapy is urgently needed.

We used an ELISA test to quantify the release of Hsp 70 into the serum of cancer-bearing mice and to test whether heat-shock proteins are involved in the positive anticancer reaction of mice exposed to EMF–BEMER. The level of Hsp 70 in the serum taken 4 days before the experiments represented a control. Serum samples were then taken from individual mice on day 0, i.e. before transplantation of malignant EL4 cells, on day 9 after the transplantation, i.e. at the time when solid cancer is already palpable, on day 16, i.e. at the time of aggressive growth of the tumor, and on day 30, i.e. in the terminal state of the disease. Using sensitive ELISA test, we repeatedly failed to determine *in vivo* measurable levels of Hsp 70 in serum samples. The reason could be quantitative as the positive effect of EMF on the expression of the heat-shock protein genes *HSP27, HSP60,* and *HSP70* was documented *in vitro* in tissue culture of human cells, malignant as well as normal, exposed to a wide range of environmental stimuli, including EMFs alone or in combination with thermal stress (Dressel & Günther, 1999; Lin et al., 1999).

Using a combination of low electric field cancer treatment and chemotherapy with 5-FU, Plotnikov et al. (2004) reported a significant tumor size reduction and a prolongation of survival time in mice bearing murine colon carcinoma CT-26. Tumor growth inhibition was accompanied by an initiation of antitumor immune reaction probably due to the antigenic material released from the deteriorating cancer cells.

Thus, we tested the formation of specific anti-EL4 antibodies in mice suffering from EL4 T-cell lymphoma and exposed or non-exposed (controls) to EMF–BEMER. The antibodies were detected by indirect ELISA and their maximal level was seen between days 9 and 16 (Tables 1 and 2). Then the free antibodies from serum disappeared, probably due to their binding to solid tumor and to metastasizing cells in peripheral blood and solid lymphatic tissues, such as lymph nodes and spleen (Říhová et al., 2002). Anti-EL4 antibodies detected in experimental animals before their first contact with EL4 cells (negative control) represent cross-reacting natural antibodies taken as a baseline. The sera of mice immunized five times with 5×10^5 dead EL4 cells incorporated in a CFA were used as a positive control. In the end, no difference was recorded between experimental groups exposed to EMF–BEMER and that without EMF intervention.

In several studies, the exposure to EMF was combined with different anticancer drugs, such as 5-FU (Plotnikov et al., 2004), anthracyclines (Liang et al., 1997; Orel et al., 2005), or methotrexate (Laqué-Rupérez et al., 2003). Liang et al. (1997) report the enhancement of direct *in vitro* cytotoxicity of daunomycin by a pulsed magnetic field using multidrug resistant subline KB-ChR-8-5-11, while no such effects were seen by Laqué-Rupérez et al. (2003) in MCF-7 breast cancer cells treated with methotrexate. The rare animal studies explain a positive effect of EMF given simultaneously with anticancer drugs by enhancing the drug delivery across biological barriers (Murthy, 1999).

The original reason for the conduction of this study was to document the effect, if any, of EMF–BEMER on the growth of cancer cell line EL4 *in vitro* and on experimental EL4 cancer model *in vivo*. The data presented in

Table 1. Serum level of anti-EL4 antibodies; antigen = EL4 cells.

Day	EMF				
	30 min/10.5 µT/4 h	30 min/21 µT/4 h	30 min/35 µT/4 h	perm/3.5 µT	0
-4	6.0[a,b]	4.5	3.0	7.0	6.0
0	6.0	4.5	6.5	6.0	6.0
9	8.5	7.5	8.5	8.0	7.5
16	10.5	10.5	10.0	9.0	10.0
30	5.5	5.0	5.0	7.5	5.0

[a]The numbers represent $\log_2$ of serum dilution.
[b]Positive control > 24, negative control (natural antibodies) 4.5–6.0.

Table 2. Serum level of anti-EL4 antibodies; antigen = EL4 cell lysate.

Day	EMF				
	30 min/10.5 µT/4 h	30 min/21 µT/4 h	30 min/35 µT/4 h	perm/3.5 µT	0
-4	9.5[a,b]	8.0	7.0	10.0	9.5
0	9.5	8.5	9.5	10.0	10.0
9	10.5	10.5	9.0	9.5	10.5
16	12.5	13.5	11.5	14.5	13.0
30	8.5	8.0	7.0	9.5	8.5

[a]The numbers represent $\log_2$ of serum dilution.
[b]Positive control > 22, negative control (natural antibodies) 8.5–10.5.

Figures 3A, 3B, 4A, and 4B, which document slight but undoubted anticancer effect of EMF, substantiated the study of a hypothetical combinatorial effect of EMF-BEMER and a cytostatic drug. We decided to use its polymeric form, as anticancer drugs bound to different polymeric carriers represent an advanced approach for anticancer treatment. Such derivatives have long-term peripheral blood circulation, increased tumor accumulation, a decrease of side-toxicity (Kopecek 2010; Kopecek & Kopeckova, 2010), and have also been extensively used for combination therapies (Krinick et al., 1994; Greco & Vicent, 2009; Lammers, 2010). In addition, in those based on N-(2-hydroxypropyl)methacrylate (HPMA) carrier was repeatedly documented therapy-dependent activation of the immune system (Říhová & Kovář, 2010).

We used a suboptimal dose (15 mg of Dox eq./kg) of doxorubicin bound to N-(2-hydroxypropyl)methacrylamide (HPMA) carrier through a hydrazone bond (DOX^{HYD}-HPMA; Figure 1). It is a formulation which was repeatedly shown to have an exceptional anticancer effect based on the direct cytotoxicity and therapy-activated anticancer-immune response (Říhová & Kovář, 2010; Šírová et al., 2010). The decreased growth of tumor was recorded in all experimental groups. About 60% (5/8) of cured mice, when treated with DOX^{HYD}-HPMA only, correspond to the fact that a suboptimal dose of the drug derivative was used. Similar percentage of LTSs was seen when mice were simultaneously exposed to EMF of the intensity of 10.5 µT (30 min every 4 h; 60% of LTS; 6/10) or permanently to 3.5 µT (70% of LTS; 7/10). Results definitely proving the effect of EMF were obtained in mice exposed to EMF-BEMER of the intensity of 21 µT (30 min every 4 h; 80% of LTS; 8/10) or 35 µT (30 min every 4 h; 80% of LTS; 8/10) (Figure 5A and B). The survival of athymic nude (nu/nu) mice was also

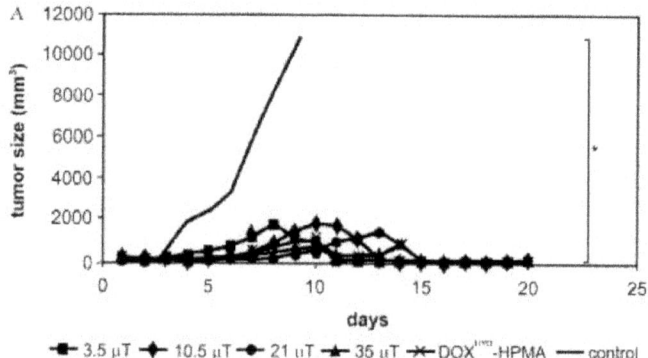

Figure 5A. The combinatory effect of pulsed EMF-BEMER and DOX^{HYD}-HPMA (15 mg DOX eq./kg) on the growth of EL4 mouse T-cell lymphoma in conventional C57BL/6 mice exposed to EMF for 30 min every 4 h (intensity of 10.5 µT, 21 µT, or 35 µT) or permanently (intensity of 3.5 µT). The exposure to EMF started 4 days before cancer cell transplantation; *$p < 0.001$.

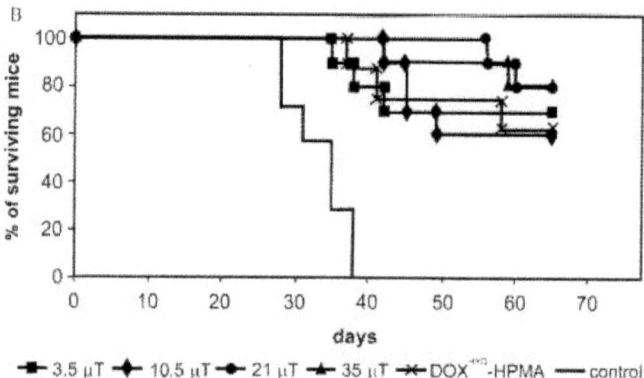

Figure 5B. The combinatory effect of pulsed EMF-BEMER and DOX^{HYD}-HPMA (15 mg DOX eq./kg) on the survival of conventional C57BL/6 mice exposed to EMF for 30 min every 4 h (intensity of 10.5 µT, 21 µT or 35 µT), or permanently (intensity of 3.5 µT). The exposure to EMF started 4 days before cancer cell transplantation.

prolonged when the animals were treated with the same dose of DOX^{HYD}-HPMA as conventional animals (15 mg of Dox eq./kg) and exposed to the EMF-BEMER. In addition, the higher intensities (21 µT and 35 µT) were more efficient (Figure 6). Unexpectedly, one mouse survived more than 4 months. It could not be recorded as a LTS as tumor, even if considerably shrunken, was still there (see "The case report").

We have seen a clear EMF dose-response, which implies that higher doses are more effective. Barbault et al. (2009) suggest that tumor-specific frequencies have to be used for the treatment of patients with advanced tumors. Such studies could be the basis for the design of strategic and clinical application of selected EMF sources for the treatment of different diseases.

Immunocompetent cells involved in the defense mechanisms are those preferentially acting in native (natural) immunity, such as macrophages and natural killer (NK) cells, and those effective in acquired (specific) immunity, such as NKT, and different subpopulations of T- and B-cells. The NK cells have an important role, though not decisive, in anticancer response where CTL cells are the major player in the game. The possibility of the effects of EMF on activity of the immune functions in living organisms has already been hypothesized and tested (Arafa et al., 2003; Di Giampaolo et al., 2006; Tuschl et al., 2006; Boscolo et al., 2007; Akan et al., 2010; Kleijn et al., 2011) but never directly demonstrated *in vivo*. For instance, Rossi et al. (2007) report that ELF-EMFs (source SEQEX) reduce the oxidative stress and the side effects of chemotherapy, and specifically myelodepression (myelotoxicity), in patients with Hodgkin's lymphoma. As oxidative stress may be, at least in part, responsible for secondary malignancies, they conclude that SEQEX with its ability to reduce an oxidative stress induced by treatment with chemo-radiotherapy may reduce the risk of late toxicities. The EMF was reported as both increasing and decreasing the activity/number of circulating NK cells or no effect at all (Gobba et al., 2009a; 2009b). However, it has to be stressed, that serious scientific data are so far still extremely limited.

In all our experimental systems, we routinely proved the activation of the immune system during anticancer therapy by re-transplantation of LTS with a lethal dose of cancer cells. As no therapy is provided after such a re-transplantation, the only explanation for the eventual eradication of re-injected cancer cells is the activation of defense mechanisms of the cancer-bearing host during the primary treatment (Říhová & Kovář, 2010). Figure 7A and B document a high cancer resistance in experimental

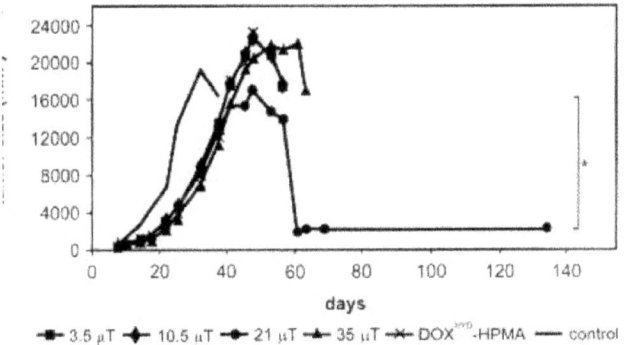

Figure 6A. The combinatory effect of pulsed EMF-BEMER and DOX^{HYD}-HPMA (15 mg DOX eq./kg) on the growth of EL4 mouse cell lymphoma in nu/nu CD-1 mice exposed to EMF for 30 min every 4 h (intensity of 10.5 µT, 21 µT, or 35 µT) or permanently (intensity of 3.5 µT). The exposure to EMF started 4 days before cancer cell transplantation; *$p < 0.001$.

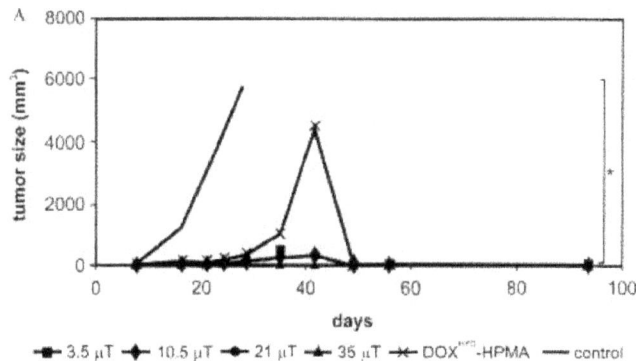

Figure 7A. The growth of EL4 mouse T-cell lymphoma in EL4-cured LTS (see Figure 5B) re-transplanted with a lethal dose (1×10^5) of EL4 cancer cells; *$p < 0.001$.

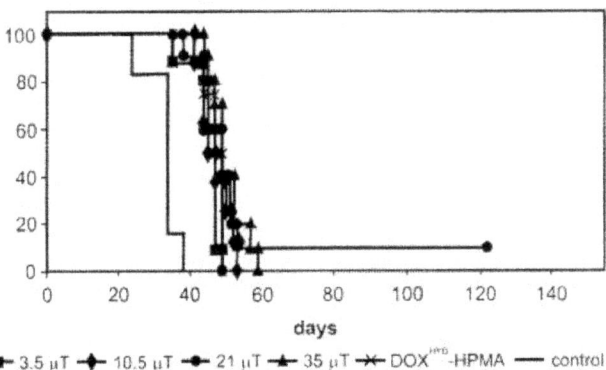

Figure 6B. The combinatory effect of pulsed EMF-BEMER and DOX^{HYD}-HPMA (15 mg DOX eq./kg) on the survival of nu/nu CD-1 mice exposed to EMF for 30 min every 4 h (intensity of 10.5 µT, 21 µT, or 35 µT) or permanently (intensity of 3.5 µT). The exposure to EMF started 4 days before cancer cell transplantation.

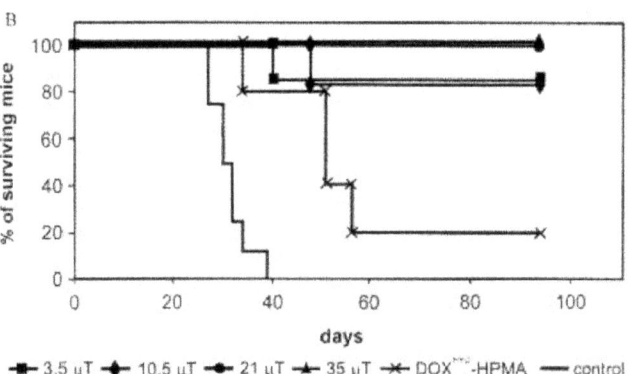

Figure 7B. Survival of EL4-cured LTS (see Figure 5B) re-transplanted with a lethal dose (1×10^5) of EL4 cancer cells.

groups exposed simultaneously to DOX^{HYD}-HPMA and EMF–BEMER. While 20% of re-transplanted LTS (1/5) survived when treated with DOX^{HYD}-HPMA only, up to 100% of them survived if simultaneously exposed to EMF–BEMER. Around 86% (6/7) of primary LTS survived, when permanently exposed to 3.5 μT; 84%; 5/6 when exposed to 10.5 μT, and 100% (8/8) when exposed either to 21 μT or to 35 μT given 30 min every 4 h. To our knowledge, it is the first direct *in vivo* documentation the immune-stimulating effect of EMF.

The case report

One nude mouse treated with DOX^{HYD}-HPMA and exposed to EMF–BEMER of an intensity of 21 μT survived more than 4 months, which is quite exceptional (Figure 6). As a rule for conventional or nude mice, immediately after the treatment with polymeric drugs the growth of experimental cancer stops. In a week or so the cancer shrinks. After another few days the tumors disappear (mice are cured) or their aggressive growth starts again. However, in that one mouse the size of the tumor (about 15 mm^3) and health condition stayed unchanged for more than 4 months. About 140 days from the beginning of the experiment and 122 days after "stabilization" of the cancer size it was decided to re-transplant the mice with a lethal dose of cancer cells similarly as we have routinely done for conventional mice to test the mechanisms responsible for the control of cancer growth. Here, mainly innate immunity could be involved in cancer eradication as the number of T-cells responsible for adaptive anticancer immunity in nude mice is very limited. Rather surprisingly, no cancer growth was observed at the site of secondary re-injection, i.e. on the left side on the back of mice. However, immediately after such "a second cancer cell attack" we have detected aggressive growth of previously stabilized primary cancer (solid EL4 thymoma) on the right side of the mouse back. The growth was almost exponential until day 38 (Figure 8). Then, from day to day, a substantial decrease in the size of tumor was observed which is usual in tumor-exhausted experimental models. We decided to end the experiment and to test (i) the sensitivity/resistance of EL4 cells isolated from the tumor to original DOX^{HYD}-HPMA conjugate, (ii) the ability of spleen cells to respond to activation with Con A (T-cell response), LPS (B cell response), and anti-CD3 plus IL-2, (iii) different immune cell subpopulations in blood, and finally (iv) to perform histopathological examination of different organs (tumor, liver, spleen, lung, heart, and bone marrow). The drug sensitivity of EL4 cancer cells isolated from the tumor was comparable with that of original cancer cell line EL4 (IC$_{50}$ = 0.44 μg/mL versus 0.53 μg/mL) and so was the ability of spleen cells to respond to different activation stimuli. Histopathological analyses did not reveal substantial metastatic cancer cell infiltration. Unfortunately, there was not enough material to precisely determine the immune cell subpopulations in the blood. However, we consider the case interesting

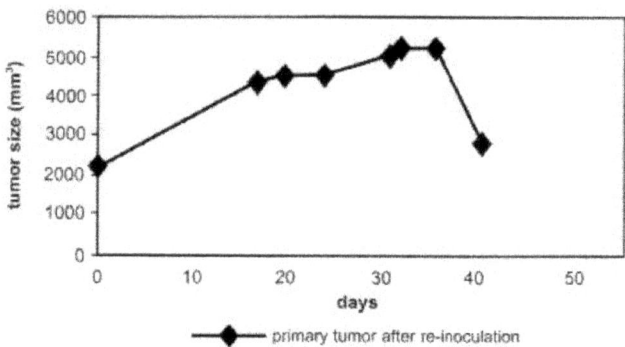

Figure 8. The growth of primary solid EL4 T-cell lymphoma injected s.c. on the right back of experimental mouse (see Figure 6B); after its s.c. re-transplantation with a lethal dose (1 × 10^5) of the same cancer cells on the left back.

enough to share it with others as hypothetical documentation of "immunoediting" (Dunn et al., 2004; Prestwich et al., 2008).

Acknowledgments

We should like to express our appreciation for the excellent technical assistance of Miss Pavlína Jungrová and Mrs. Helena Mišurcová.

Declaration of interest

This research was supported by the Institutional Research Concept AV0Z50200510, BEMER International AG, Lichtenstein and by the Grant Agency of the Academy of Sciences of the Czech Republic (grant IAA 400 200 702).

References

Akan Z, Aksu B, Tulunay A, Bilsel S, Inhan-Garip A. (2010). Extremely low-frequency electromagnetic fields affect the immune response of monocyte-derived macrophages to pathogens. Bioelectromagnetics, 31, 603–612.

Arafa HM, Abd-Allah AR, El-Mahdy MA, Ramadan LA, Hamada FM. (2003). Immunomodulatory effects of L-carnitine and q10 in mouse spleen exposed to low-frequency high-intensity magnetic field. Toxicology, 187, 171–181.

Barbault A, Costa FP, Bottger B, Munden RF, Bomholt F, Kuster N, Pasche B. (2009). Amplitude-modulated electromagnetic fields for the treatment of cancer: Discovery of tumor-specific frequencies and assessment of a novel therapeutic approach. J Exp Clin Cancer Res, 28, 51.

Beneduci A, Chidichimo G, De Rose R, Filippelli L, Straface SV, Venuta S. (2005). Frequency and irradiation time-dependant antiproliferative effect of low-power millimeter waves on RPMI 7932 human melanoma cell line. Anticancer Res, 25, 1023–1028.

Beniashvili D, Avinoach'm I, Baasov D, Zusman I. (2005). The role of household electromagnetic fields in the development of mammary tumors in women: Clinical case-record observations. Med Sci Monit, 11, CR10–CR13.

Blank M, Goodman R. (1999). Electromagnetic fields may act directly on DNA. J Cell Biochem, 75, 369–374.

Boscolo P, Di Gioacchino M, Di Giampaolo L, Antonucci A, Di Luzio S. (2007). Combined effects of electromagnetic fields on immune and nervous responses. Int J Immunopathol Pharmacol, 20, 59–63.

Busljeta I, Trosic I, Milkovic-Kraus S. (2004). Erythropoietic changes in rats after 2.45 GHz nonthermal irradiation. Int J Hyg Environ Health, 207, 549–554.

Cameron IL, Sun LZ, Short N, Hardman WE, Williams CD. (2005). Therapeutic Electromagnetic Field (TEMF) and gamma irradiation on human breast cancer xenograft growth, angiogenesis and metastasis. Cancer Cell Int, 5, 23.

de Vocht F. (2010). "Dirty electricity": What, where, and should we care? J Expo Sci Environ Epidemiol, 20, 399-405.

Dressel R, Günther E. (1999). Heat-induced expression of MHC-linked HSP70 genes in lymphocytes varies at the single-cell level. J Cell Biochem, 72, 558-569.

Di Giampaolo L, Di Donato A, Antonucci A, Paiardini G, Travaglini P, Spagnoli G, Magrini A, Reale M, Dadorante V, Iannaccone U, Di Sciascio MB, Di Gioacchino M, Boscolo P. (2006). Follow up study on the immune response to low frequency electromagnetic fields in men and women working in a museum. Int J Immunopathol Pharmacol, 19, 37-42.

Dunn GP, Old LJ, Schreiber RD. (2004). The immunobiology of cancer immunosurveillance and immunoediting. Immunity, 21, 137-148.

Erren TC. (2001). A meta-analysis of epidemiologic studies of electric and magnetic fields and breast cancer in women and men. Bioelectromagnetics, Suppl 5, S105-S119.

Etrych T, Mrkvan T, Chytil P, Koňák Č, Říhová B, Ulbrich K. (2008). N-(2-hydroxypropyl)methacrylamide-based polymer conjugates with pH-controlled activation of doxorubicin. I. New synthesis, physicochemical characterization and preliminary biological evaluation. J Appl Polym Sci, 109, 3050-3061.

Forssén UM, Rutqvist LE, Ahlbom A, Feychting M. (2005). Occupational magnetic fields and female breast cancer: A case-control study using Swedish population registers and new exposure data. Am J Epidemiol, 161, 250-259.

Gabrys M. (2004). Pulsierende Magnetfeldtherapie bei zytostatisch bedingter Polyneuropathie. Deutsche Zeitschrift für Onkologie 3, 154-156.

Gapeyev AB, Kulagina TP, Aripovsky AV, Chemeris NK. (2011). The role of fatty acids in anti-inflammatory effects of low-intensity extremely high-frequency electromagnetic radiation. Bioelectromagnetics, 32, 388-395.

Girgert R, Schimming H, Körner W, Gründker C, Hanf V. (2005). Induction of tamoxifen resistance in breast cancer cells by ELF electromagnetic fields. Biochem Biophys Res Commun, 336, 1144-1149.

Gobba F, Bargellini A, Bravo G, Scaringi M, Cauteruccio L, Borella P. (2009a). Natural killer cell activity decreases in workers occupationally exposed to extremely low frequency magnetic fields exceeding 1 microT. Int J Immunopathol Pharmacol, 22, 1059-1066.

Gobba F, Bargellini A, Scaringi M, Bravo G, Borella P. (2009b). Extremely low frequency-magnetic fields (ELF-EMF) occupational exposure and natural killer activity in peripheral blood lymphocytes. Sci Total Environ, 407, 1218-1223.

Grassi C, D'Ascenzo M, Torsello A, Martinotti G, Wolf F, Cittadini A, Azzena GB. (2004). Effects of 50 Hz electromagnetic fields on voltage-gated Ca^{2+} channels and their role in modulation of neuroendocrine cell proliferation and death. Cell Calcium, 35, 307-315.

Greco F, Vicent MJ. (2009). Combination therapy: Opportunities and challenges for polymer-drug conjugates as anticancer nanomedicines. Adv Drug Deliv Rev, 61, 1203-1213.

Chen C, Ma X, Zhong M, Yu Z. (2010). Extremely low-frequency electromagnetic fields exposure and female breast cancer risk: A meta-analysis based on 24,338 cases and 60,628 controls. Breast Cancer Res Treat, 123, 569-576.

Jian W, Wei Z, Zhiqiang C, Zheng F. (2009). X-ray-induced apoptosis of BEL-7402 cell line enhanced by extremely low frequency electromagnetic field in vitro. Bioelectromagnetics, 30, 163-165.

Jiménez-García MN, Arellanes-Robledo J, Aparicio-Bautista DI, Rodríguez-Segura MA, Villa-Treviño S, Godina-Nava JJ. (2010). Anti-proliferative effect of extremely low frequency electromagnetic field on preneoplastic lesions formation in the rat liver. BMC Cancer, 10, 159.

Jin M, Blank M, Goodman R. (2000). ERK1/2 phosphorylation, induced by electromagnetic fields, diminishes during neoplastic transformation. J Cell Biochem, 78, 371-379.

Kafka WA. (1998). Vorrichtung und elektrisches oder elektromagnetisches Signal zur Beeinflussung biologischer Systeme. Europäische Patentanmeldung 98119944.1 v 21.10.98.

Kafka WA, Spodaryk K. (2003). Effects of extremely weak BEMER 3000 type pulsed electromagnetic fields on red blood cell metabolism and hemoglobin oxygen affinity, Fizoterapia, 11, 24-31.

Kafka WA, Schütze N, Walther M. (2005). Einsatz extrem niederfrequent (BEMER typisch) gepulster schwacher elektromagnetischer Felder im Bereich der Orthopädie (Application of extreme low frequent (BEMER type) pulsed electromagnetic fields in orthopedics). Orthopädische Praxis, 41, 1, 22-24.

de Kleijn S, Bouwens M, Verburg-van Kemenade BM, Cuppen JJ, Ferwerda G, Hermans PW. (2011). Extremely low frequency electromagnetic field exposure does not modulate toll-like receptor signaling in human peripheral blood mononuclear cells. Cytokine, 54, 43-50.

Kopecek J, Kopecková P. (2010). HPMA copolymers: Origins, early developments, present, and future. Adv Drug Deliv Rev, 62, 122-149.

Kopecek J. (2010). Biomaterials and drug delivery: Past, present, and future. Mol Pharm, 7, 922-925.

Krinick NL, Sun Y, Joyner D, Spikes JD, Straight RC, Kopecek J. (1994). A polymeric drug delivery system for the simultaneous delivery of drugs activatable by enzymes and/or light. J Biomater Sci Polym Ed, 5, 303-324.

Lammers T, Ulbrich K. (2010). HPMA copolymers: 30 years of advances. Adv Drug Deliv Rev, 62, 119-121.

Lacy-Hulbert A, Metcalfe JC, Hesketh R. (1998). Biological responses to electromagnetic fields. FASEB J, 12, 395-420.

Lange S, Viergutz T, Simkó M. (2004). Modifications in cell cycle kinetics and in expression of G1 phase-regulating proteins in human amniotic cells after exposure to electromagnetic fields and ionizing radiation. Cell Prolif, 37, 337-349.

Lin H, Blank M, Goodman R. (1999). A magnetic field-responsive domain in the human HSP70 promoter. J Cell Biochem, 75, 170-176.

Liang Y, Hannan CJJr, Chang BK, Schoenlein PV. (1997). Enhanced potency of daunorubicin against multidrug resistant subline KB-ChR-8-5-11 by a pulsed magnetic field. Anticancer Res, 17, 2083-2088.

Laqué-Rupérez E, Ruiz-Gómez MJ, de la Peña L, Gil L, Martínez-Morillo M. (2003). Methotrexate cytotoxicity on MCF-7 breast cancer cells is not altered by exposure to 25 Hz, 1.5 mT magnetic field and iron (III) chloride hexahydrate. Bioelectrochemistry, 60, 81-86.

Lammers T. (2010). Improving the efficacy of combined modality anticancer therapy using HPMA copolymer-based nanomedicine formulations. Adv Drug Deliv Rev, 62, 203-230.

Murthy SN. (1999). Magnetophoresis: An approach to enhance transdermal drug diffusion. Pharmazie, 54, 377-379.

Orel VE, Kudryavets YI, Satz S, Bezdenezhnih NA, Danko ML, Khranovskaya NN, Romanov AV, Dzyatkovskaya NN, Burlaka AP. (2005). Mechanochemically activated doxorubicin nanoparticles in combination with 40 MHz frequency irradiation on A-549 lung carcinoma cells. Drug Deliv, 12, 171-178.

Phillips JL, Singh NP, Lai H. (2009). Electromagnetic fields and DNA damage. Pathophysiology, 16, 79-88.

Plotnikov A, Fishman D, Tichler T, Korenstein R, Keisari Y. (2004). Low electric field enhanced chemotherapy can cure mice with CT-26 colon carcinoma and induce anti-tumour immunity. Clin Exp Immunol, 138, 410-416.

Pollán M, Gustavsson P, Floderus B. (2001). Breast cancer, occupation, and exposure to electromagnetic fields among Swedish men. Am J Ind Med, 39, 276-285.

Porock D, Gentry J. (2002). Re: Night shift work, light at night, and risk of breast cancer. J Natl Cancer Inst, 94, 530-1; author reply 533.

Prestwich RJ, Errington F, Hatfield P, Merrick AE, Ilett EJ, Selby PJ, Melcher AA. (2008). The immune system–Is it relevant to cancer development, progression and treatment? Clin Oncol, 20, 101–112.

Rannug A, Holmberg B, Ekström T, Mild KH. (1993). Rat liver foci study on coexposure with 50 Hz magnetic fields and known carcinogens. Bioelectromagnetics, 14, 17–27.

Rossi E, Corsetti MT, Sukkar S, Poggi C. (2007). Extremely low frequency electromagnetic fields prevent chemotherapy induced myelotoxicity. Electromagn Biol Med, 26, 277–281.

Richard D, Lange S, Viergutz T, Kriehuber R, Weiss DG, Myrtill S. (2002). Influence of 50 Hz electromagnetic fields in combination with a tumour promoting phorbol ester on protein kinase C and cell cycle in human cells. Mol Cell Biochem, 232, 133–141.

Ronchetto F, Barone D, Cintorino M, Berardelli M, Lissolo S, Orlassino R, Ossola P, Tofani S. (2004). Extremely low frequency-modulated static magnetic fields to treat cancer: A pilot study on patients with advanced neoplasm to assess safety and acute toxicity. Bioelectromagnetics, 25, 563–571.

Ruiz-Gómez MJ, Martínez-Morillo M. (2009). Electromagnetic fields and the induction of DNA strand breaks. Electromagn Biol Med, 28, 201–214.

Ríhová B, Strohalm J, Kubácková K, Jelínková M, Hovorka O, Kovár M, Plocová D, Sírová M, St'astný M, Rozprimová L, Ulbrich K. (2002). Acquired and specific immunological mechanisms co-responsible for efficacy of polymer-bound drugs. J Control Release, 78, 97–114.

Ríhová B, Kovár M. (2010). Immunogenicity and immunomodulatory properties of HPMA-based polymers. Adv Drug Deliv Rev, 62, 184–191.

Scarfí MR, Sannino A, Perrotta A, Sarti M, Mesirca P, Bersani F. (2005). Evaluation of genotoxic effects in human fibroblasts after intermittent exposure to 50 Hz electromagnetic fields: A confirmatory study. Radiat Res, 164, 270–276.

Scott A, Dana KM, Stewens RY. (2002). Residential magnetic fields and risk of breast cancer. Am J Epidemiol, 155, 446–454.

Sommer AM, Streckert J, Bitz AK, Hansen VW, Lerchl A. (2004). No effects of GSM-modulated 900 MHz electromagnetic fields on survival rate and spontaneous development of lymphoma in female AKR/J mice. BMC Cancer, 4, 77.

Sommer AM, Bitz AK, Streckert J, Hansen VW, Lerchl A. (2007). Lymphoma development in mice chronically exposed to UMTS-modulated radiofrequency electromagnetic fields. Radiat Res, 168, 72–80.

Sirova M, Mrkvan T, Etrych T, Chytil P, Rossmann P, Ibrahimova M, Kovar L, Ulbrich K, Rihova B. (2010). Preclinical evaluation of linear HPMA-doxorubicin conjugates with pH-sensitive drug release: Efficacy, safety, and immunomodulating activity in murine model. Pharm Res, 27, 200–208.

Tofani S, Cintorino M, Barone D, Berardelli M, De Santi MM, Ferrara A, Orlassino R, Ossola P, Rolfo K, Ronchetto F, Tripodi SA, Tosi P. (2002). Increased mouse survival, tumor growth inhibition and decreased immunoreactive p53 after exposure to magnetic fields. Bioelectromagnetics, 23, 230–238.

Tokalov SV, Gutzeit HO. (2004). Weak electromagnetic fields (50 Hz) elicit a stress response in human cells. Environ Res, 94, 145–151.

Trosic I, Busljeta I, Pavicic I. (2004). Blood-forming system in rats after whole-body microwave exposure; reference to the lymphocytes. Toxicol Lett, 154, 125–132.

Tuschl H, Novak W, Molla-Djafari H. (2006). *In vitro* effects of GSM modulated radiofrequency fields on human immune cells. Bioelectromagnetics, 27, 188–196.

Vijayalaxmi J, Prihoda TJ. (2009). Genetic damage in mammalian somatic cells exposed to extremely low frequency electro-magnetic fields: A meta-analysis of data from 87 publications (1990–2007). Int J Radiat Biol, 85, 196–213.

Weiderpass E, Vainio H, Kauppinen T, Vasama-Neuvonen K, Partanen T, Pukkala E. (2003). Occupational exposures and gastrointestinal cancers among Finnish women. J Occup Environ Med, 45, 305–310.

Williams CD, Markov MS, Hardman WE, Cameron, I.L. (2001). Therapeutic electromagnetic field effects on angiogenesis and tumor growth. Anticancer Res, 21, 3887–3891.

Zheng T, Holford T, Mayne S. (2000). Exposure to electromagnetic fields from use of electric blankets and other in-home electrical appliances and breast cancer risk. Am J Epidemiol, 151, 1103–1111.

BEMER Electromagnetic Field Therapy Reduces Cancer Cell Radioresistance by Enhanced ROS Formation and Induced DNA Damage

Katja Storch, Ellen Dickreuter, Anna Artati, Jerzy Adamski, and Nils Cordes
PLoS One. 2016; 11(12): e0167931.
Published online 2016 Dec 13. doi: 10.1371/journal.pone.0167931
PMCID: PMC5154536 Kerstin Borgmann, Editor

Abstract

Each year more than 450,000 Germans are expected to be diagnosed with cancer subsequently receiving standard multimodal therapies including surgery, chemotherapy and radiotherapy. On top, molecular-targeted agents are increasingly administered. Owing to intrinsic and acquired resistance to these therapeutic approaches, both the better molecular understanding of tumor biology and the consideration of alternative and complementary therapeutic support are warranted and open up broader and novel possibilities for therapy personalization. Particularly the latter is underpinned by the increasing utilization of non-invasive complementary and alternative medicine by the population. One investigated approach is the application of low-dose electromagnetic fields (EMF) to modulate cellular processes. A particular system is the BEMER therapy as a Physical Vascular Therapy for which a normalization of the microcirculation has been demonstrated by a low-frequency, pulsed EMF pattern. Open remains whether this EMF pattern impacts on cancer cell survival upon treatment with radiotherapy, chemotherapy and the molecular-targeted agent Cetuximab inhibiting the epidermal growth factor receptor. Using more physiological, three-dimensional, matrix-based cell culture models and cancer cell lines originating from lung, head and neck, colorectal and pancreas, we show significant changes in distinct intermediates of the glycolysis and tricarboxylic acid cycle pathways and enhanced cancer cell radiosensitization associated with increased DNA double strand break numbers and higher levels of reactive oxygen species upon BEMER treatment relative to controls. Intriguingly, exposure of cells to the BEMER EMF pattern failed to result in sensitization to chemotherapy and Cetuximab. Further studies are necessary to better understand the mechanisms underlying the cellular alterations induced by the BEMER EMF pattern and to clarify the application areas for human disease.

Introduction

Modern multimodal anticancer strategies consist of surgery, chemotherapy and radiotherapy. The combination of intrinsic and acquired therapy resistances, normal tissue toxicities and lack of biological personalization remain obstacles to overcome for a significant improvement in cancer patient survival rates [1–4]. While our increasing understanding of tumor biology by means of various "omics" technologies and molecular biology provides a wealth of possibilities for the development of molecular-targeted agents, therapeutic strategies falling in the field of complementary and alternative medicine gradually enter the conventional cancer therapy field without clear mechanistic insight. Based on the increasing demand by the population and the unexploited potential of such approaches, we investigated the potential of a particular electromagnetic field (EMF) therapy for cancer cell therapy sensitization shown to effectively normalize tissue microcirculation.

Reviewing the literature indicated an impact of cellular functions and response to cancer therapies upon application of EMF [5]. EMF therapies reduced proliferation [6–9] and induced apoptosis [8,10–13] in different cancer cells such as osteosarcoma, breast cancer, gastric cancer, colon cancer, and melanoma. Marchesi and colleagues also showed that autophagy is induced upon EMF exposure in neuroblastoma cells [14]. Interestingly, tumor vascularization was diminished in vitro and in vivo in breast cancer treated with EMF therapy [15,16]. In line, EMF therapy decreased tumor growth in mouse models of malignant melanoma, colon carcinoma and adenocarcinoma [9,17]. Baharara and colleagues showed that extremely low EMF therapy restored the sensitivity of cisplatin resistant human ovarian carcinoma cells by increased apoptosis rates [18]. In combination with radiotherapy, EMF improved survival of mice bearing hepatoma as compared with EMF or radiotherapy alone [19]. Similarly, Cameron and colleagues showed this for breast cancer xenografts including decreased lung metastasis [20]. These studies clearly illustrate the potential of EMF therapy in combination with conventional cancer therapies as new approach for sensitizing tumors. Importantly, the applied EMF patterns show great differences in intensity, direction and frequency as well as wave forms, ranging from sinusoidal to square-wave to pulsed-wave forms across studies [5,21]. Mainly pulsed EMFs with low frequency were used.

In this study, we applied the Bio-Electro-Magnetic-Energy-Regulation (BEMER) system, which uses a low-frequency, pulsed magnetic field (max. 35 µT) with a series of half-wave-shaped sinusoidal intensity variations and was shown to increase vasomotion and microcirculation for improved organ blood flow, supply of nutrients and removal of metabolites [22,23]. In multiple sclerosis (MS) patients, BEMER therapy decreased the levels of fatigue in a randomized, double-blinded pilot study [24]. A follow-up long-term study demonstrated beneficial effect of long-term BEMER therapy on MS fatigue [25]. In the field of cell biology, Walther and colleagues showed altered gene expression of a limited number of gene products associated with e.g. energy metabolism, cytoskeleton stabilization and vesicle transport in human mesenchymal stem cells and human chondrocytes upon BEMER therapy [26]. A second study revealed BEMER therapy to delay EL4 mouse T-cell lymphoma growth and prolong survival of mice [27]. Interestingly, simultaneous BEMER therapy and synthetic HPMA copolymer-based doxorubicin showed a synergizing antitumor effect [27].

By focusing on cells from solid tumors, we explored how the BEMER EMF pattern affects the metabolome in terms of glycolysis and tricarboxylic acid (TCA) cycles and the sensitivity to radiotherapy, chemotherapy and Cetuximab. To better address this question, we utilized a more physiological 3D laminin-rich extracellular matrix (lrECM)-based cell culture model. We found a significant radiosensitization of cancer cells by the BEMER therapy mechanistically derived from higher levels of reactive oxygen species and increased numbers of DNA double strand breaks (DSBs).

Materials and Methods

Cell culture and irradiation

Human head and neck squamous carcinoma (HNSCC) cell line UTSCC15 was kindly provided by R. Grenman (Turku University Central Hospital, Finland), human lung carcinoma cell line A549, human colorectal carcinoma cell line DLD1 and human pancreatic ductal adenocarcinoma cell line MiaPaca2 were purchased from American Tissue Culture Collection. Cells were cultured in Dulbecco's modified Eagle's medium (DMEM; PAA, Cölbe, Germany) containing glutamax-I supplemented with 10% fetal calf serum (FCS; PAA) and 1% non-essential amino acids (PAA) at 37°C in a humidified atmosphere containing 8.5% CO_2. In all experiments, asynchronously growing cells were used. Three (3D)-dimensional cell cultures were accomplished by imbedding cells in 0.5 mg/ml lrECM (Matrigel; BD, Heidelberg, Germany) [28–30]. Irradiation was performed at room temperature using single doses of 200 kV X-rays (Yxlon Y.TU 320; Yxlon; dose rate ~1.3 Gy/min at 20 mA) filtered with 0.5 mm Cu. The absorbed dose was measured using a Duplex dosimeter (PTW).

BEMER therapy

BEMER (Bio-Electro-Magnetic-Energy-Regulation) therapy uses a low-frequency pulsed magnetic field [22,23] which was applied for 8 min, 1 h or 24 h. The detailed physical properties of this device are reviewed in the following patents: EP 0995463 A1, WO 2008025731 A1; WO 2011023634 A1 [31–33]. The electromagnetic field (EMF) with a pulse-duration of 30 ms and a pulse-frequency of 30 Hz was generated by a commercially available control unit B.Box Classic (BEMER AG Int.; Fig 1A) with 10 different levels of magnetic field intensity (from 0 µT to 35 µT) and a mattress applicator (Fig 1B) with a flat coil system (Bio-Electromagnetic- Energy-Regulation, BEMER International AG, Triesen, Liechtenstein). The pulse generator is fed with a mains voltage of 230 V AC / 50 Hz. Based on the commercially available construction, this mattress applicator was specifically designed for cell culture use with a maximum operating voltage of 12 V DC. Additionally, different signal intensities were used at level 1 (~2.7 µT), level 4 (~13 µT), level 7 (~23 µT) and level 10 (~35 µT). The signal is a sequence of individual pulses with a pulse width of approximately 33 milliseconds in the altitude of 3 to 35 µT within a predetermined time period of 18 to 22 seconds. The preferred exponential function described in detail in EP 0995463 A1 is $y = (x^3 \cdot e^{\sin(x3)}):c$ (with y as amplitude) [31]. The amplitudes of the single pulses correspond to an e-function and are then summarized as a group of pulses. As shown in fig 1C, BEMER-treated cells were placed within the labeled area above the flat coil on the mattress, and then stimulated with indicated intensities for 8 min, 1 h or 24 h. BEMER therapy was conducted at 37°C in a humidified atmosphere containing 8.5% CO_2 for pH 7.4. Control cells were sham-treated by placing them on the BEMER applicator for the respective time without applying the BEMER signal. BEMER signal intensity was measured using a 3D teslameter (PCE-G28, PCE, Germany) and cells were placed in the same area of the BEMER applicator for each treatment.

Samples collection for non-targeted metabolomic analysis

For metabolome analysis, A549 cells were cultured for 24 h in 3D lrECM followed by BEMER therapy (~13 µT, 8 min; sham-treated cells served as control). After 1 h, cells were harvested with 200 µl pre-cooled 80% MeOH containing 4 recovery standards to monitor extraction efficiency. The extraction solvent and cellular material were transferred into a 2 ml microtube (Sarstedt, Nümbrecht, Germany). Then, the wells were washed with 200 µl extraction solvent, which was collected in the same microtube. The samples were immediately stored in -80°C until analysis.

Non-targeted metabolomics analysis

Non-targeted metabolomics analysis was conducted at the Genome Analysis Center, Helmholtz Zentrum München. Prior to analysis, all samples were stored at -80°C. Prior to homogenization, 160 mg of 0.5 mm glass beads (Precellys, Berlin, Germany) were placed into the tubes with the cell lysates, which were collected in 80% v/v methanolic extraction solvent spiked with 4 recovery standards. The lysates were then homogenized for 2 times 25 s at 5500 rpm, with a 5 s break. The homogenization was done using a Precellys 24 homogenizer (PEQLAB Biotechnology GmbH, Erlangen, Germany) equipped with an integrated cooling unit to maintain a temperature of 4°C. After homogenization, the cell lysates were centrifuged for 5 min at 11,000 x g at 4°C and the clear extract supernatants were used thereafter. Each sample was loaded onto a 96-well 350-µl PCR plates by splitting it into 2 aliquots, 105 µl each aliquot. The first aliquot was used for LC-MS/MS analysis in positive electrospray ionization mode and the second aliquot was used for that in negative mode.

In addition to the study samples, a pool of all cell homogenates was prepared and aliquoted into the 96-well PCR plate, 105 µl per well, 3 wells for each ionization mode. Furthermore, 100 µl of a pooled human reference plasma sample (Seralab, West Sussex, United Kingdom) was extracted independently and the extract was loaded into the 96-well PCR plate, a well for each ionization mode, 105 µl in each well. A similar procedure was performed for pure lrECM as additional control for measurement and normalization to background. These samples served as control replicates throughout the study to assess process variability. Besides the reference plasma sample, 100 µl water was extracted independently and the extract was aliquoted into a 96-well plate, 3 wells per ionization mode, 105 µl in each well. These samples served as blanks. The samples were then dried in a TurboVap 96 (Zymark, Sotax, Lörrach, Germany).

Before LC-MS/MS in positive ion mode, the samples were reconstituted with 50 µl 0.1% formic acid. Those samples analyzed in negative ion mode were reconstituted with 50 µl 6.5 mM ammonium bicarbonate (pH 8.0). Reconstitution solvents for both ionization modes contained internal standards that allowed monitoring of instrument performance and also served as retention markers. LC-MS/MS analysis was performed on a linear ion trap LTQ XL mass spectrometer (Thermo Fisher Scientific GmbH, Dreieich, Germany) coupled with a Waters Acquity UPLC system (Waters GmbH, Eschborn, Germany). Two separate columns (2.1 x 100 mm Waters BEH C18, 1.7 mm particle-size) were used for acidic (solvent A: 0.1% formic acid in water, solvent B: 0.1% formic acid in methanol) and for basic (solvent A: 6.5 mM ammonium bicarbonate (pH 8.0), solvent B: 6.5 mM ammonium bicarbonate in 95% methanol) mobile phase conditions, optimized for positive and negative electrospray ionization, respectively. After injection of the sample extracts, the columns were developed with a gradient of 99.5% A to 98% B over an 11 min run time at a flow rate of 0.35 ml/min. The eluent flow was directly routed through the electrospray ionization source of the LTQ XL mass spectrometer. The full MS scan was performed from 80 to 1000 m/z and alternated between MS and MS/MS scans using a dynamic exclusion technique, which enables a wide range of metabolite coverage.

Metabolites were annotated by curation of the LC-MS/MS data against proprietary Metabolon's chemical database library (Metabolon, Inc., Durham, NC, USA) based on retention index, precursor mass and MS/MS spectra. In this study, 315 metabolites, 240 compounds of known identity (named biochemicals) and 75 compounds of unknown structural identity (unnamed biochemicals) were identified. The unknown chemicals are indicated by a letter X followed by a number as the compound identifier. The metabolites were assigned to cellular pathways based on PubChem, KEGG, and the Human Metabolome Database.

3D colony formation assay

3D colony formation assays (CFA) were applied for measurement of clonogenic cell survival as published [28,34]. For 3D CFA cells were imbedded in 0.5 mg/ml 3D lrECM in 96-well plates (BD). After 23 h, cells were treated with BEMER therapy applying different levels and durations. Irradiation occurred at different time points after BEMER therapy. In most experiments, radiotherapy was carried out 1 h after BEMER therapy. After 8–10 days, cell colonies (>50 cells) were counted microscopically. Images of representative colonies were acquired using an Axiovert 40 CFL (Zeiss, Jena, Germany). Each point on the survival curve represents the mean surviving fraction from at least three independent experiments.

3D microtumor assay

3D microtumors originated from single cells embedded in 0.5 mg/ml 3D lrECM in 96-well plates (BD) over a time period of 3 days. After 3 days, cells were treated with BEMER therapy applying different levels and durations. Irradiation occurred at different time points after BEMER therapy. After 8–10 days, cell colonies (>50 cells) were counted microscopically. Each point on the survival curve represents the mean surviving fraction from at least three independent experiments.

Cetuximab, Cisplatin and Gemcitabine treatment

At 24 h after seeding cells were treated with Cetuximab (Erbitux[L], Merck, Darmstadt, Germany; 5 µg/ml; IgG as control), Cisplatin (Teva, Ulm, Germany; 0.1 µM) or Gemcitabine (Medac, Wedel, Germany; 10 nM). After 23 h of incubation, cells were treated with BEMER therapy (~13 µT, 8 min) and irradiated 1 h later as described above. Cetuximab remained in the cell culture medium for the entire growth period, Cisplatin and Gemcitabine treated cells were washed with cell culture medium 48 h after treatment.

Foci assay

4 x 10⁵ cells per well were grown in 3D lrECM for 23 h, then treated with different levels of BEMER therapy (~13 µT and ~35 µT; 8 min) and irradiated 1 h later with 6 Gy or left unirradiated. After 24 h, cells were isolated using PBS and trypsin (PAA), fixed with 3% formaldehyde/PBS (Merck, Darmstadt, Germany), permeabilized with 0.25% Triton-X-100/PBS (Roth, Karlsruhe, Germany) and stained with specific antibodies for γH2AX and 53BP1. Samples were spread on a slide and covered with Vectashield/DAPI mounting medium. γH2AX/53BP1-positive foci were counted microscopically with an Axioscope 2 plus fluorescence microscope (Zeiss) and defined as residual DSB [34]. Immunofluorescence images were sustained using LSM 510 meta (Zeiss).

ROS scavenger analysis

Three different scavengers (Thermo Fisher Scientific (Darmstadt, Germany)), i.e. sodium pyruvate (hydrogen radicals, 10 µM), MnTBAP (superoxide anion) and Carboxy-PTIO (nitric oxid) and (both 50 µM), were applied (complete culture medium served as control) and clonogenicity and DSB measurement were performed in 3D cell cultures. Cells were treated with scavengers for 10 min. prior to BEMER therapy (~35 µT, 8 min). One hour later, cells were irradiated with 6 Gy. For foci assays, cells were isolated and fixed 24 h after irradiation, for CFA, cells were grown several days, cell line dependently.

Data analysis

Means ± standard deviation (SD) of at least three independent experiments were calculated with reference to non-treated (n.t.) samples defined in total numbers or 1.0. For statistical significance, Student t-test was performed using Microsoft®Excel 2003. P-value of less than 0.05 was considered statistically significant.

Results

BEMER treatment modulates cancer cell metabolism

Based on previous data, EMF application is likely to influence cell metabolism [7,35]. Evaluation of A549 cancer cell metabolism by the BEMER system showed metabolites of different pathways (Fig 2A) and, particularly and of the glycolysis and TCA cycle pathways to be significantly altered relative to non-treated cells (Fig 2B–2D). The levels of pyruvate, succinate, aspartate and adenosindiphosphate (ADP) were significantly downregulated after BEMER therapy whereas serine showed significant upregulation (Fig 2B–2D). These data demonstrate that the specific low-frequency pulsed BEMER EMF pattern leads to changes in certain part of the cellular metabolism.

BEMER treatment fails to alter basal tumor cell survival but radiosensitizes tumor cells in a time-dependent manner.

Next, we analyzed basal tumor cell survival of a panel of four cell lines (A549, UTSCC15, MiaPaCa, DLD1) after BEMER treatment. Interestingly, BEMER therapy did not alter basal cell survival of all tested cell lines (Fig 3A and 3B). In combination with X-ray irradiation, 3D lrECM grown cancer cell cultures, however, responded with radiosensitization when BEMER-pretreated for 8 min (Fig 3C and 3D). Upon longer BEMER exposure times, the radiosensitization was lost (Fig 3D).

Interestingly, the radiosensitizing potential of a pretreatment with the BEMER signal was confirmed in 3D grown microtumors A549, UTSCC15, MiaPaCa and DLD1 in a time-dependent manner relative to sham-treated microtumors (Fig 4A and 4B). An 8 minute pretreatment with BEMER therapy radiosensitized all tested cell lines, while longer treatment time of BEMER therapy were less or not effective (Fig 4C).

These observations evidently demonstrate that the cellular radiosensitivity of human cancer cells grown in a physiological environment can be increased by the specific BEMER EMF pattern in a time-dependent manner.

BEMER therapy/radiotherapy time interval and BEMER EMF frequency determine BEMER therapy-induced radiosensitizing potential

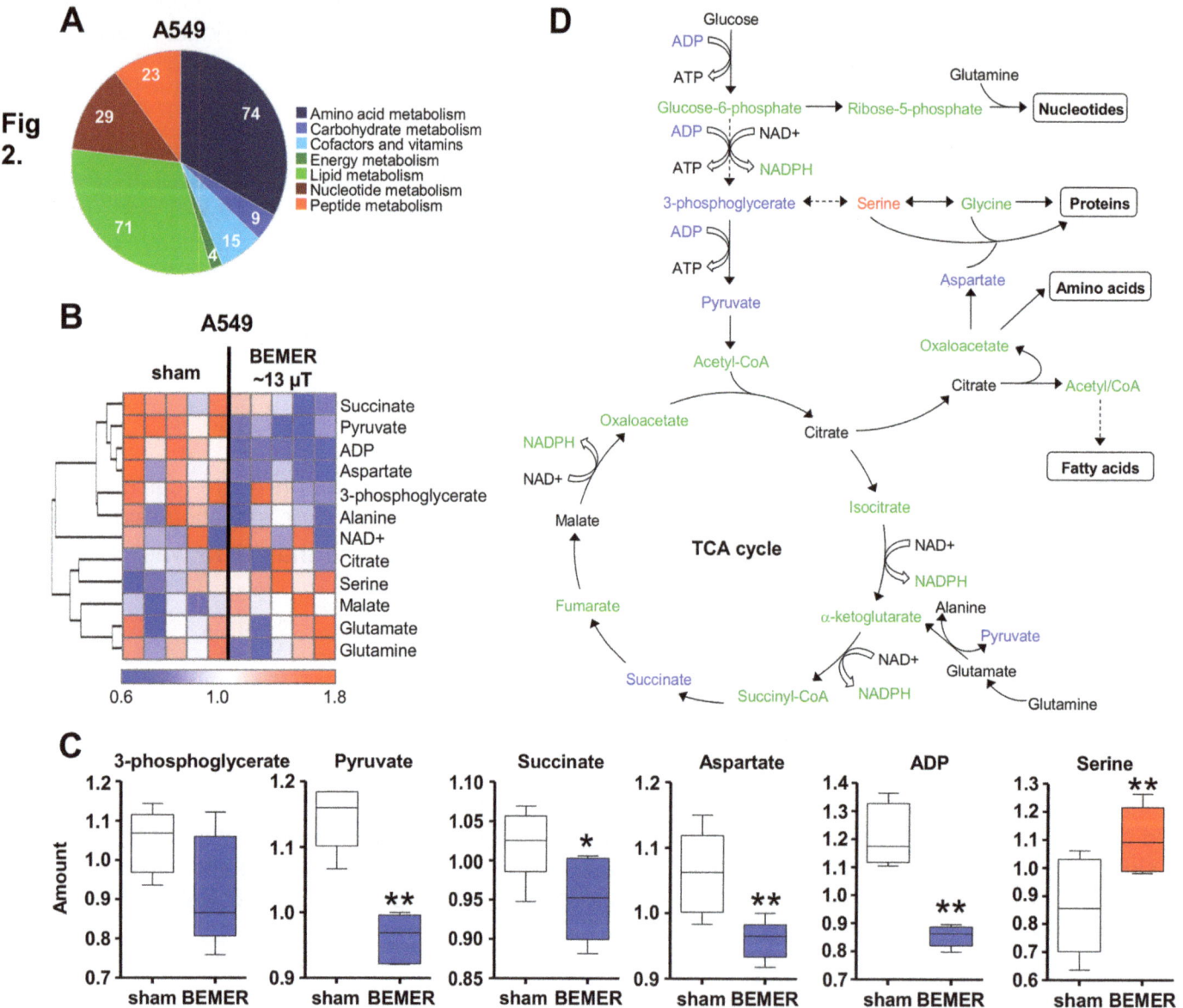

The specific BEMER EMF pattern impacts on cancer cell metabolism.

(A) Pie chart showing the number of detected metabolites categorized by pathways (Σ 225). (B) Heatmap comparing levels of metabolites in BEMER signal treated (~13 µT, 8 min) and BEMER sham-treated (sham) A549 cells. Red and blue indicate up- and downregulation, respectively. Cells were cultured in 3D lrECM for 24 h prior to BEMER treatment. (C) Amount of indicated metabolites in A549 cells without (sham) and with BEMER EMF exposure. (D) Scheme of glycolysis and TCA cycle. Metabolites in blue were downregulated, in red upregulated and in black unaffected upon BEMER therapy compared with sham-treated controls. Metabolites depicted in green were not measured in the metabolome analysis. All results represent mean ± SD. Student's t-test. n = 5. * $P < 0.05$; ** $P < 0.01$.

To further characterize the radiosensitizing effect elicited by a pretreatment with BEMER therapy, we modulated the time interval between BEMER and radiotherapy (Fig 5A) and found that the surviving fraction of 6 Gy-irradiated cells is clearly different between the tested time intervals (Fig 5B). With increasing time between BEMER treatment and radiotherapy, the radiosensitizing effect was diminished and completely abolished at the 24 h interval (Fig 5B).

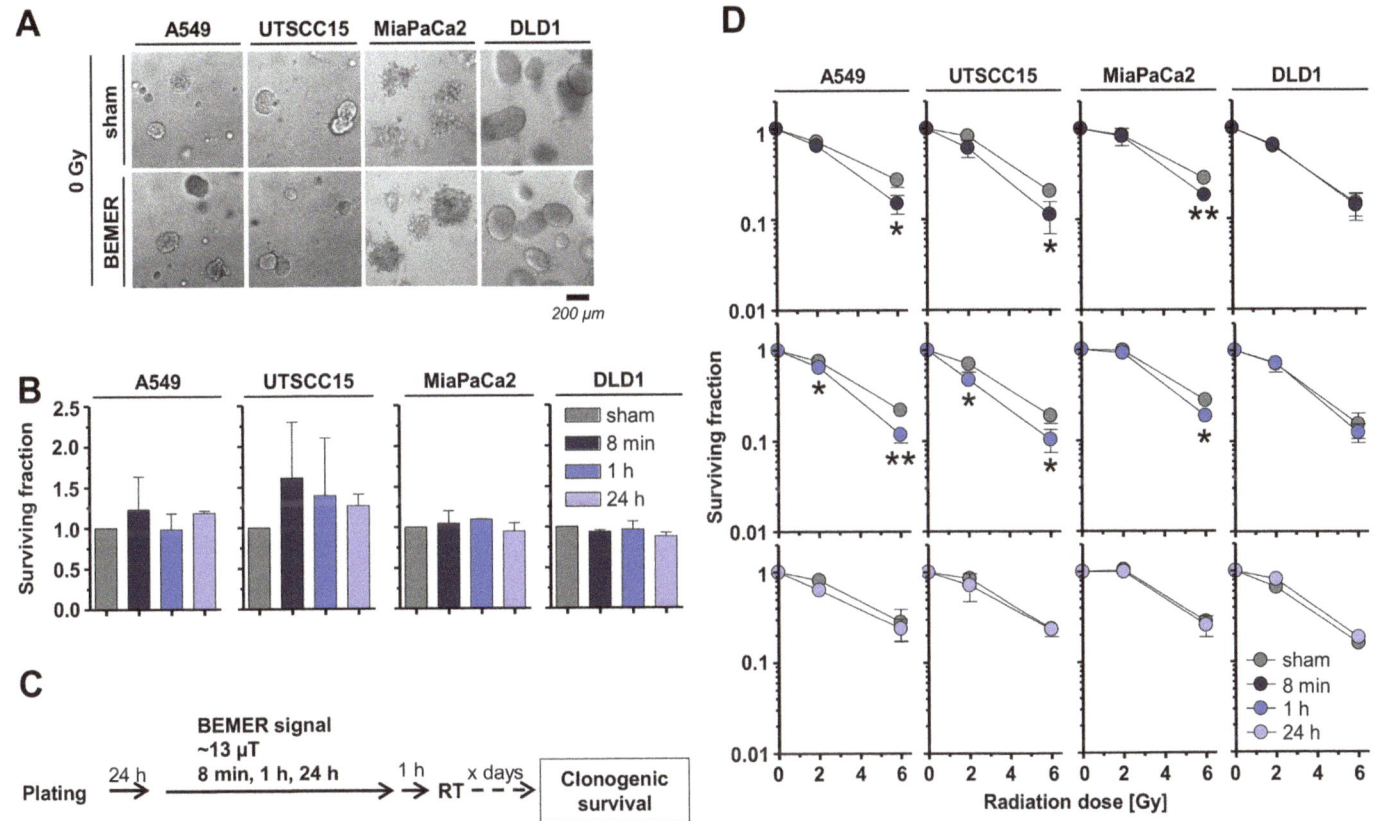

Fig 3. *BEMER therapy mediates radiosensitization of cancer cells.*
*(A) Phase contrast images and (B) basal surviving fraction of 3D grown colonies of BEMER treated (~13 μT, 8 min, 1 h, 24 h) and BEMER sham-treated (sham) cancer cell lines. (C) Flow chart of colony formation assay. (D) Clonogenic cell survival after BEMER therapy (~13 μT, 8 min, 1 h, 24 h) combined with radiotherapy (2 and 6 Gy). All results represent mean ± SD. Student's t-test. n = 3. * P < 0.05; ** P < 0.01.*

Next, we analyzed if the frequency of BEMER treatments influences cancer cell radioresistance (Fig 5C and 5D). In general, BEMER application is recommended twice a day every 12 h [22,24]. Consequently, 3D grown cells were treated either once with the BEMER signal (~13 μT, 8 min) at 1 h prior to irradiation or twice where a 12-h time interval was between the two BEMER treatments followed by irradiation after 1 h (Fig 5C). Only A549 cells were significantly radiosensitized after one-time and two-time BEMER therapy (Fig 5D). In UTSCC15 and MiaPaCa2 cells, only the one-time BEMER therapy led to radiosensitization (Fig 5D). DLD1 cells remained resistant to BEMER treatment as shown in fig 3D (Fig 5D). These data indicate that a one-time BEMER therapy followed by radiotherapy within a short time interval is most effective for radiosensitization of tumor cells with respect to the different treatment schedule tested in this study.

BEMER treatment has no additional effect on radiochemosensitivity

Due to radiochemotherapy being standard of care for the tumor types investigated in this study, we sought to determine clonogenic survival after respective radiochemotherapy (Figs [6](Figs6) and [7](and7).7). According to the treatment schedules (Figs [6A](Figs6A6A) and [7A](and7A),7A), the chemotherapeutics Cisplatin and Gemcitabine or the anti-epidermal growth factor receptor (EGFR) antibody Cetuximab were tested. Cisplatin and Gemcitabine either alone or in combination with BEMER therapy resulted in significantly decreased clonogenic cell survival in all tested cell lines ([Fig 6B and 6C](Fig 6B and 6C)). Cetuximab treatment with or without BEMER therapy led to reduced basal survival in UTSCC15 but not A549, MiaPaCa2 or DLD1 cells ([Fig 6D](Fig 6D)).

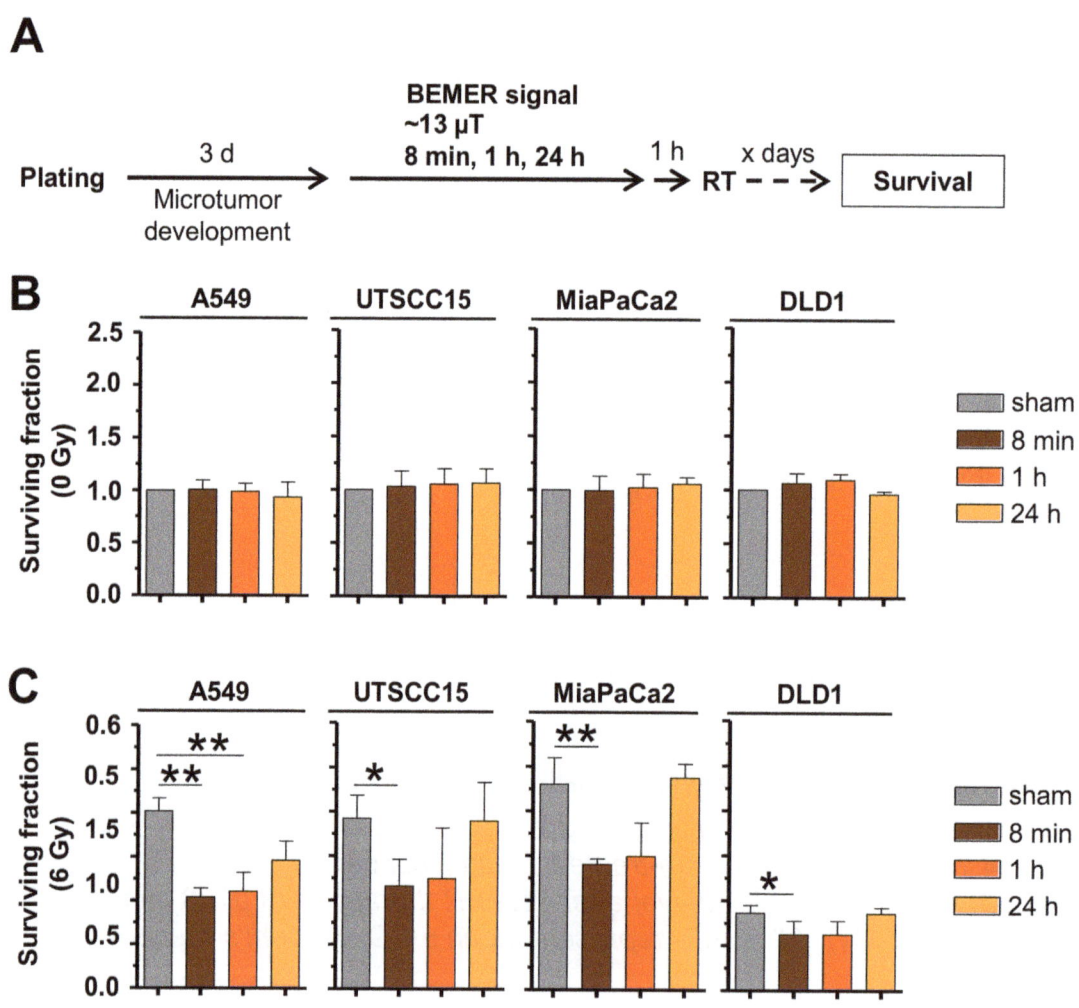

Fig 4. *BEMER therapy radiosensitizes microtumors.*

*(A) Flow chart of colony formation assay. (B) Basal surviving fraction of BEMER (~13 µT, 8 min, 1 h, 24 h) treated and BEMER sham-treated (sham) microtumors. (C) Clonogenic survival after BEMER therapy (~13 µT, 8 min, 1 h, 24 h) combined with radiotherapy (2 and 6 Gy). All results represent mean ± SD. Student's t-test compares BEMER therapy versus sham samples. n = 3. * P < 0.05; ** P < 0.01.*

The combination of Cisplatin, radiotherapy and BEMER therapy remained equitoxic to Cisplatin/radiotherapy for clonogenic survival of A549 and UTSCC15 cells ([Fig 7B](Fig 7B)). In MiaPaCa2 cells, the combination of Gemcitabine and radiotherapy showed no effect on cell survival whereas the Gemcitabine/radiotherapy/BEMER combination elicited a significantly decreased survival relative to BEMER sham-treated, irradiated controls ([Fig 7C](Fig 7C)). Cetuximab plus radiotherapy led to significantly reduced clonogenic survival of A549 and MiaPaCa2 cells with no further enhancement of the effect upon application of BEMER therapy (Fig 7D). In UTSCC15 and DLD1 cells, neither Cetuximab plus radiotherapy alone nor in combination with BEMER therapy impacted on clonogenic cell survival (Fig 7D). Thus, the combination of BEMER therapy and radiochemotherapy failed to generally enhance cancer cell sensitization.

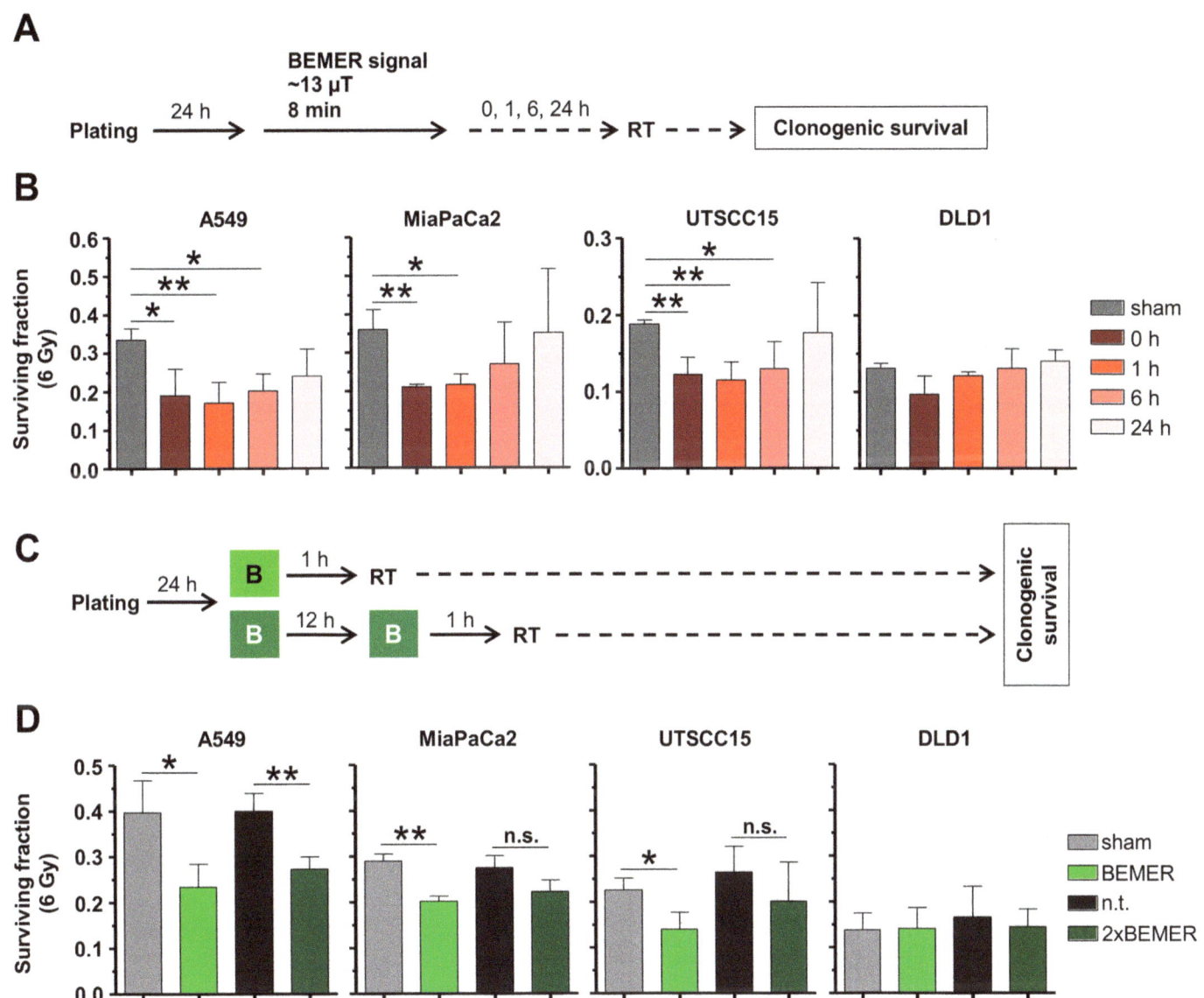

Fig 5. BEMER therapy-mediated radiosensitization depends on treatment intervals and frequency.

(A) Flow chart of colony formation assay. (B) Clonogenic survival after BEMER therapy (~13 µT, 8 min) combined with 6-Gy irradiation of indicated cell lines. BEMER sham-treated (sham) and irradiated cells served as control. Time intervals of 0, 1, 6, and 24 h between BEMER therapy and radiotherapy were applied. (C) Flow chart of colony formation assay. (D) Clonogenic survival of one time or two time BEMER therapy (~13 µT, 8 min) combined with 6-Gy irradiation of indicated cell lines (BEMER sham-treated (sham), irradiated cells as control). All results represent mean ± SD. Student's t-test. n = 3. * P < 0.05; ** P < 0.01. n.s., not significant.

BEMER therapy decreases radioresistance and increases DSB numbers dependent on BEMER signal intensity

To elucidate whether the radiosensitizing effect of BEMER therapy is related with increased signal intensity and increased number of radiation-induced DNA double strand breaks (DSBs), we applied the BEMER signal with varying intensities between 2.7 and 35 µT 1 h after 6-Gy X-ray irradiation (Fig 8A). In A549, UTSCC15 and MiaPaCa2 but not DLD1 cells, BEMER therapy accomplished radiosensitization in a signal intensity-dependent manner compared with BEMER sham-treated, irradiated controls (Fig 8B). Accordingly, DSB numbers of A549 and UTSCC15 cells were significantly elevated by BEMER EMF exposure intensity-dependently compared to controls (Fig 8C and 8D).

These results suggest a connection between BEMER therapy-mediated radiosensitization and DSB induction.

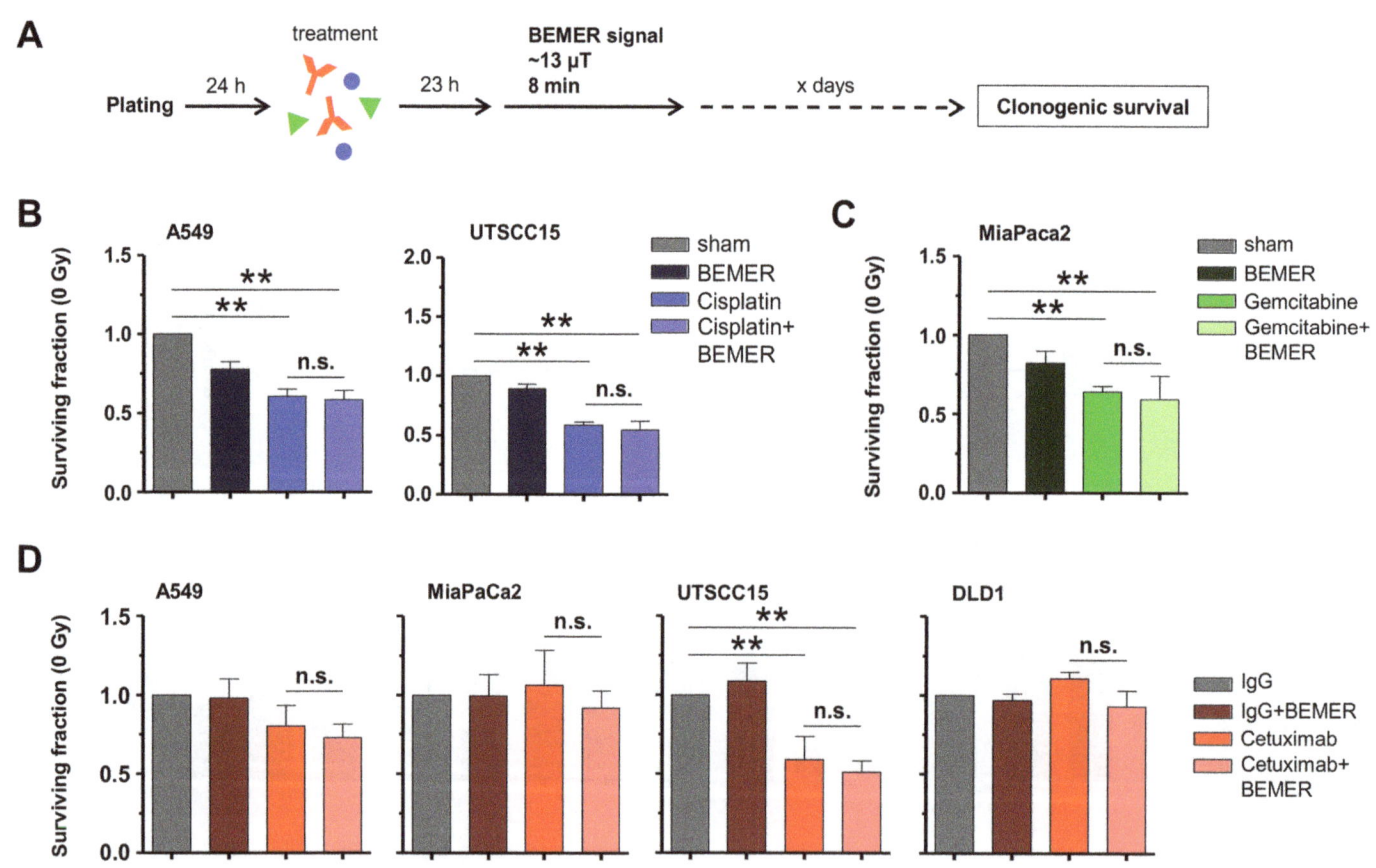

Fig 6. Sensitivity to chemotherapy and Cetuximab is not influenced by BEMER therapy.
(A) Flow chart of colony formation assay. Cells were plated in 3D lrECM, treated with respective agents followed by BEMER therapy 23 h later. (B) Basal surviving fraction after Cisplatin (0.1 µM; DMEM as control) treatment and BEMER therapy (~13 µT, 8 min). (C) Basal surviving fraction after Gemcitabine (10 nM; DMEM as control) treatment and BEMER therapy (~13 µT, 8 min). BEMER sham-treated (sham) cells served as control. (D) Basal surviving fraction after Cetuximab (5 µg/ml; IgG as control) treatment and BEMER therapy (~13 µT, 8 min). IgG-treated cells served as control. All results represent mean ± SD. Student's t-test. n = 3. * $P < 0.05$; ** $P < 0.01$. n.s., not significant

BEMER therapy increases ROS levels leading to radiosensitization via increased induction of DSBs

Connecting ROS as essential regulator of metabolomic processes and DNA damaging factor, we tested for different ROS scavengers (here sodium pyruvat, MnTBAP, Carboxy-PTIO) given prior to BEMER therapy (Fig 9A). While sodium pyruvate only abolished the effect of BEMER therapy in UTSCC15 but not in A549 cells (Fig 9B), the ROS scavengers MnTBAP and Carboxy-PTIO abrogated the BEMER-mediated radiosensitization in both cell lines leading to similar clonogenic survival as observed for BEMER sham-treated, irradiated controls (Fig 9B). Next, we tested the effect of MnTBAP and Carboxy-PTIO pretreatment on DSB induction upon BEMER treatment and irradiation and found that both scavengers reduced DSB numbers to a level similar to controls (Fig 9C). These findings indicate that the radiosensitization mediates by the BEMER therapy elicits from increased ROS levels and subsequent generation of DSBs.

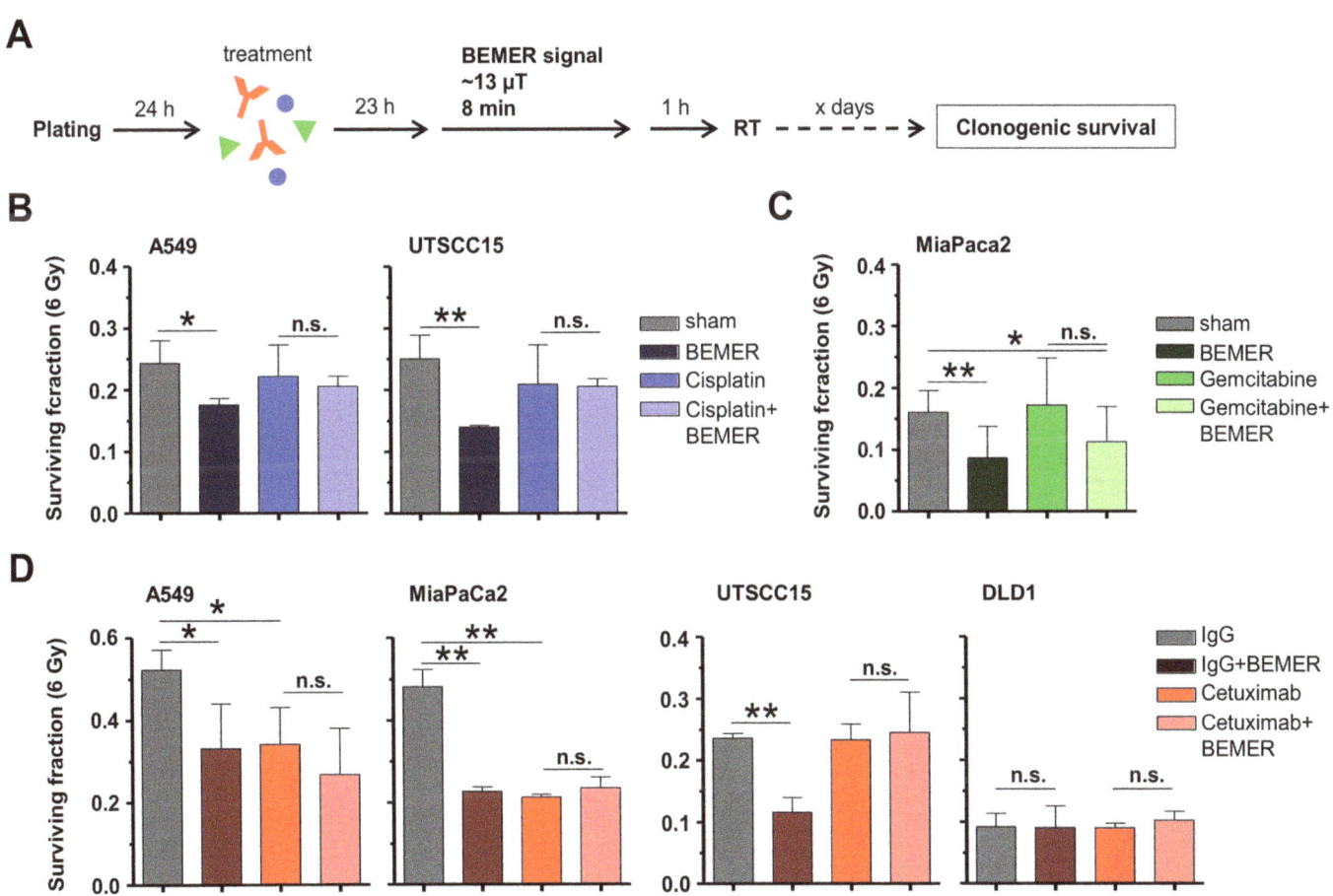

Fig 7. *BEMER therapy-mediated radiosensitization remains unaltered upon chemotherapy and Cetuximab.*

*(A) Flow chart of colony formation assay. (B) Clonogenic survival after 6-Gy irradiation combined with BEMER therapy (~13 µT, 8 min) and Cisplatin (0.1 µM; DMEM as control). (C) Clonogenic survival after 6-Gy irradiation combined with BEMER therapy (~13 µT, 8 min) and Gemcitabine (10 nM; DMEM as control). Sham-treated (sham) but irradiated cells served as control. (D) Clonogenic survival after 6-Gy irradiation combined with BEMER therapy (~13 µT, 8 min) and Cetuximab (5 µg/ml; IgG as control). IgG-treated, irradiated cells served as control. All results represent mean ± SD. Student's t-test. n = 3. * $P < 0.05$; ** $P < 0.01$. n.s., not significant.*

Discussion

Different studies showed the influence of EMF exposure on various functions of tumor cells, which beneficially impact on therapy response and tumor growth. On this basis, we hypothesized BEMER therapy to exhibit radio- and chemosensitizing potential in tumor cells. Here we show radiosensitization of cancer cell lines upon pretreatment with the particular low-frequency, pulsed EMF pattern of the BEMER system as compared with radiotherapy alone. Mechanistically, this effect is mediated through elevated ROS levels that are critically involved in the generation of DSBs.

Reviewing the literature for effects of EMF therapy in tumor cells, one has to take into consideration large differences in EMF application devices and exposure set-ups. Variations in EMF signal pulsation, strength, amplitude and frequency are highly likely to fundamentally accomplish a differential impact on cell behavior and degree of investigated effects. Using the BEMER system had the clear advantage of reported observations about improved blood flow, vasomotion and microcirculation [22,23]. Testing the BEMER EMF pattern in conjunction with conventional tumor therapies was conducted to identify the therapy-sensitizing potential of this specific EMF pattern.

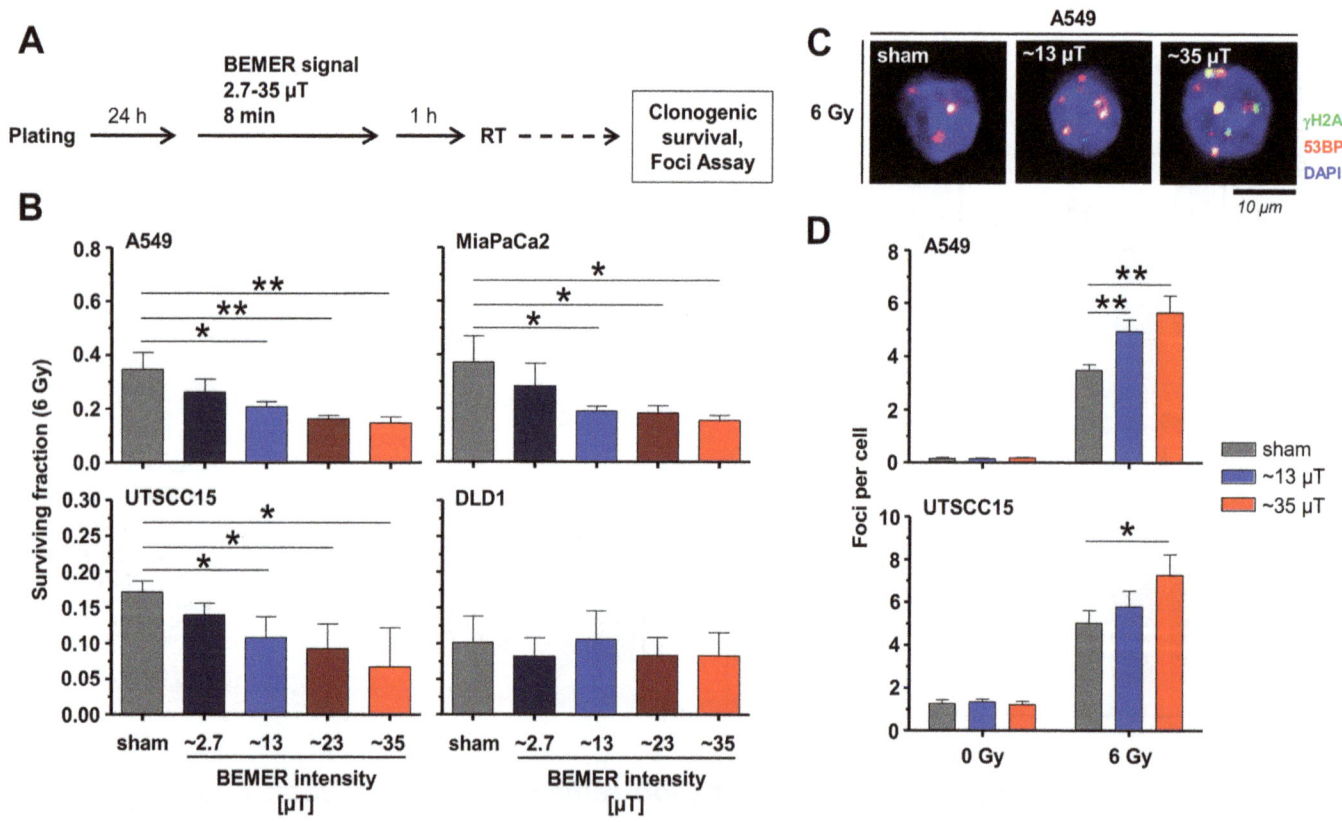

Fig 8. *BEMER signal intensity determines radiosensitization and DSB numbers.*
*(A) Flow chart of colony formation assay and foci assay. (B) Clonogenic survival after 6-Gy irradiation combined with BEMER therapy (2.7–35 µT; 8 min) of A549 and UTSCC15 cells. (C) Immunofluorescence images show nuclei with γH2AX/53BP1-positive foci after 6-Gy irradiation with (~13 or ~35 µT; 8 min) and without BEMER therapy in A549 cells. (D) Number of γH2AX/53BP1-positive DSBs 24 h after irradiation in A549 and UTSCC15 cells. BEMER sham-treated (sham), irradiated cells served as control. All results represent mean ± SD. Student's t-test. n = 3. * P < 0.05; ** P < 0.01.*

(Discussion cont)

As first step, we performed a broad metabolome analysis as EMF exposure is reported to alter physiological and metabolic processes [7,35,36]. Cancer cells exhibit a deregulated metabolism and produce their energy mainly via glycolysis [37,38]. Interestingly, we found decreased levels of metabolites of the glycolysis and the TCA cycle upon BEMER therapy. While the identification of such changes is difficult to test in-vitro, it was of utmost importance to demonstrate that the BEMER therapy does not induce cancer cell proliferation and enhanced survival of either single cells as well as microtumors.

Intriguingly, we found cells originating from lung, head and neck and pancreas to be radiosensitized by BEMER EMF exposure. As approximately 60% of cancer patients are receiving radiotherapy alone or as part of a radiochemotherapeutic regimen, this result provides the first basis describing a therapeutic potential for applying the BEMER therapy to cancer patients briefly before radiotherapy. By means of more physiological cell culture models intensively validated to in-vivo growth conditions [34,39], our results indicate a differential impact of the BEMER EMF in different tumor types. Why cells from colorectal cancers, taking into account that only one cell line was examined, demonstrated resistance to BEMER therapy warrants further analysis. Moreover, we found the radiosensitization generated by BEMER therapy to depend on (i) the duration of the treatment, (ii) the interval between BEMER therapy and radiotherapy, and (iii) the signal intensity of the EMF. Although highly speculative concerning clinical usage, it becomes obvious that the BEMER therapy is most efficient for radiosensitization when applied 1 h prior to radiotherapy with certain intensity.

Addressing the potential of the BEMER therapy to chemo- or radiochemotherapy, we observed no changes in clonogenic cancer cell survival upon chemotherapy alone or upon radiochemotherapy. This result strongly suggests that chemotherapy confers cytotoxicity via molecular mechanisms independent from BEMER therapy-related changes in cell physiology in contrast to X-ray radiation. Moreover, this could be due to our treatment schedule with a 23-h drug pretreatment before BEMER signal application. Ruiz-Gómez and colleagues showed that the EMF therapy is more efficient when cells are simultaneously exposed to EMF and cytostatic agents [40]. In our hands, administering cisplatin on top of BEMER/radiotherapy, the radiosensitizing effect caused by BEMER was even abolished. Discussing these observations on a clinical background is highly challenging and speculative. In-vivo studies are clearly required administering clinically applied radiochemotherapy regimens to identify the translational bench-to-bedside potential of BEMER EMF exposure for cancer patients.

To further explore the radiation-related mechanisms contextually linked to the BEMER therapy, we measured ROS levels and DSBs as most life-threatening DNA lesions produced by X-ray irradiation [41]. Interestingly, the application of scavengers for superoxide anions (MnTBAP) and nitric oxides (Carboxy-PTIO) abolished BEMER-related radiosensitization, which strongly proposes that the specific BEMER EMF pattern considerable increases ROS levels by yet to be discovered mechanisms. Despite the fact that our observations are in line with other cancer research studies showing EMF exposure to indirectly provoke DNA strand breaks via free radicals [5,42,43], the induction of DNA damage by EMF is quite controversially discussed. Other studies reported changes of the redox status and increased DNA damage in EMF-treated neuroblastoma [44] or leukemia cells [45,46]. Mechanistically, EMF therapy reduced antioxidant enzyme activity and enhanced nitrogen intermediates in leukemia cells [45] and increased ROS levels in neuroblastoma cells [46]. Kim and colleagues published repetitive EMF exposure of cervical cancer cells and normal lung fibroblasts to result in an increase of γH2AX phosphorylation indicative of DSBs [47]. In accordance, Winker and colleagues found increased chromosomal aberrations and elevated numbers of micronuclei upon exposure to EMF [48]. These studies support our view that BEMER therapy induces higher levels of ROS converted into elevated DSB numbers by X-ray irradiation finally detectable as radiosensitization.

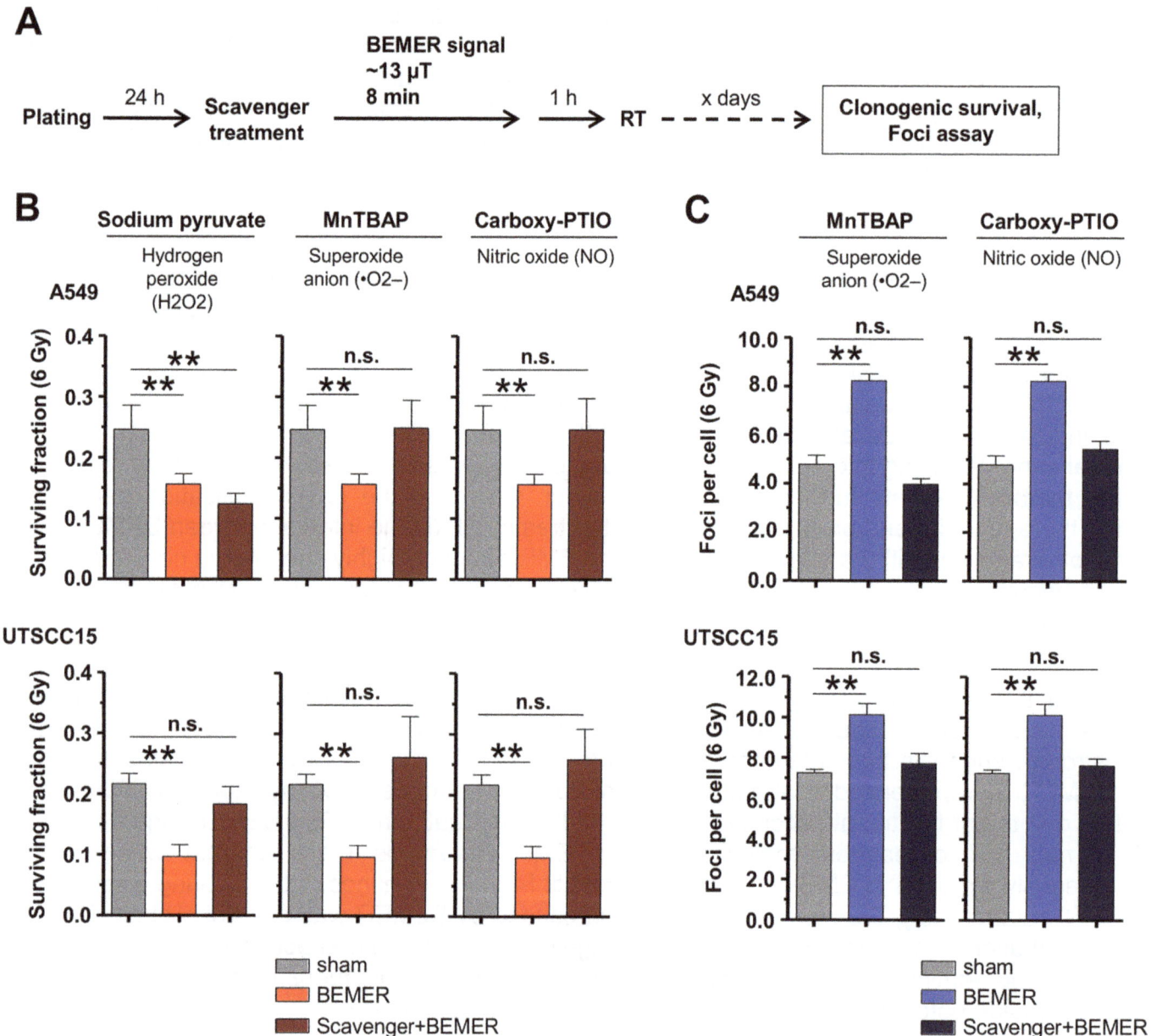

Fig 9. BEMER therapy induces elevated ROS levels resulting in increased DSB numbers.
(A) Flow chart of colony formation assay and foci assay. (B) Surviving fraction of indicated cell lines treated with sodium pyruvate (10 µM), MnTBAP (50 µM) or Carboxy-PTIO (50 µM) in combination with BEMER therapy and radiotherapy. (C) Number of γH2AX/53BP1-positive DSBs 24 h after irradiation in A549 and UTSCC15 cells. Cells were treated with indicated scavenger agents and BEMER therapy (~35 µT, 8 min). BEMER sham-treated (sham), irradiated cells served as control. All results represent mean ± SD. Student's t-test. n = 3. ** P < 0.01. n.s., not significant.

In conclusion, our data suggest that the BEMER therapy radiosensitizes cancer cells via ROS in a time- and intensity-dependent manner. Future studies are required in animal tumor models treated with conventional radiochemotherapy to evaluate the reasonable and safe benefit and bench-to-bedside transferability.

Acknowledgments

The research and authors were in part supported by the BEMER Int. AG (Liechtenstein) and grants from the Deutsche Krebshilfe (108976 to N.C.), the European Union (RADIATE; GA No.642623 to N.C.) and the EFRE Europäische Fonds für regionale Entwicklung, Europa fördert Sachsen (100066308). This work was also supported in part by a grant from the German Federal Ministry of Education and Research (BMBF) to the German Center for Diabetes Research (DZD e.V.). We are grateful to R. Grenman for providing UTSCC15 cell line.

Funding Statement

The research and authors were in part supported by the BEMER Int. AG (Liechtenstein) and grants from the Deutsche Krebshilfe (108976 to N.C.), the European Union (RADIATE; GA No. 642623 to N.C.) and the EFRE Europäische Fonds für regionale Entwicklung, Europa fördert Sachsen (100066308). This work was also supported in part by a grant from the German Federal Ministry of Education and Research (BMBF) to the German Center for Diabetes Research (DZD e.V.). The funders had no role in study design, data collection and analysis, decision to publish, or preparation of the manuscript.

References

1. Eke I, Cordes N. Focal adhesion signaling and therapy resistance in cancer. Semin Cancer Biol. 2015;31: 65–75.

2. Al-Dimassi S, Abou-Antoun T, El-Sibai M. Cancer cell resistance mechanisms: A mini review. Clin Transl Oncol. 2014;16: 511–516.

3. Tannock IF. Tumor physiology and drug resistance. Cancer Metastasis Rev. 2001;20: 123–132.

4. Vaupel P, Thews O, Hoeckel M. Treatment resistance of solid tumors: role of hypoxia and anemia. Med Oncol. 2001;18: 243–259.

5. Artacho-Cordón F, del M Salinas-Asensio M, Calvente I, R'ios-Arrabal S, León J, Román-Marinetto E, et al. Could radiotherapy effectiveness be enhanced by electromagnetic field treatment? Int J Mol Sci. 2013;14: 14974–14995.

6. Buckner CA, Buckner AL, Koren SA, Persinger MA, Lafrenie RM. Inhibition of cancer cell growth by exposure to a specific time-varying electromagnetic field involves T-type calcium channels. PLoS One. 2015;10: e0124136

7. Destefanis M, Viano M, Leo C, Gervino G, Ponzetto A, Silvagno F. Extremely low frequency electromagnetic fields affect proliferation and mitochondrial activity of human cancer cell lines. Int J Radiat Biol. Taylor {&} Francis; 2015;91: 964–972.

8. Miao X, Yin S, Shao Z, Zhang Y, Chen X. Nanosecond pulsed electric field inhibits proliferation and induces apoptosis in human osteosarcoma. J Orthop Surg Res. 2015;10: 104

9. Tofani S, Barone D, Cintorino M, De Santi MM, Ferrara A, Orlassino R, et al. Static and ELF magnetic fields induce tumor growth inhibition and apoptosis. Bioelectromagnetics. 2001;22: 419–428.

10. Chenguo Y, Yan M, Xiaoqian H, Chengxiang L, Caixin S, Junying T, et al. Experiment and mechanism research of SKOV3 cancer cell apoptosis induced by nanosecond pulsed electric field. Eng Med Biol Soc 2008 EMBS 2008 30th Annu Int Conf IEEE. 2008; 1044–1047.

11. Crocetti S, Beyer C, Schade G, Egli M, Fröhlich J, Franco-Obregón A. Low intensity and frequency pulsed electromagnetic fields selectively impair breast cancer cell viability. PLoS One. 2013;8: e72944

12. Reubold TF, Eschenburg S. A molecular view on signal transduction by the apoptosome. Cell Signal. 2012;24: 1420–1425.

13. Gorczynska E, Wegrzynowicz R. Structural and functional changes in organelles of liver cells in rats exposed to magnetic fields. Environ Res. 1991;55: 188–198.

14. Marchesi N, Osera C, Fassina L, Amadio M, Angeletti F, Morini M, et al. Autophagy Is Modulated in Human Neuroblastoma Cells Through Direct Exposition to Low Frequency Electromagnetic Fields. J Cell Physiol. 2014;229: 1776–1786.

15. Cameron IL, Markov MS, Hardman WE. Optimization of a therapeutic electromagnetic field (EMF) to retard breast cancer tumor growth and vascularity. Cancer Cell Int. 2014;14: 125

16. Delle Monache S, Angelucci A, Sanità P, Iorio R, Bennato F, Mancini F, et al. Inhibition of angiogenesis mediated by extremely low-frequency magnetic fields (ELF-MFs). PLoS One. 2013;8: e79309

17. Kirson ED, Gurvich Z, Schneiderman R, Kirson ED, Gurvich Z, Schneiderman R, et al. Disruption of Cancer Cell Replication by Alternating Electric Fields. Cancer Res. 2004;64: 3288–3295.

18. Baharara J, Hosseini N, Farzin TR. Extremely low frequency electromagnetic field sensitizes cisplatin-resistant human ovarian adenocarcinoma cells via P53 activation. Cytotechnology. Springer Netherlands; 2015

19. Wen J, Jiang S, Chen B. The effect of 100 Hz magnetic field combined with X-ray on hepatoma-implanted mice. Bioelectromagnetics. 2011;32: 322–324.

20. Cameron IL, Sun L-Z, Short N, Hardman WE, Williams CD. Therapeutic Electromagnetic Field (TEMF) and gamma irradiation on human breast cancer xenograft growth, angiogenesis and metastasis. Cancer Cell Int. BioMed Central; 2005;5: 23.

21. Elson E. I. The little explored efficacy of magnetic fields in cancer treatment and postulation of the mechanism of action. Electromagn Biol Med. 2009;28: 275–82.

22. Bohn W, Hess L, Burger R. The effects of the "physical BEMER® vascular therapy", a method for the physical stimulation of the vasomotion of precapillary microvessels in case of impaired microcirculation, on sleep, pain and quality of life of patients with different clinical pictur. J Complement Integr Med. 2013;10: S5–12, S5–13.

23. Bohn W. The technological development history and current significance of the "physical BEMER® vascular therapy" in medicine. J Complement Integr Med. 2013;10: S1–3.

24. Piatkowski J, Kern S, Ziemssen T. Effect of BEMER magnetic field therapy on the level of fatigue in patients with multiple sclerosis-A randomised, double-blind controlled trial. Mult Scler. 2009;15: S255–S256.

25. Ziemssen T, Piatkowski J, Haase R. Long-term effects of Bio-Electromagnetic-Energy Regulation therapy on fatigue in patients with multiple sclerosis. Altern Ther Health Med. 2011;17: 22–28.

26. Walther M, Mayer F, Kafka W, Schütze N. Effects of weak, low-frequency pulsed electromagnetic fields (BEMER type) on gene expression of human mesenchymal stem cells and chondrocytes: an in vitro study. Electromagn Biol Med. 2007;26: 179–190.

27. Říhová B, Etrych T, Šírová M, Tomala J, Ulbrich K, Kovář M. Synergistic effect of EMF-BEMER-type pulsed weak electromagnetic field and HPMA-bound doxorubicin on mouse EL4 T-cell lymphoma. J Drug Target. 2011;19: 890–9.

28. Eke I, Hehlgans S, Sandfort V, Cordes N. 3D matrix-based cell cultures: Automated analysis of tumor cell survival and proliferation. Int J Oncol. 2016;48: 313–21.

29. Eke I, Deuse Y, Hehlgans S, Gurtner K, Krause M, Baumann M, et al. β$_1$Integrin/FAK/cortactin signaling is essential for human head and neck cancer resistance to radiotherapy. J Clin Invest. 2012;122: 1529–1540.

30. Eke I, Hehlgans S, Zong Y, Cordes N. Comprehensive analysis of signal transduction in three-dimensional ECM-based tumor cell cultures. J Biol methods. 2015;2: e31

31. Kafka WAP. Vorrichtung und elektrisches oder elektromagnetisches Signal zur Beeinflussung biologischer Abl{ä}ufe [Internet]. Google Patents; 2000.

32. Gleim P, Klopp R. Vorrichtung zur erzeugung eines pulsierenden elektromagnetischen feldes mit impulssteuerung [Internet]. Google Patents; 2008.

33. Gleim P, Klopp R. Vorrichtung zur stimulierung autoregulativer mechanismen der hom{ö}ostase des organismus [Internet]. Google Patents; 2011.

34. Storch K, Eke I, Borgmann K, Krause M, Richter C, Becker K, et al. Three-dimensional cell growth confers radioresistance by chromatin density modification. Cancer Res. 2010;70: 3925–3934.

35. Jiang Y, Gou H, Wang S, Zhu J, Tian S, Yu L. Effect of Pulsed Electromagnetic Field on Bone Formation and Lipid Metabolism of Glucocorticoid-Induced Osteoporosis Rats through Canonical Wnt Signaling Pathway. Evid Based Complement Alternat Med. 2016;2016: 4927035

36. Duan Y, Wang Z, Zhang H, He Y, Fan R, Cheng Y, et al. Extremely low frequency electromagnetic field exposure causes cognitive impairment associated with alteration of the glutamate level, MAPK pathway activation and decreased CREB phosphorylation in mice hippocampus: reversal by procyanidins extracted from t. Food Funct. Royal Society of Chemistry; 2014;5: 2289–97

37. Vander Heiden MG, Cantley LC, Thompson CB. Understanding the Warburg effect: the metabolic requirements of cell proliferation. Science. 2009;324: 1029–1033.

38. Tennant D a, Durán R V, Gottlieb E. Targeting metabolic transformation for cancer therapy. Nat Rev Cancer. Nature Publishing Group; 2010;10: 267–277.

39. Eke I, Schneider L, Forster C, Zips D, Kunz-Schughart LA, Cordes N. EGFR/JIP-4/JNK2 Signaling Attenuates Cetuximab-Mediated Radiosensitization of Squamous Cell Carcinoma Cells. Cancer Res. 2013;73: 297–306.

40. Ruiz-Gómez MJ, De La Peña L, Prieto-Barcia MI, Pastor JM, Gil L, Martínez-Morillo M. Influence of 1 and 25 Hz, 1.5 mT Magnetic Fields on Antitumor Drug Potency in a Human Adenocarcinoma Cell Line. Bioelectromagnetics. 2002;23: 578–585.

41. Karagiannis TC, El-Osta A. DNA damage repair and transcription. Cell Mol Life Sci. Birkhäuser-Verlag; 2004;61: 2137–2147.

42. Ruiz-Gomez MJ, Martinez-Morillo M. Electromagnetic Fields and the Induction of DNA Strand Breaks. Electromagn Biol Med. 2009;28: 201–214.

43. Phillips JL, Singh NP, Lai H. Electromagnetic fields and DNA damage. Pathophysiology. 2009;16: 79–88.

44. Falone S, Grossi MR, Cinque B, D'Angelo B, Tettamanti E, Cimini A, et al. Fifty hertz extremely low-frequency electromagnetic field causes changes in redox and differentiative status in neuroblastoma cells. Int J Biochem Cell Biol. 2007;39: 2093–2106.

45. Patruno A, Pesce M, Marrone A, Speranza L, Grilli A, De Lutiis MA, et al. Activity of matrix metallo proteinases (MMPs) and the tissue inhibitor of MMP (TIMP)-1 in electromagnetic field-exposed THP-1 cells. J Cell Physiol. 2012;227: 2767–2774.

46. Wolf FI, Torsello A, Tedesco B, Fasanella S, Boninsegna A, D'Ascenzo M, et al. 50-Hz extremely low frequency electromagnetic fields enhance cell proliferation and DNA damage: possible involvement of a redox mechanism. Biochim Biophys Acta. 2005;1743: 120–129.

47. Kim J, Ha CS, Lee HJ, Song K. Repetitive exposure to a 60-Hz time-varying magnetic field induces DNA double-strand breaks and apoptosis in human cells. Biochem Biophys Res Commun. 2010;400: 739–744.

48. Winker R, Ivancsits S, Pilger A, Adlkofer F, Rüdiger HW. Chromosomal damage in human diploid fibroblasts by intermittent exposure to extremely low-frequency electromagnetic fields. Mutat Res. 2005;585: 43–49.

BEMER Therapy Applied in Gynaecology

Pregnancy Studies, Magnetic Fields, Stress Proteins and Teratogenesis

Jelinek R (2002); Charles University, Prague, 3rd Department for Internal Medicine, Faculty of Medicine

SUMMARY: In a controlled study, it was possible to prove (using the scientifically recognized biological chick embryo model) that treatment with BEMER-typically pulsed low-energy electromagnetic fields not only have not negative effects on the development of embryos, but in fact protects embryos from embryotoxic influences. This may be explained by the occurrence of special chaperonins, known as Heat Shock Proteins (specifically HSP 70), under the influence of the BEMER treatment. This hypothesis has been investigated in numerous experiments.

Magnetic Fields, Stress Proteins and Teratogenesis

Summary: Magnetic fields (MF) can protect chick embryos against subsequence embryotoxic treatments. In many studies, it has been shown over the last 10 years that short-term treatments with weak, low-frequency electromagnetic fields (EMF) not only protect unprotected embryos against ultraviolet and X-ray waves (Dicarlo et al., 1999, Pafkova, Jarabek, 1994), but also protect them against harmful treatments with various chemical teratogens (Pafkova et al., 1996).

The discovery of a human Heat Shock Protein (HSP 70) promoter (Lin et al., 1999) consistent with the protective effects of the magnetic field first established greater clarity. As the positive effects of the BEMER therapy potentially were also due to the influence of such Heat Shock Proteins, which protect living cells against a large spectrum of disruptions, the BEMER effects were studied using the well-known and easily applied biological model to text teragonicity in chick embryos under precisely defined experimental conditions. The design of the experiment and the initial results are described below.

Introduction

Over the last ten years, a number of studies have documented that short-term, weak, low-frequency electromagnetic fields (EMF) can protect embryos against UV light (4), ionizing gamma rays (17) and the destructive effect of various chemical teratogens (18). The mechanisms of this protective effect remained unclear for a long time, until the existence of an electromagnetically sensitive region in the human Heat Shock Protein (HSP 70) was proved (13). As the therapeutically positive effect of the BEMER 3000 treatment (20) conforms to the basis of this explanation, i.e. that it induces the formation of Heat Shock Proteins, which in turn protect living cells against various types of injury, an experimental procedure was developed to study the mechanisms of the BEMER 3000 effect more closely. The procedure is based on the well-known and easily applied biological model of the chick embryo under precisely defined and controlled experimental conditions. The procedure and the initial results are presented here.

Stress proteins and their characteristics

Living organisms are known to react to stress by selectively induced synthesis of polyproteins. Once this discovery was known in connection with hyperthermia, these polypeptides were named Heat Shock Proteins (HSP).

One of the first assumptions was that these proteins are involved in the formation of abnormalities in chick embryos. It was soon clear that induction to form Heat Shock Proteins (HSP) is influenced by a number of environment- related factors – including chemicals and viruses. Furthermore, it was possible to identify HSPs of all types in almost all stressed cells. HSPs act on polypeptides within the cells and prevent them decomposing or (in genesis) forming incorrectly. In short, they play the role of highly efficient intracellular chaperonins. HSPs are divided into five main groups by size:

HSP 110: This protein is found in the nucleolus and is synthesized in the cells of mammals. It is assumed that HSP 110 facilitates the restoration of nucleolus activity.

HSP 90: This protein is linked to hormone receptors and at least two glucose- related proteins. Its chaperonin function primarily relates to a series of protein interactions that operate without ATP hydrolysis. It also occurs in unstressed cells, but it quantity can increase five-fold in response to heat stress. HSP 90 interacts with a series of steroid receptors and protein kinases.

HSP 70: The HSP 70 family consists of a complex of 21 proteins. One of them, HSP 73, is one of the first constitutive gene expressions on zygotic activation of the genome during the early embryo stage (14). A further, closely related protein, HSP 72, reinforces the expression (gene-related characteristic formation) as a result of stress and the transfer of oncogene such as c-Myc.

(**Oncogenes**: Gene sequences into tumor viruses that cause biosynthesis of proteins after infection of a cell, which in turn cause a malignant transformation, e.g. the src gene of the Rous sarcoma virus (RSV), the myc gene of myelocytomatosis virus and the abl gene of the Abelson murine leukemia virus).

HSPs with intermediate molecular weight: Such proteins are formed in low quantities when cells are not under stress. They are localized in mitochondria and at cell membranes.

HSPs with low molecular weight: Such proteins, including hemoxygenase stathmin and a small polypeptide ubiquitin (8kDa), form a separate group from the other HSPs, with a protein structure denatured for non-lysosomal transport.

Lysosomes: Cell organelles enclosed by a basic membrane (lipoproteins), formed in the Golgi apparatus and that contain abundant hydrolases. Location of intracellular digestion of core acids, glycogen, proteins, mucopolysaccharides and lipids; on the release of enzymes (e.g. cell death from medicines), autolysis of the cells occurs.

EPF, an early pregnancy factor, was recently identified as a protein homologous to chaperonin 10 with immunosuppressing and growth-influencing characteristics. In this respect, it should be included in the family of HSPs, but, in contrast to the other HSPs, it was found outside the cell (15). It now seems clear that the formation of Heat Shock Proteins or their increase in quantity should primarily be understood as a reaction to a number of damaging effects, such as hyperthermia, free oxygen radicals, heavy metals, ethanol, analogues of amino acids, inflammations and infections and that they are involved in a large number of processes essential to cell function (16). It therefore seems appropriate to refer to them as Stress Proteins rather than Heat Shock Proteins.

Induction of Stress Proteins by (electro) magnetic fields

In many cases it has been assumed that the effect of electromagnetic fields (EMF) is related initially to the membranes of the cells and, in particular, to the Na- / Ka-ATPase of electromagnetic signal transduction. However, these mechanisms are not the only possible mechanisms (1). Electromagnetic fields clearly also influence transcription (i.e. synthesis – controlled by transcriptases and the nucleotide sequence of the codogenic DNA strand – of a complementary single-stranded m, t and ribosomal RNA, respectively corresponding to the second DNA strand; as "transcription" of the DNA into an RNA text as the first Step in the realization of genetic information in the biosynthesis of proteins) at specific location, e.g. the regulating range of the c- Fos gene of the DNA (19). It should be noted here that magnetic fields (MF) penetrate the body without significant, substantial loss of field strength. However, in contrast, the field strength of electric fields (EF) is reduced by at least one millionth and is therefore hardly capable of overcoming the naturally existing electric fields caused by thermal fluctuations (3). It is therefore relevant to consider magnetic field effects below. (Separation into EMF and MFN seems unnecessary, particularly considering the Maxwell's law of induction (every change of the electric field induces the formation of a magnetic field and vice versa)).

Stimulation with a 60 Hz EMF causes the HSP 1 factor, which mediates the transcription of the stress gene HSP 70 and the formation of HSP 70 (11). After investigating the c-myc protein binding to the HSP 70 promoter (i.e. section of the DNA chain of an operon at which the RNA polymerase binds and synthesis of the m-RNA (see transcription) begins), Lin et al. have inferred that, as a consequence of electromagnetic stimulations, endogenously increased myc protein quantities could contribute to HSP 70 induction (12).

The systematic and careful investigations by this working group led to the discovery of an electromagnetically sensitive area in the area of the human HSP 70 promoter.
There are some defined and very important differences between electromagnetically and thermally (heat shock) inducted HSP 70 gene expressions:

1. The stress protein is induced by EMF at an energy level 14 orders of magnitude lower than heat shock induction (5).
2. EMF stimulation does not inhibit normal, basal cellular protein synthesis (6, 2).

On that basis, it can be maintained that at least some of the therapeutically positive effects arise from the induction of Stress Proteins.

However, this hypothesis must be verified. The two last statements imply that the electromagnetic BEMER 3000 stimulation in typically, well-suited organisms does not cause damage, but improves and stabilizes the functions of an exhausted, tired, damaged and diseased tissue – as per the findings from clinical studies.

Materials and methods

For the purpose of testing the above hypothesis, we have developed an experimental device that may be used to investigate the mechanisms of the BEMER stimulation at different levels of bio-organization. It requires a sensitive, easily controllable organism that allows for well-defined exposures and injures, as well as extensive and unambiguous statements. The developing chick meets all these requirements. During development, the following basic technical problems had to be solved:

1. Development of a pair of reference incubators, one placed under typical magnetic field conditions and the other additionally placed under the influence of the electromagnetic BEMER field.
2. Development of computer-controlled and programmed temperature regulation in a stability range of 37.5+/-0.2 Celsius for both incubators.

Two fully non-magnetic incubators, heated by warm air via units emitting extremely weak electromagnetic fields, were developed. A special regulation algorithm provided the necessary precision and stability in the field and temperature conditions. The system therefore made it possible to incubate an untreated control group (C) and a treated test group (E) as required for the results to be reliable and reproducible.

Fresh eggs from white leghorn hens from the Institute of Molecular Genetics at Academy of Sciences of the Czech Republic were used. The experiment consisted of two phases: During phase 1 (0-4 days), a total of 45 eggs from the experimental group (E) were exposed to the electromagnetic BEMER field (level 10, 3x20 mins./day at 8h intervals). The incubator of the (comparison) control group (C) with the same number of eggs was not exposed to electromagnetic BEMER stimulation. At the fourth day, the eggs were opened at the top following standard methods (8) and an Olympus preparation microscope was used to test the normality of the stage of development. The eggs were categorized in terms of development as per Hamburger and Hamilton (HH stages) (7). By comparing the distribution of early embryonal death, abnormal development and HH stages, we gathered data about the possible influence of the electromagnetic BEMER treatment within the first 96 hours of incubation. At the same time, we prepared for the start of phase 2, during which the consequences of tetratogen treatment both in the BEMER- treated and in the non-BEMER-treated eggs was to be investigated.

Cyclophosphamide (Endoxan®, ASTA Medica AG, Frankfurt, Germany) was used as tetratogen, after determining the standard dose-response relationship. In the first experiment, two micrograms were injected into each embryo of both groups intra-amniotically using a special glass capillary. After wetting the vascular region with a 0.7% salt solution and closing the window in the egg shell (approx. 4 mm^2) with small glass plates attached to a paraffin frame, the eggs were put back into their respective incubators. During the subsequent incubation phase of 5 days, the eggs were observed through the windows and the transparent walls of the incubator. Dead embryos were removed, investigated under the preparation microscope for visible abnormalities and possible causes of death and the results were recorded. On the ninth day of incubation, the eggs were removed again, the embryos were collected, weighted and checked for defects in the following organs: Central nervous system, eyes, exterior shape, appendages, body wall and trunk. A routine section of the hearts provided information about abnormalities in the major arteries and the cardiac chambers. STATISTICA® (Statsoft), an evaluation and statistics program (including descriptive statistics, contingency tables, t- test, multiple regression etc.) was used to evaluate the data.

Results

The results of the first phase are summarized in two charts. The first (B001a) displays the outcome of the investigations from phase 1, i.e. comparing BEMER-treated and non-BEMER-treated control embryos on day 4 (before treatment with cyclophosphamide). The second (B001b) compares the two groups on day 9. Five days after treatment with cyclophosphamide (phase 2).

Abbreviations: n - number of eggs, O - unfertilized eggs or early dead embryos, N - normal embryos, D - dead embryos, M - misformed embryos; organ damage in surviving embryos: CNS - central nervous system, BW - body wall; C - control group, E - experimental (BEMER-treated) group.

There were no statistically significant differences between the experimental and the control groups. The number of abnormalities among the BEMER- treated animals does not exceed the number to be expected during a standard text (10) in phase 1 and the subliminal cyclophosphamide treatment similarly caused no significant difference in phase 2.

Conclusions
1. The device developed to test the electromagnetic BEMER stimulation is fit for purpose.
2. The electromagnetic BEMER stimulations caused no negative effect on the chick embryos during their most sensitive phase of development.
3. The BEMER stimulation had no effect when a subliminal dose of cyclophosphamide (a well-known teratogen) was applied in the development stage with the greatest sensitivity to embryotoxic effect

References
1. Blank M., Goodman R.: Do electromagnetic fields interact directly with DNA?
2. Bio electromagnetics 1997, 18:111-5
3. Blank M., Khorkova O., Goodman R.: Changes in polypeptide distribution stimulated by different levels of electromagnetic and thermal stress. Bioelectochem Bioenerg. 1994, 33:109-14
4. Brent R., Gordon WE., Bennett WR., Beckmann DA.: Reproductive and teratologic effects of electromagnetic fields. Reprod Toxicol, 1993, 7:535-80
5. Dicarlo AL., Hargis MT., Penafiel LM., Litovitz TA.: Short-term magnetic field exposures (60Hz) induce protection against ultraviolet radiation damage. Int. J Radiat Biol. 1999, 75:1541-9
6. Goodman R., Blank M.: Magnetic fields stress induced expression of hsp70. Cell Stress Chaperones 1998, 3:79-88
7. Goodman R., Henderson A.: Exposure of salivary gland cells to low-frequency electromagnetic fields alters polypeptide synthesis. Proc Natl Acad Aci USA 1988, 85:3928-32
8. Hamburger V., Hamilton HL.: a series of normal stages in the development of the chick embryo. J. Morphol. 1951, 88:429-33
9. Jelinek R., Peterka M.: Method used in our laboratory in Prague for the Chick Embryo toxicity Screening Test (CHEST), pp. 599- 602.
10. In Neubert D., Merker H-J., (eds) Culture Techniques: Applicability for Studies on Prenatal Differentiation and Toxicity, Walter de Gruyter, Berlin (GER) 1983
11. Jelinek R., Peterka M., Rychter Z.: Chick embryo toxicity screening test – 130 substances tested. Indian Exp Biol. 1985, 23:588-95
12. Lin H., Li Han, Blank M., Head M., Goodman R.: Magnetic field activation of protein-DNA binding. J. Cell Biochem. 1998, 70:297-303
13. Lin H., Head M., Blank M., Li Han, Jin M., Goodman R., Myc- mediated transactivation of HSP 70 expression following exposure to magnetic fields. J. Cell Biochem. 1998, 69:181-8
14. Lin H., Blank M., Goodman R.: A magnetic field-responsive domain in the human HSP 70 promoter. J.Cell Biochem. 1999, 75:170-6
15. Manejwala FM, Logan CY, Schultz RM: Regulation of hsp 70 mRNA levels during oocyte maturation and zygotic gene activation in the mouse. Dev Biol. 1991, 114:301-8
16. Morton H.: Early pregnancy factor: an extracellular chaperonin ten homologue. Immunol Cell Biol., 1998, 76, 483-96
17. Neuer A., Spandorfer SD, Giraldo P., Dieterle S., Rosenwaks Z., Witkin SS: The role of heat shock proteins in reproduction. Hum Reprod Update. 2000, 6:149-59
18. Pafkova H., Jerabek J.: Interaction of MF 50Hz, 10 mT with high dose of X-rays: evaluation of embryo toxicity in chick embryos. Rev Environ Health. 1994, 10:235-41
19. Pafkova H., Jerabek J., Teynorova I., Bednar V.: Developmental effects of magnetic field (50 Hz) in combination with ionizing radiation and chemical teratogens. Toxicol Lett. 1996, 88:313-6
20. Rao S., Henderson AS: Regulation of c-fos is affected by electromagnetic fields. J. Cell Biochem. 1996, 63:358-65
21. Kafka W.A. (1999) extremely low, wide frequency range pulsed electromagnetic fields for therapeutically use (WFR-ELF-PEMS) International Association for the Research of the physiological effects of electromagnetic fields under normal and extreme (space) conditions (Emphyspace), Emphyspace Report 1:1-20

Figures

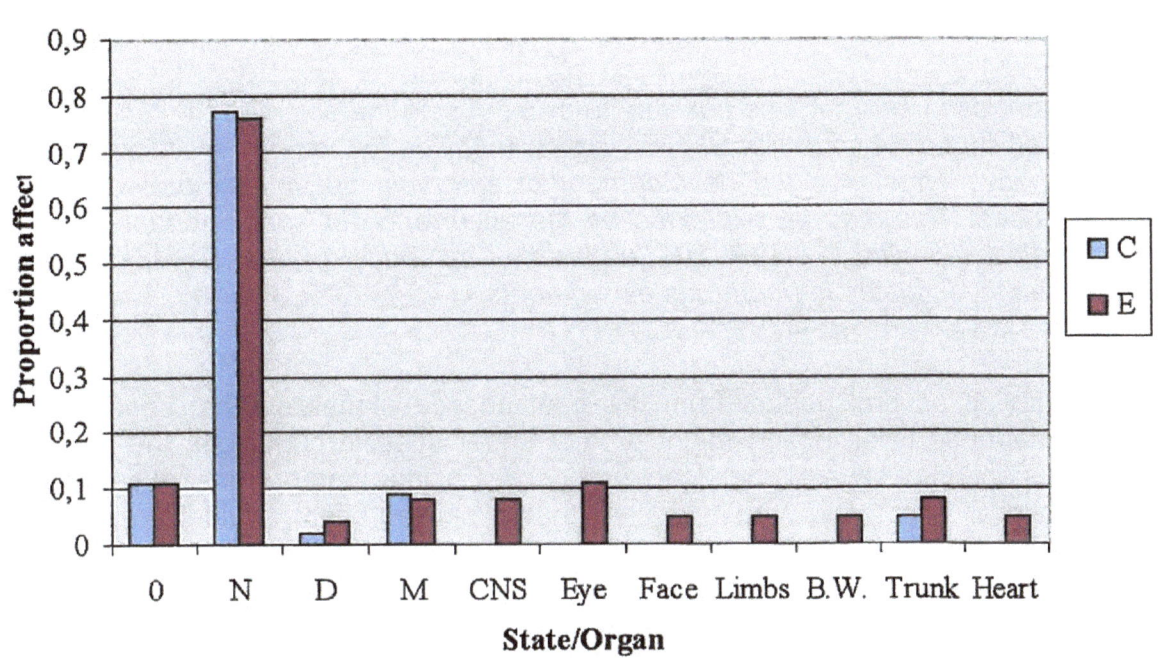

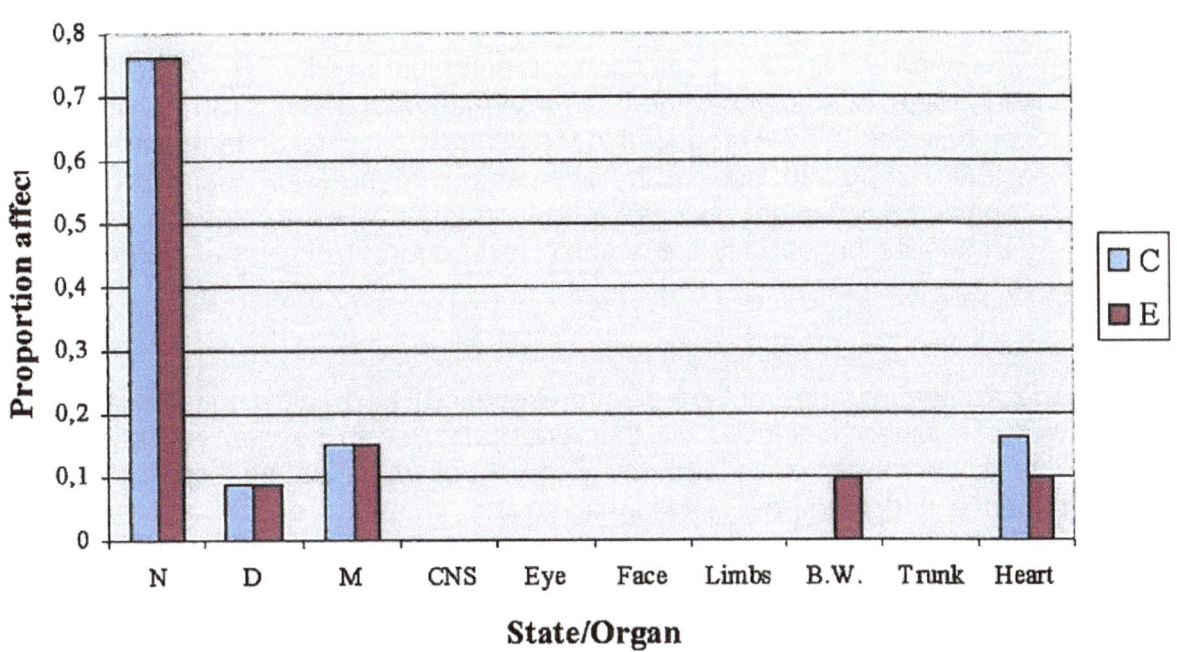

The Eectromagnetic BEMER Signal Modifies Response to Teratogens

Lecture at the 3rd BEMER World Congress in Bad Windsheim 2002

Jelinek Richard, Blaha Jiri, Dbaly Jaroslav; Charles University Prgaue, 3rd Faculty of Medicine

SUMMARY: In a controlled study, it was possible to prove (using the scientifically recognized biological chick embryo model) that treatment with BEMER-typically pulsed low-energy electromagnetic fields not only have not negative effects on the development of embryos, but in fact protects embryos from embryotoxic influences. This may be explained by the occurrence of special chaperonins, known as Heat Shock Proteins (specifically HSP 70), under the influence of the BEMER treatment. This hypothesis has been investigated in numerous experiments.

Abstract
Background: Results of several papers from the past decade signalized that short-term weak low-frequency electromagnetic fields (EMF) might protect under specific conditions the exposed progeny from the deleterious action of several chemical teratogens. Basing upon our past experience it could be expected that a similar effect could be expected that a similar effect could be expected from the electromagnetic BEMER 3000 signal.

Method: An experimental system was developed with the aim to study the mechanism of BEMER action. The system employs the well-Known and easy available biological model – the chick embryo, under precisely controlled conditions. The eggs were exposed from the beginning of incubation to BEMER signal (3x daily 20 minutes, grade 10). On day 4 the externally normal embryos were injected intraamniotically with mounting doses of a well-known teratogenic agent – Cyclophosphamide (CP) – (Endoxan) used for cancer therapy. Embryos were incubated further in the normal geomagnetic field were harvested on day 9 and checked for the presence of malformations and other manifestations of embryo toxicity. Control groups comprised similarly treated embryos that were not exposed to BEMER signal.

Results: Initial experiments were focused on approximating a no-effect level, i.e. the basal incidence of embryo toxicity phenomena within the population of embryos used. The proportion of dead and malformed foetuses in groups of embryos without CP treatment reached 0.3 (30%), which is considered a normal value. Doses between 2-8 CP produced in the controls a typical dose-response curve, which in BEMER-treated specimens appeared modified by a remarkable depression, situated below ED 50. This phenomenon, accompanied by relevant changes in malformation spectra supports the hypothesis that exposure to BEMER modifies beneficially the embryo toxic effect in the lower segment of an overall dose-response curve.

Introduction
Extremely low, wide frequency range pulsed electromagnetic (EMF) fields under BEMER 3000 signal configuration have been widely employed for therapeutically use in several indications [5]. Although many beneficial effects have been described, the well-controlled clinical studies are still missing. The action of EMF is gentle and moderate, lacking acute and dramatic effects, so that very sensitive, complex and sophisticated detection systems should be used. Such a system is offered by developing vertebrate embryos. Several papers have already documented that EMF protected under specific conditions the exposed progeny from the deleterious action of several chemical teratogens [6, 7].Basing upon our past experience we could expect that a similar effect might be exerted by the electromagnetic BEMER 3000 signal. However, working with embryos needs special knowledge, skills and experience

concerning both exposure and assessment. Therefore we decided to start our paper with a brief excursion in teratology.

Modern teratology is a science dealing with poor pregnancy outcome. The poor pregnancy outcome comprises all phenomena except normally developed foetus delivered in term. To wit, from one hundred successfully fertilized human ova, only 30-50 healthy babies are born. The rest are either lost mainly during the first weeks of pregnancy, or develop abnormally, manifesting either intrauterine growth retardation (IUGR), or the least frequent event – developmental defect. Mechanisms of abnormal development can hardly be studied in humans. Many experimental models are therefore used – each for special purposes.

Most difficulties arise from the fact that we deal with two, to a certain extent independent biological units: the mother and the fetus. When a mammalian female is exposed to a deleterious agent, the final outcome depends largely on pharmacokinetic properties of the maternal organism. To avoid this complication, sub-mammalian species (e.g. birds) are often used. Investigation on such objects resulted in the past in disclosure of several basic principles of teratology formulated concisely already by Wilson in 1977 [8]:
1. Susceptibility to teratogenic agents varies with the developmental stage at the time of exposure.
2. The final manifestations of abnormal development (embryo toxicity phenomena) are death, malformation, growth retardation and functional disorder.
3. Manifestation of deviant development increase in degree as dosage increases from the no-effect to the totally lethal one.
4. More recently, two additional rules were added [3]:
5. With increasing dose, the embryo toxicity phenomena transform one into another. For this reason, to obtain a usual S-Shaped dose- response curve, one must sum the manifestations of deviant development (at least malformation and death) into one parameter of embryo toxicity. As teratogen such agent should be labeled, which increases significantly the overall incidence of embryo toxicity phenomena within the exposed population over the basal frequency present in the unexposed one. In the experiment, this basal frequency contributes to the so-called-no-effect level.

Respecting the principles mentioned above, we start to verify the hypothesis that BEMER 3000 signal decreases the incidence of embryo toxicity phenomena induced by administration of a standard teratogen.

Material and Method
An experimental system was developed with the aim to study the mechanism of BEMER action [2]. Fresh laid eggs of random-bred stock of White Leghorn Fowl purchased from the Institute of Molecular Genetics, Academy of Sciences of the Czech Republic were used. The experiment consisted of two phases. In the course of Phase 1 (1-4 days) the experimental (E) group of 45 eggs was exposed to BEMER 3000® (step 10, 3 x 20 minutes per day, at eight-hour intervals). The flat circular coil was placed 10cm below the shelf carrying about 31 eggs, the resting to the amount of 45 were kept on the other side of the incubator where the intensity of BEMER-induced magnetic fields appeared negligible. Embryos kept in the latter compartment were used as the second additional control.

The control (C) group of the same size was placed in the reference incubator without exposure. On day 4 the eggs were candled and opened using the conventional window technique (see, for instance, [4]). Using the Olympus preparation microscope, embryos were examined for normality and staged according to Hamburger and Hamilton (HH stages) [1]. By comparing the distribution of early embryonic death, abnormal specimens and HH stages, we established information on the possible influence of BEMER during the first 96 hours of incubation. At the same time, we gained a starting point for the

Phase 2 in which consequences of teratogen administration was studied in the BEMER exposed and unexposed groups. Altogether 453 selected embryos in HH stages 21-24 were used. As a teratogen, Cyclophosphamide (CP) (Endoxan®, ASTA Medica AG, Frankfurt, Germany) was chosen after establishing the standard dose-response relationships. Two initial experiments served for establishing the no-effect level. In the main experimental series 2 to 8 of pure substance known to exert embryo toxic effects were injected intraamniotically to each embryo in both groups using a special glass canule. After moistening the vascular area by 0.7% saline and after closing windows in the shell with glass slides on paraffin frames, the eggs were put back to the appropriate oven. In course of the 5-day re-incubation period, embryos were checked through the windows and transparent walls of the incubators. Dead specimens were removed, inspected under the preparation microscope for visible malformation and probable cause of death and the findings recorded. On day 9 of incubation the eggs were reopened, the embryos were harvested, weighed and checked for defects of the following organs: central nervous system, eyes, face, limbs, body wall and trunk. A routine dissection of the heart allowed us to include defects of great arteries and heart septation. A BEMER-treated group was compared to its relevant control group in any evaluation that, besides the descriptive statistics and t-test, included contingency table analysis and distribution test following Smirnov-Kolmogorov.

Results and Discussion

Initial experiments were focused on approximating a no-effect level, i.e. the basal incidence of embryo toxicity phenomena within the population of embryos used. The proportion of dead and malformed foetuses in groups without CP treatment reached 0.3 (30%), which is considered a normal value in testing for embryo toxicity and corresponds to the historical controls [4].

Doses between 2-8 CP produced in the controls a typical dose-response curve, which in BEMER pretreated specimens appeared modified by a remarkable depression, situated below the point where Cyclophosphamide affected adversely 50& embryos above the no-effect level (the so-called ED50). This finding is not surprising because in interactions other than those based on a chemical reaction between the teratogen and a modifying agent, the beneficial effects is regularly found only in doses that allow the majority of embryos to survive. The final embryo toxicity profile comparing the incidence of particular embryo toxicity phenomena and organ malformations in BEMER-treated and no.-treated groups is shown on Fig. 2. The graph columns document the decreased incidence of both malformed and dead embryos and relevant changes in the individual organ affliction, which occurred under the influence of BEMER.

Conclusion

Significant depression of the dose-response curve observed after administration of Cyclophosphamide to embryos pretreated by BEMER 3000, accompanied by the relevant change in malformation spectra, supports the hypothesis that exposure to BEMER modifies beneficially the embryo toxic effect in the lower segment of an overall dose-response curve.

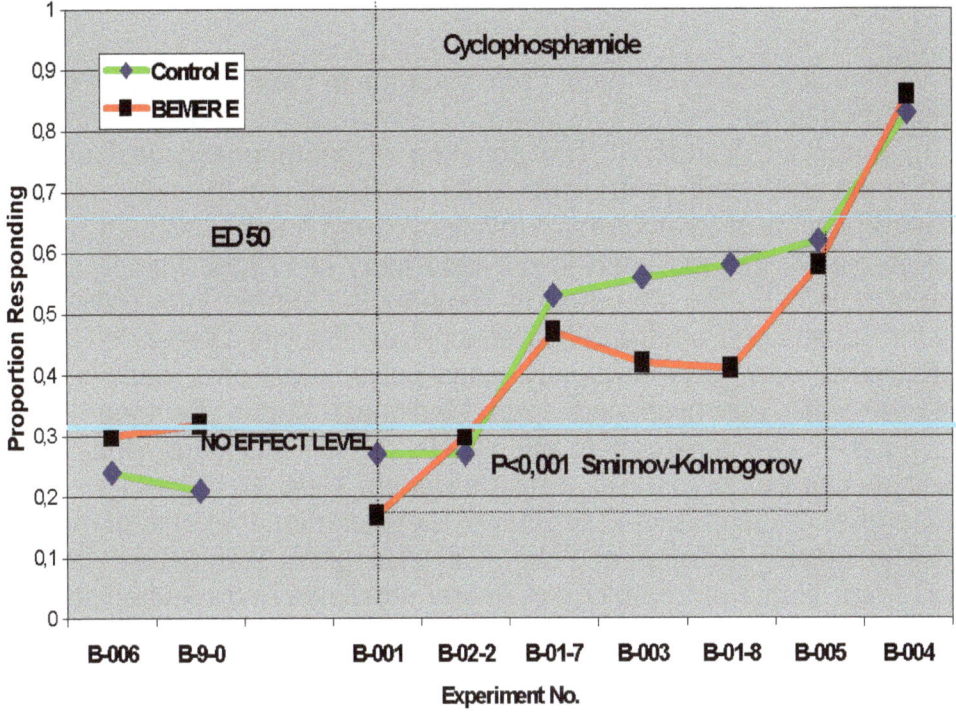

Fig. 1: Dose-response relationships for Cyclophosphamide injected to chick embryos on day 4 in doses 2-4ug/embryo. Control E – in embryos unexposed to BEMER 3000, BEMER E – in embryos exposed to BEMER prior to administration of Cyclophosphamide. The BEMER values are plotted against the control one in any particular experiment.

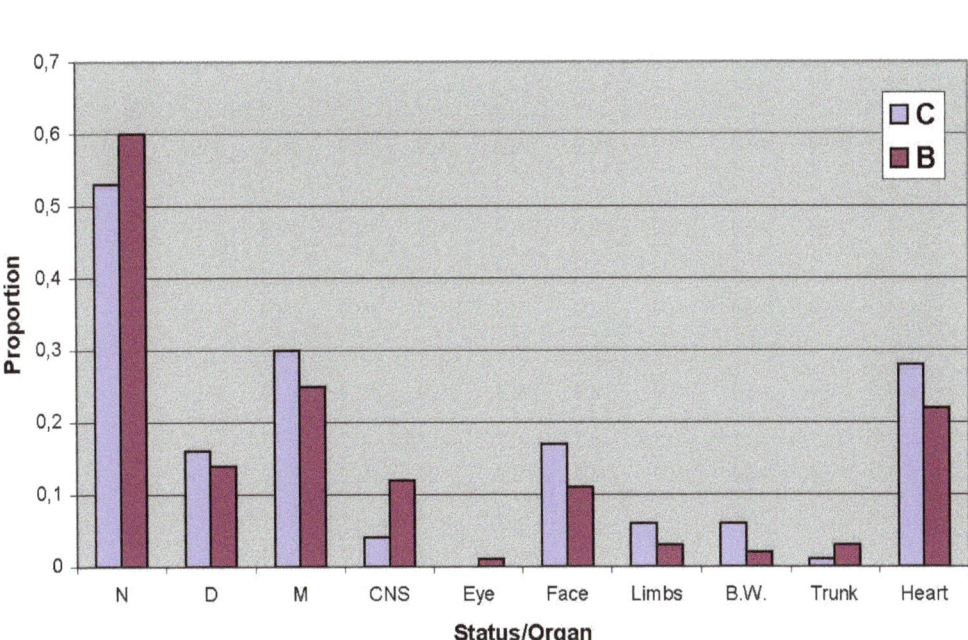

Fig. 2: Embryo toxicity profile of Cyclophosphamide effect in the lower part of the dose-response curve in BEMER pretreated (B) and non-pretreated (C) embryos. N - proportion of normal, D - proportion of dead, M - proportion of malformed embryos. The resting columns depict the proportion of malformed organs.

References

1. Hamburger V., Hamilton HL: A series of normal stages in the development of the chick embryo. J. Morphol. 1951, 88:429-33
2. Janoutova J., Blaha J., Jelinek R: The absence of geomagnetic field does not influence the development of the chick embryo. Biologia 1999, 54 (Suppl. 6): 151-156
3. Jelinek R: The principles of teratogenesis revisited. Cong Anom. 1988, 28:S145-S155
4. Jelinek R., Peterka M: Method used in our laboratory in Prague for the Chick. Embryo toxicity Screening Test (CHEST). Pp. 599-602. In Neubert D., Merker H-J. (eds). Culture Techniques: Applicability for Studies on Penetral Differentiation and Toxicity. Walter de Gruyter, Berlin 1983.
5. Kafka WA: Extremely low, wide frequency range pulsed electromagnetic fields for therapeutically use (WFR-ELF-PEMS). Emphyspace Report. Mediquat – Verlag, Sevelen (Swiss) 2000, pp.20
6. Pafkova H., Jerabek J: Interaction of MF 50 Hz, 10 mT with high dose X-rays; evaluation of embryo toxicity in chick embryos. Rev. Environ Health. 1994, 10: 235-41
7. Pafkova H., Jerabek J., Tejnorova I., Bednar V: Developmental effects of magnetic field (50Hz) in combination with ionizing radiation and chemical teratogens. Toxicol Lett. 1996, 88: 313-6. In
8. Wilson JG: Current status of teratology (General principles and mechanism derived from animal studies) pp. 47-74. In Wilson JG., Fraser FC (eds), Handbook of teratology Vol. 1. General Principles and Etiology. Plenum Press, N.Y., London, 1977

BEMER Therapy Applied in Otorhinolaryngology

Experience with Bio-Electro Magnetic Energy Regulation (BEMER) Therapy in Patients with Subjective Tinnitus.

(From the journal Hals-, Nasen- und Ohrenheilkunde [Otorhinolaryngology] No. 56 (4)/ 2010. Received for release on 2/26/2009 Dr. Bugyi István Hospital in Szentes Matrix Department of Otolaryngology and Urology.)

Dr. Imre Szilágyi
Szilagyi I. (2010); Otorhinologica Hungaria 56(4), 2010, 251-260

SUMMARY: The author presents the method with which he treats subjective tinnitus. It is Bio-Electro-Magnetic Energy Regulation (BEMER therapy in short), which uses the positive physiological effects of a pulsed magnetic field on the human body. The treatment has a positive effect on the nervous system as well as on microcirculation in various organs. The cases analyzed in the study were treated in hospital, a control group was additionally formed, which enabled a randomized, double-blind clinical study.

The patients in one group received a daily infusion of 200 mg pentoxiphylin, plus 2 x 1,200 mg piracetam per os as well as BEMER treatment. The other group received the same therapy. In these patients, however, the BEMER therapy device was not effectively on, i.e., the treatment was only simulated. The treatments were arranged so that for each actually treated patient, a placebo-treated patient followed. Both the examinations and their evaluations were performed by two persons independently of each other. The healing results of the two groups and their evaluation were statistically analyzed by the author. The computational results show that in patients additionally treated with BEMER, the decrease in complaints was significantly greater than in patients in the control group.

Introduction

As a practicing ear, nose and throat doctor, you frequently encounter patients in both outpatient and inpatient treatment who complain about tinnitus.

To be honest, we must admit that these patients are dissatisfied with the outcome of their treatment, their symptoms frequently remain unchanged.

Regarding the frequency of occurrence of tinnitus, very different data are available, several assume that 15-35% of the population have already experienced inconveniences related to tinnitus and this difficult to tolerate symptom presents an ongoing, unresolved problem for 5-8% of people. (2, 20, 24). It is a common experience that the number of people suffering from tinnitus patients displays a rising trend. Presumably there are several reasons. The fact that people are now living in a time where hearing organs are increasingly burdened and are surrounded by an increasingly tense, edgy environment at breakneck speed is certainly a pathological factor. As a result, the number of stressed, distressed and depressed people has increased.

According to our statistics, the number of patients treated in our department as a result of subjective tinnitus has gradually increased in the last twenty years. During this period, that number has tripled.

Table no. 1. Presentation of the number of inpatients treated in our department due to subjective tinnitus in the last twenty years.

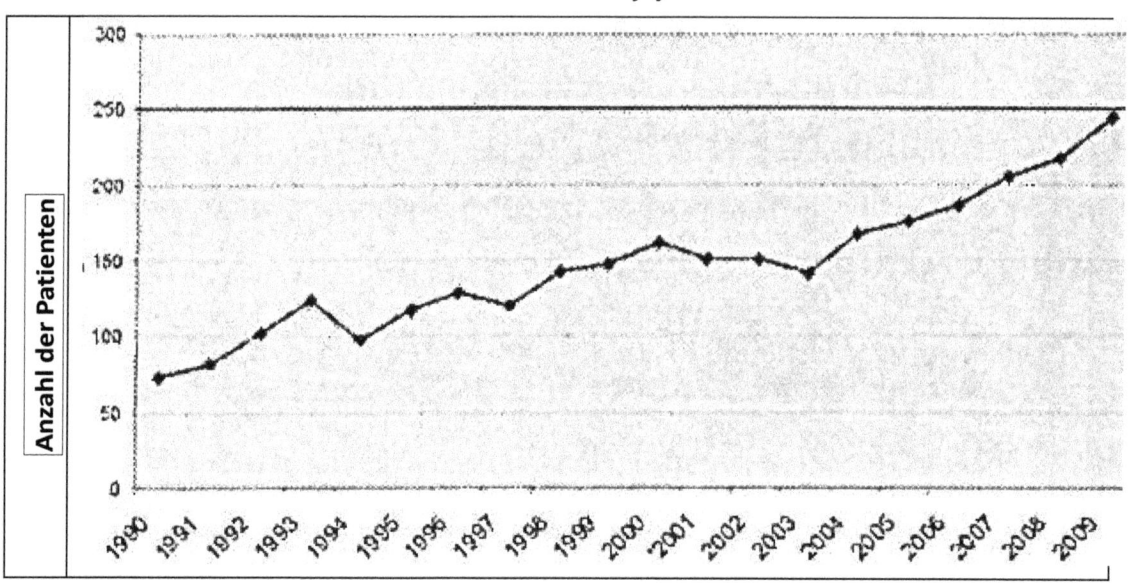

Tinnitus is defined as a listening experience that arises without an acoustic stimulus. Various authors have grouped tinnitus according to several views, but all share the opinion that tinnitus can be divided into two basic groups, such as objective and subjective tinnitus. In the case of objective tinnitus, the examining physician also hears the patient's tinnitus. In subjective tinnitus, only the patient perceives these sounds (2, 4, 15, 16, 19, 20, 24). With respect to everyday activities in otolaryngology, objective tinnitus is rare, a true task and challenge is the treatment of the group of patients suffering from subjective tinnitus with many patients for the otolaryngologist.

Tinnitus is a symptom that can be caused by the abnormal function of the organ of Corti or the brain. For this reason, the patient suffering from tinnitus must be thoroughly examined (2, 4, 15, 20, 24). Once the changes in the organs are excluded as a possible cause of tinnitus, many authors use the term idiopathic subjective tinnitus. It must be noted that although the doctor very often finds no organic reason for the occurrence of tinnitus, a sign of functional organ damage, injury to the inner ear or the auditory pathway is often found in the organ, for example: Noise damage, presbycusis, or other nerve-induced hearing loss.

Especially in recent years, experts have pointed out that not only the diseases of the ear, but also diverse, emotionally related disease states (depression, distress, panic disease) can cause tinnitus or in other words, these conditions are accompanied by tinnitus (4, 6, 20, 24, 25). Regarding pathophysiology, there is no uniform, generally accepted point of view. Even the question is disputed as to whether tinnitus comes from the ear at all (resulting from damage to a hair cell or the withering away of an auditory nerve fiber) or is formed in the brain (4, 6, 24). Most accept the last-mentioned consideration and hold the increase of morbid activity of the auditory cortex responsible for the development of tinnitus. It is also supported by clinical experience that tinnitus often does not automatically stop, but also persists when the auditory nerve is cut for whatever reason (4, 24). One can argue that damage to the inner ear to whatever extent is confirmed in most cases when tinnitus is existent (4, 20, 24).

Often the doctors are witnesses as to how this problem, this difficult-to-affect symptom is becoming more and more serious, moving ever closer to the patient's personality and putting him or her into greater despair. Here, processes can combine with each other that reinforce, generate and act on each other and the different processes can be combined in a vicious circle (6, 20).

Figure No. 1

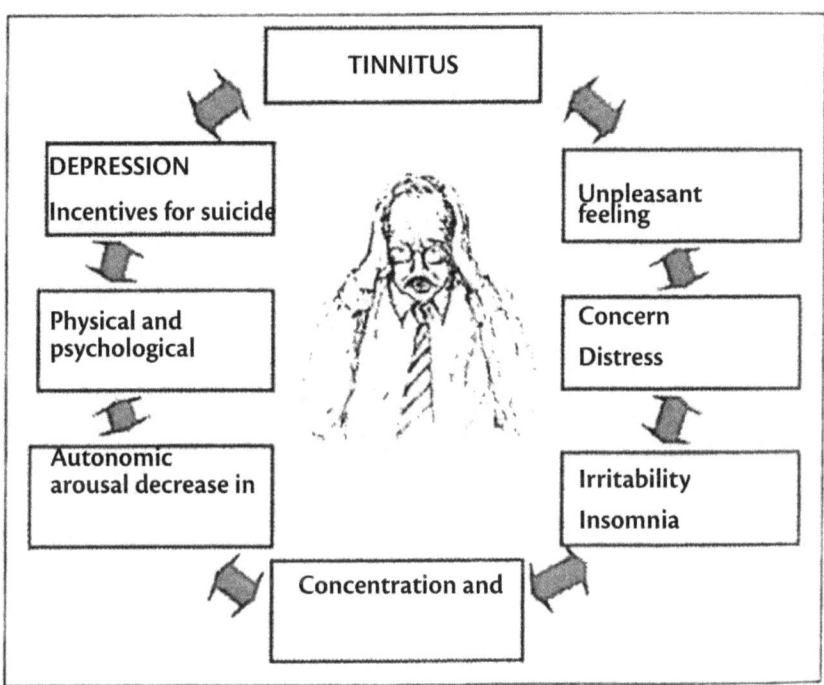

Material and method

In patients suffering from tinnitus, a therapy is applied that has already been very successful for several years in various fields of medicine, but has little experience with use in tinnitus. The method we use is Bio-Electro-Magnetic Energy Regulation, abbreviated as BEMER therapy. We have been treating patients for almost three years with the method mentioned above. We use the aforementioned therapy for both outpatient and in-patient treatment. Because of previous clinical experience, a randomized, placebo-controlled, double-blind clinical investigation for the purpose of convincing evidence of the effectiveness of the method was performed in the period between 07.01.2009 and 6.30.2010 (12 months).

The patients were examined before the start of treatment according to the guidelines of the instructions for otorhinolaryngology (20). For each patient, neurological and psychiatric examinations were carried out to uncover potential symptoms of the soul and psyche hidden in the background (distress, depression, panic disease). The result of these studies was summarized in the table of the accompanying diseases (Table 11).

We have compiled a questionnaire to analyze the patients' tinnitus, determine the level of difficulty and be able to measure the situation as to how far tinnitus has influenced the patients' life, work, their interpersonal contacts in conducting recreational activities. (Table no. 2)

The questionnaire has apparently 8 questions. The first question refers to the period of the existence of tinnitus. Here we would like to clarify whether this is acute, subacute or chronic tinnitus. The second question relates to the type of sounds that occur. Defining the above is important for the reason that a conclusion can be made concerning tinnitus in the case of Meniere's disease or Purulens labyrithis. The intention is to clarify the type of tinnitus and the properties of the interfering sound before the start of therapy because they may change during therapy, be less uncomfortable, or become more tolerable.

For this reason it is advisable to document the characteristics of the tinnitus- named sound. The results of the tinnitometric investigations provide important information as well.

In the questionnaire for the assessment of tinnitus, all questions can be answered with three possible answers starting with the third question. The order of the answers may be associated with the difficulty of tinnitus. Starting with this question you receive points for the answers. One point for the first answer, 2 points for the second answer and 3 points for the third answer. The tinnitus patient could thus receive 6 to 18 points. Accordingly, tinnitus is divided into 3 different difficulty levels, levels I, II and III, which are summarized in the following table.

Table no. 2. Questionnaire No. 1 for the evaluation of tinnitus

Name:		Insurance no.:		
Underline the correct answer!				
1. Since when do you have ringing in your ears?		0-3 months	3-6 months	longer than 6 months
2. What kind of noise do you hear?	Monotonous Ringing	Roar	Wind-like roar	Whisper
	Drumming	Clatter	Knocking	Rattling
	Engine noise	Metal clanking	Composite sound	
	Other……………………………..			
Classification of the severity of the ringing in your ears		1 point	2 points	3 points
3. Do you constantly hear ringing in your ears or only alternately?		rarely	often	constantly
4. To what extent does it bother you when performing work?		not at all	slightly	very much
5. To what extent does it bother you in your lifestyle? (e.g.: Communicating with your fellow human beings, during recreation, entertainment, watching television)		not at all	slightly	very much
6. To what extent does it affect your nervous state, your mood?		not at all	slightly	very much
7. Does it affect your sleep? Do you wake up because of the ringing in your ears?		not at all	rarely	often
8. Is the ringing in your ears accompanied by other symptoms? (e.g.: Dizziness, headaches, crampedness and tension of the neck muscles)		not at all	rarely	often

On the questionnaires completed by the patients, the line for issuing points was not listed. It has been integrated in the table above for the purpose of better presentation.

Table no. 3. The emergence of different levels of tinnitus as a result of the answers to the questions of the previous table.

Tinnitus Level I	1-6 points
Tinnitus Level II	7-12 points

| Tinnitus Level II | 13-18 points |

In the previously mentioned period (from 07.01.2009 to 6.30.2010), a randomized, double-blind clinical study was conducted. During this period, 245 patients were treated in our department for tinnitus. 214 patients agreed to participate in a clinical trial. The patients participating in the study were given an infusion of 1x200mg Pentoxiphylin in 250 ml (in physiological saline) and 2x1,200 Pyracetam mg per os daily. In addition, these patients received BEMER treatment daily. Patients with odd serial numbers received real treatment, the other patients with even serial numbers received placebo BEMER treatment. Each patient receiving real BEMER treatment was followed by a patient with placebo BEMER treatment. Treatment lasted for 8 days. The person carrying out the treatment, the specialist assistant, secretly managed the data on the patients' changing condition.

BEMER treatments were performed with the BEMER 3000 signal plus device. The treatment consists of two phases. In the first phase, pulsating magnetic field treatment is applied to the whole body surface whereby the patient lies on a mattress with rolls for 8 minutes. In the second phase, the so-called intensive applicator of the device was placed on the temporal region of the skull. This is a cuboid-shaped, 7 cm long, 6 cm wide and 3 cm thick treatment unit. The intensive applicator stimulated the temporal region of the brain with much larger (adjustable) intensity. This treatment period lasted for 20 minutes. The device was switched on even in the placebo treatments. The patient could see the flashing lights and hear the signal when switching the device on and off. The treatment was ineffective because of insufficient connection of the intensive applicator. BEMER treatment was therefore simulated. The patient could not know that he or she received ineffective treatment.

To determine the effect of the applied therapy, a questionnaire was compiled and is shown in Table 4: The evaluation of the question is presented in the following Table no. 5.

Table no. 5

Ringing stopped.	The answer to the 1st question was yes.
Ringing decreased.	The answer to questions 2, 3, 4 and 5 was yes.
Ringing remained unchanged.	The answer to the 6th question was yes.
Ringing became stronger.	The answer to questions 7 and 8 was yes.

Two patient groups arose due to the difference of BEMER treatment.

The people classified under patient group I were given drug treatment and real BEMER treatment. Their number amounted to 108.

The people classified under patient group II were also given drug treatment and placebo BEMER treatment. Their number amounted to 106.

Table no. 4. Questionnaire No. 2 for the evaluation of tinnitus

How do you rate your symptoms in comparison with your condition before treatment?	Underline the matching answer!	
1. The ringing is completely gone.	yes	no

2. The ringing is less strong.	yes	no
3. The ringing is gone in one ear or has been reduced.	yes	no
4. The ringing has temporarily stopped, appears less frequently than prior to treatment.	yes	no
5. The ringing has changed and I can tolerate it better.	yes	no
6. The strength and character of the ringing did not change.	yes	no
7. The ringing has become stronger.	yes	no
8. The ringing has become more unpleasant.	yes	no

In one of the patients included in the treatment, tinnitus treatment had to be discontinued because of other symptoms, which is why patients are not represented in the two groups in equal numbers.

The patient groups were compared according to the difficulty level of their tinnitus, their age, hearing and the accompanying diseases occurring in addition to tinnitus.

The results are shown in Tables 6, 7 and 8.

Table no. 6. The distribution of the patients belonging to patient group I according to the difficulty level of the tinnitus (n = 108)

Tinnitus Level I	45	41,6%
Tinnitus Level II	37	34,2%
Tinnitus Level III	26	24,2

Table no. 7. The distribution of the patients belonging to group II patients according to the difficulty level of the tinnitus (n = 106)

Tinnitus Level I	44	41,7%
Tinnitus Level II	40	38,5%
Tinnitus Level III	22	19,8%

Table no. 8. The distribution of the patients by age in patient group I and II

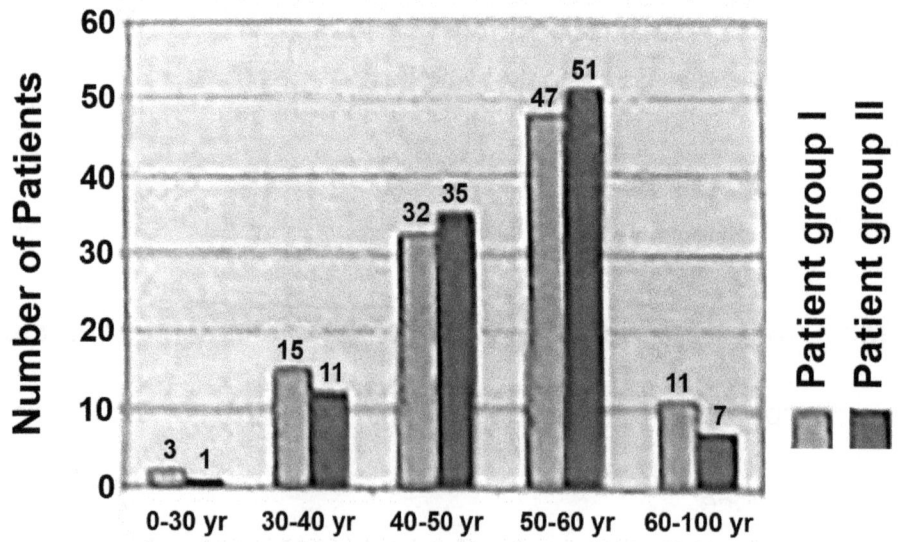

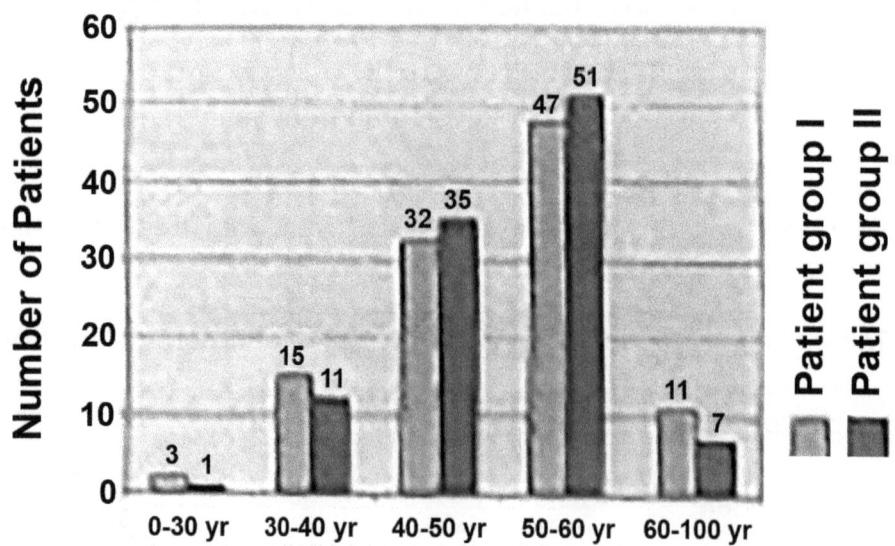

In the patient group I the youngest patient was 15 years old and the oldest patient was 88 years old. Distribution according to gender: 64 men (59.5%) and 44 women (40.5%). In the patient group II the youngest patient was 19 years old and the oldest patient was 86 years old. Distribution according to gender: 59 men (55.7%) and 47 women (44.3%). The tables show that age distribution is similar in the two groups. There was no significant difference in the proportion of the sexes and in both groups the number of men was a little higher.

Table no. 9. The results of the hearing test of patients belonging to patient group I (N=108)

Normal hearing	14	13.0%
Perceived deterioration of hearing	66	61.1%
Deterioration of hearing	9	8.4%
Mixed-type deterioration of hearing	19	17.5%

Table no. 10. The results of the hearing test of patients belonging to patient group II (N=106)

Normal hearing	18	16.9%
Perceived deterioration of hearing	60	56.5%
Guided deterioration of hearing	13	12.3%
Mixed-type deterioration of hearing	15	14.3%

Table no. 11. The more frequently occurring comorbidities apart from tinnitus

Comorbidities	Group I (n=108)		Group II (n=106)	
Diabetes mellitus	25	23.2%	28	26.3%
Cervical spondylosis	51	47.4%	55	51.7%
Hypertension	22	20.7%	17	16.0%
Ischemic heart disease	12	11.2%	9	8.5%
COPD	21	19.5%	13	12.2%
Bronchial asthma	8	7.4%	10	9.4%
GERD	27	25.1%	36	33.9%
Distress	72	66.9%	64	60.1%
Depression	35	32.6%	39	36.7%
Panic disease	11	10.2%	9	8.5%
Anaemia	4	3.7%	6	5.6%
Hypercholesterolemia	21	19.5%	15	14.1%
Hyperlipidemia	14	13.0%	12	11.3%
Hyperuricaemia	5	4.6%	3	2.8%

Based on the data above, it is evident that there was no substantial difference between the two groups from any tested standpoint. The patients in the two groups can be considered as practically identical.

The essence of BEMER therapy is that a phenomenon from physics is used for treating patients that is naturally present in the Earth's environment and acts on the living beings. This phenomenon in physics is the magnetic field. Life originated in the magnetic field of the earth, which is the natural environment for living things. If this field were no longer present, living things on Earth would probably die. The intensity of the magnetic field is different at various points of the globe.

This value generally varies between 50 and 100 µT (micro tesla). Earth's magnetic field has changed with the passage of time. According to some calculations, it has halved since our era (1). This value is an average of 50-60 µT in Budapest.

The control unit of the BEMER treatment unit generates an electric pulsating electromagnetic field. This pulsating magnetic field generated by the device has specific physical properties and a wide frequency range. The magnetic signal device was specially developed. This allows this treatment to stand out against the electromagnetic therapies with its physiological effects on living organisms. The intensity of the magnetic field generated by the device can be set between 3.5 µT and 100 µT. The greatest intensity that is generated by the device does not exceed the maximum value of the magnetic field occurring on Earth. It is the explanation for the fact that the BEMER treatment has no harmful side effects.

The main physiological effects of BEMER therapy can be summarized as follows:

- The BEMER therapy increases blood circulation in the capillaries in the human body, opens the lumen of closed capillaries not participating in circulation and accelerates the blood stream. As a result of better circulation, the nutrient and oxygen supply to the cells improves, the metabolism of the cells is more active, their energy generation increases, and their ATP content increases. The effect of BEMER therapy on microcirculation could be made visible and confirmed with the micro cameras implanted into the gums and endothelial lining of the intestines and with the use of a special vital microscope. The experiments and scientific investigations of R.C. Klopp and his colleagues were performed at the Institute for Microcirculation in Berlin (10, 11).

- Due to the increase of the energy content of the cells, the protein synthesis increases as well. It is important that the amount of some protecting proteins (such as heat shock protein 70) is very high (3).

- The amount of supplied oxygen in the blood increases (the partial pressure of oxygen is increased) (7, 10, 11, 12, 14).

- Due to the pulsating magnetic field, the sticking together of red blood cells and their tendency for rouleaux formation decreases. For this reason, the viscosity of the blood is low, blood circulation is accelerated, the risk of thrombosis in various organs is reduced, the separated red blood cells can easily penetrate into the small capillaries with a thin diameter. (10, 11, 12).

- The therapy accelerates the movement of white blood cells, and sticking to the artery wall. This way they quickly reach the tissues, enabling them to better provide their protective functions, which results in the more effective functioning of the immune system (1, 10, 11).

- After BEMER treatment, the glutathione reductase content of the red blood cells could be increased, which helps the neutralization of certain aggressive molecules (e.g. peroxide, nitric oxide). As a result, the cell-damaging, destructive effect of the aforementioned molecules can be blocked (1, 11).

- The therapy exerts a broad effect on the nervous system, reduces stress-related tension, and has a beneficial effect on distress and depression. It relaxes tense, tight and painful muscles and promotes peaceful sleep at night (1, 13, 18).

Results

The evaluation of the results was performed by the author, who received the list of patients participating in treatments and/or placebo treatments only after the completion of the clinical investigation. In assessing the effect of the therapy, a statistical analysis was carried out while the χ^2 sample with use of the SPSS program was applied.

With the application of the previously presented therapy, we obtained the following results:

Table no. 12. The results of patient group I (n=108) (with real BEMER treatment)

Ringing stopped.	24	22.20%
Ringing improved.	51	47.30%
Ringing remains unchanged.	33	30.50%
Ringing worsened.	0	0.00%

Table no. 13. The results of patient group II (n=106) (with placebo BEMER treatment)

Ringing stopped.	9	8.5%
Ringing improved.	39	36.76%
Ringing remains unchanged.	57	53.80%
Ringing worsened.	1	0.94%

When comparing the results of these tables, it can be seen that the tinnitus of patients in the group that received real BEMER treatment (patient group I), stopped or improved in much greater numbers.

The statistical significance of the difference in the distribution of the change of condition of the two patient groups was controlled with a χ^2-test and as a result the value 0.001 was obtained. Based on the information above, it can be argued that the difference in therapy results of the two groups of patients is highly significant.

The statistical analysis thus confirmed that the application of BEMER therapy significantly improved the results obtained with drug treatment only.

The effectiveness of the therapy was observed in the various stages of tinnitus in the individual patient groups, of which the following is to be emphasized: In both patient groups in tinnitus level I and II, the proportion of patients responding positively to the therapy was higher than in patients in level III. At this point, we desist from the presentation of the detailed calculations and table because of the volume.

It is worth noting that the difficulty level of patients (no matter which group of patients) whose symptoms were unaffected by the treatment mostly did not change after treatment.

No harmful side effect occurred during the BEMER treatment.

Review

Many drugs are used nowadays to cure tinnitus and many treatment methods are tried in order to alleviate the symptoms of tinnitus patients. Without the right to a fully comprehensive picture, here we provide an overview of the drugs and treatment methods most commonly used.

The various drugs for circulatory support are mostly used in practice. From this group of drugs, the following are administered most: pentoxiphylin, vinpocetine, pyracetam. These medications can be taken or administered with an infusion, improve the circulation in the brain and inner ear and also improve microcirculation.

Lidocaine with an infusion is used abroad (e.g. in Germany, USA) but not commonly practiced in Hungary because of its cardiac side effects. In the case of tinnitus, betahistine is an often-applied drug, which reduces the sensitivity of the vestibular nuclei with an effect on H3 receptors, and through its effect on H1 receptors circulation in the inner ear increases. Its application for tinnitus is reported and mentioned in several therapeutic instructions. Nicergoline, which is a semi-synthetic ergoline derivative, is also used for the purpose of promoting blood circulation, and mainly as a peripheral means for vasodilatation in various vascular disorders. According to various experiences, this drug was also effective in the treatment of tinnitus. Several authors report on the favorable effect of the so-called calcium antagonist drugs such as: cinnarizine, flunarizine, which affect calcium metabolism. Some attempts have also been made with the use of herbal extracts such as: ginkgo biloba, vitalion.

Some authors attempted administration of an intratympanic drug, so lidocaine and steroids were used for example. The tinnitus patients still take sedatives, anti-distress substances, anti-depressants, and serotonin antagonists on the recommendation of neurologists and psychiatrists.

In addition to the drug therapies, the treatments with electrical stimulation are worth mentioning as the mastoid process, which stimulates the external auditory track and the soft palate with electricity. The method is in the experimental stage and detailed experience is not available. In ultrasonic stimulation, the mastoid process is stimulated with ultrasound at different frequencies (between 20,000 Hz and 100,000 Hz).

In Hungary, hyperbaric oxygen treatment is available in some places but opinions about it are varied. Various orthopedic methods as well as manual therapy are also used to reduce the symptoms of the patients.

Recently, opinions have been published mainly by American and German authors about the fact that favorable results were achieved with transcranial solenoid treatment in chronic tinnitus. In general, treatment of the temporal region is recommended, but some treat the frontal region, or the combination of the two. Their opinions also agree on the fact that regular repetition of the treatment is recommended.

A specific treatment method is tinnitus retraining therapy, which consists of two parts: auditory and the subsequent verbal retraining. In the case of auditory retraining, a noiser with rose noise is adjusted with open accommodation to both ears of the patient. During adjustment, the so-called "mixing point" must

be sought. This point is where the sound from the noiser and tinnitus mix. The sound of the noiser is suppressed and its intensity is set a little below this intensity. The knowledge related to the disease is discussed during verbal retraining, which is best performed by qualified psychologists.

The psychotherapist tries to steer the patient in one direction, where the tinnitus appears to be less important. The patient tries to push the disease from the center of his or her thoughts to the periphery. This therapy has also been used in our department. However, we are not satisfied with the results because it brought with it no improvement in most cases. The disadvantage of this method is that it is very time-consuming. Treatment can last for months or years and requires endurance from both the patient and the therapist.

Despite many therapeutic attempts, the recovery results of those patients suffering from subjective tinnitus remained rather modest. A large portion of patients was not satisfied with the result of the different treatments. Their tinnitus remained unchanged in many cases.

For this reason, we tried to learn and try new a method of treatment in order to reduce the most unpleasant symptoms of the patient.

As previously mentioned, subjective tinnitus is a symptom, which may hide many diseases or pathological deviations. The ideal solution would be for us to diagnose and cure the disease that caused the tinnitus. The best cure is of course treatment of the cause of the illness. Unfortunately, the current diagnostic agents do not allow us to clearly identify the reason for subjective tinnitus. Our task is also complicated by the fact that even if we suspect the reason for tinnitus such as: presbycusis or noise damage, no effective therapy is available, unfortunately.
According to our assumption, that good results achieved with the BEMER therapy can be explained principally with three reasons.

1. On the one hand, these results are due to the effect that the therapy improves microcirculation in the inner ear and the auditory center of the brain. The chemical agents used in the past (pentoxiphylin, pyracetam, vinpocentin) exerted a similar effect. The aim with the earlier drug therapy was also to improve blood circulation in the inner ear and brain. As we administered several drugs with diverse mechanisms of action to patients, we have learned in recent years that the best results could be achieved with infusion series in vasodilation for tinnitus.

2. The simultaneous use of the mentioned chemical agents (drugs) or physical agent (pulsating magnetic field) mutually increase their effectiveness and obviously make circulation in the capillaries much more powerful and thereby enable improvement of metabolism in the nerve cells, as well as increase their ATP production and protein synthesis (7, 10, 11).

3. BEMER therapy acts on the nervous system. The soothing, stress- releasing, relaxing effect is clearly demonstrated. As mentioned earlier, psychological problems, dejection and depression are in the background of tinnitus. Since the BEMER treatment affects and reduces the symptoms favorably, it apparently has an indirectly positive effect on tinnitus (1, 14, 18).

4. When applying BEMER treatment, it could be determined in most patients that their well-being, their condition and their mood improved. To a certain extent, the mentioned therapy improves physical and spiritual power (1, 12, 14). Of course this is the case if you explicitly bring about the improvement of a patient's well-being with a method. The patient will experience one of his or her previously-existing medical conditions as less unpleasant. Better well-being can alleviate the discomfort of the original symptoms and the patient is able to see them as more tolerable.

Among the advantages of BEMER treatment, you absolutely have to mention that this therapy also has a favorable impact on other accompanying diseases of patients suffering from tinnitus due to its comprehensive curative effects: A large part of our patients belonged to the older age group, so several of them are in treatment as a result of various diseases (e.g. hypertension, diabetes, cervical spondylosisischemic heart disease). In some cases, we noticed that one or more concomitant diseases of patients improved with the application of BEMER therapy.

It is generally accepted that a clear conclusion can be made on the effectiveness of the application of randomized double-blind placebo-controlled clinical study when introducing a new therapy. Our studies that were carried out in the stated method demonstrated that the BEMER therapy supplemented with drug treatment significantly reduced the symptoms of those patients suffering from tinnitus compared to patients treated with drugs only. This result was also confirmed by the statistical calculation of the χ^2-test.

Our results demonstrated our previous clinical experience that the BEMER treatment can be used successfully in patients with subjective tinnitus.

Acknowledgements

The author expresses his thanks to Andrea Patkó, specialist assistant for the implementation of the BEMER treatment applied during the double-blind trial and for accurate documentation.

Using the BEMER Therapy in the Otorhinolaryngology Departments

Habil. Kiss Géza József DPHYS, Ph.D., CSC Audiology Department, University of Szeged
Other authors: Gáborján A. *, Szirmai Á.*, Szilágyi I.**, Jarabin J.

* Semmelweis University, Otorhinolaryngology Department, Budapest

** Otorhinolaryngology Department, Szentes Hospital

BEMER therapy was tested for new indications in certain cases of tinnitus, balance disorders and impaired hearing.

We continue by summing up the findings of this study conducted at the Otorhinolaryngology Departments of Hungarian hospitals.

There were 67 patients involved in the study (mean age: 61 years). The youngest and the oldest patient were 34 and 86 years old, respectively. Two third of the patients were women, while one third were men. All participants had undergone a full clinical examination in compliance with the relevant guidelines. In many cases, medication was not sufficient, while in some cases medication was refused by the patients due to possible adverse effects.

Therefore, BEMER therapy was administered after or instead of medication.

The BEMER impulse is an internationally patented electromagnetic field that improves circulation, especially in the capillaries, activates the metabolism, stimulates the renewal of cells, provides cells with energy, improves oxygen supply and circulation, and relaxes the muscles. Tinnitus, neurosensory hearing impairment or balance disorders are frequently caused by inappropriate circulation, conditions affecting the cervical spine, muscle cramps, or nervousness, and therefore in these cases good results may be expected using the BEMER therapy. Ten sessions of treatment, 28-minutes each, were performed, which is initiated with a session of eight minutes on the mat applicator (Program P1), followed by a session of 20 minutes using the intensive applicator (Program P4) placed above the back of the neck in the occipital and retro-auricular position.

In our study, 65% of the cases showed an improvement, i.e. a decrease in complaints. In 35% of the cases complaints remained unchanged. No deterioration was observed.

During these treatment sessions, most patients have felt tingling, somnolence and relaxation. Some patients felt that they were being charged with energy. A large proportion of the patients reported an improvement in joint pain, sleeping disorders and vascular problems, and in general, an increased activity.

Hyperacusis treatment with a combination of Pulsed Electromagnetic Field, anti-oxidants and Low Level Laser Light - A clinical study

P. A. Mikael Bäckman, Nurse - Audio Laser-Kliniken, Danderyd, Sweden 2004

Abstract

A clinical study on hyperacusis treatment was carried out with a combination of "Low Level Laser Therapy", "Anti-oxidant Therapy" and "Pulsed Electromagnetic Field Therapy" in a clinical trial where all patients suffering from hyperacusis underwent the combined therapy presented in this study. Hyperacusis was evaluated both subjectively and by audiometry. The study consisted of a primary and a secondary group evaluated in two different ways.

In the first group, where the patients subjectively estimated their hyperacusis after treatment, 24 out of 27 patients felt less sensitive to sound - had milder hyperacusis or felt "cured ". Only 3 patients felt no difference at all after the treatment period consisting of 10 to 20 treatment sessions. No patients had a more aggressive hyperacusis after treatment. Some of the patients evaluated their Hyperacusis and the benefit s of the treatment as late as more than a year after finishing therapy, some of them still feeling just as good as when they ended their treatment.

In the second group, audiometric examination and evaluation was made before and after the treatment. In this group, all 24 treated patients' ears were improved due to Hyperacusis levels. All Hyperacusis patient s in this group obtained a positive effect in every dysfunctioning ear. The positive effects on hyperacusis were individually as high as 22 dB in average, counting all the frequencies where the patients experienced sensitivity to sound at levels graded as hyperacusis. An average improvement of 10.5 dB or more was measured in 16 out of 24 ears.

In both groups the patients were treated with Low Level Laser Therapy and Pulsed Electromagnetic Field Therapy for at least IO sessions, every session lasting for approximately 40 minutes. Most patients in the second group also underwent Anti-oxidant Therapy and their FORM/dROMs values (Free Oxidative Radical Metabolites) were controlled and adjusted with anti-oxidants in adequate doses.
No major complications or severe side-effects were reported from the patients. No damages or wounds in tissue were caused by the therapy. No permanent side-effects were observed.
Keywords: lllt, laser, electromagnetism, hyperacusis, anti-oxidants, dROMs

Introduction

Hyperacusis is a poorly understood disorder resulting in many theories of etiology and prognosis [I]. Hyperacusis sometimes is a severe condition for those who suffer from it. People with hyperacusis can experience discomfort at 40 to 50 decibels or lower. The disorder may be frequency-specific. Not all sounds of the same loudness (number of decibels) cause discomfort, but only sounds within a certain range, thus a small change of frequency may cause discomfort at low volume. [2]. In a survey conducted by the American Tinnitus Association, 70% of the hyperacusis patients reported some form of hearing loss. [3]. A questionnaire in a clinic population showed that 8% of tinnitus sufferers have hyperacusis [4]. There, a positive correlation was found between tinnitus and hyperacusis [5]. Among hyperacusis patients, 86% suffer from tinnitus. In such cases it is hyperacusis that is often considered the more severe of the two problems...Thus, when both conditions are present, we usually attempt to treat the hyperacusis first, and fortunately there is a potential treatment to offer the hyperacusis patient. Usually normal hearing or slight high frequency loss is present. Tolerance levels for sound of pure tone are less than 90 dB. It was found that hyperacusis strikes younger people more than tinnitus. [6]. Hyperacusis, and the combination of both hyperacusis and tinnitus, were found to be significantly more frequent among women than among men [7]. Among musicians, 56% suffered from hyperacusis. Related hearing disorders as diplacusis (3%) and distortion (17%) was measured and seemed to always be in combination with another hearing disorder which hyperacusis was not. Among rock/jazz musicians, 74% studied had hearing disorders and more than 50% had very distressing combinations of hearing disorders. Musicians suffering from hyperacusis tend to have poorer hearing thresholds than unaffected men [8].

Hyperacusis was shown to be caused by pathologic conditions of the peripheral auditory system, diseases of the central nervous system and hormonal and infectious diseases. In some cases there was no known cause. The pathophysiology of hyperacusis probably involves a central mechanism rather than a peripheral one [9]. Hyperacusis and phonophobia represent disturbances of central auditory processing without peripheral pathology, often combined with psychosomatic reactions. [10]. In the (ATA) survey patients were asked if they constantly wear ear plugs and 93% answered yes. This type of protection is false security and one way to almost surely make hyperacusis worse. Many hyperacusis patients dread going outdoors for fear of encountering loud sounds such as car horns, sirens, signals, truck noise, backfires, and so on [3].

One treatment used for hyperacusis is Auditory Integration Training (AIT). AIT lacks experimental evidence and is controversial. The treatment involves listening to modulated music with specific frequencies electively filtered.

Another problem with AIT is no training standards and guidelines for AIT trainers. Other treatments for hyperacusis include biofeedback and relaxation techniques [11]. Meyer Rosen, a hyperacusis sufferer, has tried food desensitization, exposure of nasal passages to essential oils, neurolinguistic training, rehydration of mucous membranes, correction of head-forward posture, scalp and body acupuncture, progressive relaxation of the temporomandibular joint musculature by an orthopedic mandibular repositioning device, and the use of an earplug prescription. After much study, Meyer developed an acupuncture treatment called Reflex-Correspondence Training [12]. All of these treatments lack scientific evidence. The theoretical basis for hyperacusis is not yet known. All aspects of hyperacusis need future research [1].

Laser treatment of hyperacusis as a treated disorder has rarely been mentioned in Pulsed Electromagnetic Field or Low Level Laser Therapy studies and there have been no results reported [13]. Positive results have been reported from tinnitus and inner ear studies as well as clinical experiences with Low Level Laser Therapy [14- 24]. One single tinnitus study has been carried out with Low Level Laser Therapy in combination with Electromagnetic Field Therapy and Negatively Ionized Oxygen [25]. Some studies have been made on dosimetric analysis of laser irradiation of the inner ear (26- 28). Negative studies on tinnitus treatment have also been performed with the common factor that they have used very small doses of Low Level Laser Light and have not specified desirable parameters [29- 34].

One histological inner ear study with Low Level Laser Therapy has been performed showing an instant effect on c-GMP [35]. Positive effects in nerve cells and their regeneration have been reported from laser studies [36- 52].

Regeneration of capillaries and supported microcirculation by Low Level Laser Therapy has been found [53-55]. Low Level Laser Light triggers positive mechanisms, synthesis and in cell plasma [56- 63].

Free radical occurrence and oxygen activation is found in Low Level Laser Light irradiated biological systems [64-65].

There is wide knowledge, a huge mass of scientific research and easily understandable information about Low Level Laser Therapy. The therapy is harmless and non-invasive [66].

There are several medical and biological effects reported from medical studies of the influence of electric and magnetic fields including dilation of capillaries and less blood flow resistance. [67- 77].

Tinnitus could be generated by the auditory brainstem, which is innervated by N. trigeminus [78]. There is a link between Tinnitus and cranomandibular disorders (79]. There are CMD cranomandibular disorders), TMD (tempooromandibular disorders) and TMJ (tempooromandibular joint) problems connected to tinnitus symptoms. CMD, TMD and TMJ have been successfully treated with Low Level Laser Therapy [80-89].

The following generalizations can be made:

1. Hyperacusis is not heightened hearing sensitivity (hearing thresholds are not better than normal)
2. Hyperacusis is often accompanied by tinnitus
3. The severity of hyperacusis is usually inversely proportional to the pitch of the offending noise
4. Perhaps most important, over-protection of the ears is a natural reaction of hyperacusic patients but it must be avoided as it progressively exacerbates hyperacusis.

Successful treatment for hyperacusis involves two components:

1. Training patients to use sound level meters to distinguish between truly damaging sound levels versus those which simply sound too loud.
2. Instructing them in the use of a desensitization program which involves listening to peek noise for several hours daily, starting at a low sound level and progressively increasing it over a period of several months. The longest desensitization period to date was two years; and the average is probably much closer to two years than to three months [3].

Hypothesis: "If tinnitus is positively affected by treating it with a combination of Low Level Laser Therapy and Anti-oxidant Therapy, and if Pulsed Electromagnetic Field Therapy has a positive effect on the organism, then hyperacusis could also be positively affected by a combination of all three therapies."

Material

Low Level Laser device:
The laser equipment was manufactured by the Swedish laser manufacturing company Irradia AB. The basic driver, feeding six laser probes, is a modified MID-laser device. Three different categories of laser probes were used in the hyperacusis treatment:
- 1 Ga As, 120 mW, 904 nm, 8 diodes over 50 cm2, non-col1imated, defocused pulsed light.
- 2 Ga Al As, 500 mW, 808 nm, single diode, non-collimated, defocused continuous light.
- 2 Ga Al In P, 35 mW, 650 nm, single diode, collimated, unfocused continuous light. Pulsed Electromagnetic Field device: BEMER 3000 pulsed electromagnetic field system was used including:
- BEMER 3000 basic driver.
- BEMER 3000 "bed" (mattress) 5-50 µT (micro tesla).
- BEMER 3000 standard electromagnetic intensive-applicator max. 100 µT. Free Oxidative Radical Metabolites - measurement and analysis device:
- Reactive Oxygen Metabolites (dROMs) were measured with Callegari CR2000 "FORM dROMs Free Oxygen Radicals Monitor". A sample of 20 µl capillary blood is analyzed using spectrophotometry.

Audiometry device:

- Welch Allyn AM 232 Manual Audiometer, Ref. ANSI S3.6/ISO 389, No. SIN 06604 with Welch Allyn standard earphones, TDH-39P, 296D00-9,
- SIN C 10974. Measurement was made in a sound-isolated room, not fulfilling standard acoustic requirements, but definitely totally silent and situated in an environment not affected at all by any noise.

Methods

The study included all hyperacusis patients treated in the clinic from November 1999, through March 2004 with no selections or limitations. No treated patients were excluded. Both ears were always treated during every session on every patient to minimize the risk for the appearance of dizziness after the treatment. The patients were treated in horizontal position - lying down.

Audiometry test:

The audiometric examination before and after therapy was executed with a device unable to exceed volumes more powerful than 100 dB to ensure as little risk as possible of damage to the patients' ears. The maximum test level for 250 Hz and 8000 Hz was 80 dB. If the patient didn't experience any annoyance at that level after therapy, the observation was given a value of 85 dB.

The maximum test level for 125 Hz was 60 dB and therefore the observation was given a value of 65 dB if the patient didn't feel any annoyance at that frequency after therapy. Upper limits for hyperacusis were set as shown in table 1. Pulse mode with 2.5 pulses/sec was used in the test. If a patient wasn't annoyed by sound levels higher than the "hyperacusis level" in table J, displaying audiometry levels and limits, the patient was not considered to be suffering from hyperacusis. Frequencies not measured as annoying at all before therapy were not registered and were left blank in the statistical data.

The 85 dB limit was set at this level because of the natural defense it constitutes. Even if there are no real limits for hyperacusis, this is probably an adequate sound level because feeling sensitive to that level probably prevents most ears from being damaged from more powerful sound levels. However, there are many reasons for setting hyperacusis limits individually, but that would certainly cause a lot of problems evaluating the observations, and thereby endanger a consequent evaluation of the hyperacusis treatment.

Table 1- Audiometric levels and limits

Frequency (Hz)	125	250	500	750	1000	1500	2000	3000	4000	6000	8000
Maximum test level (dB)	60	80	100	100	100	100	100	100	100	100	80
Hyperacusis limit (dB)	60	80	85	85	85	85	85	85	85	85	80

- Measurement was taken before and after treatment. They were taken for every patient in the second group. The audiometry test was conducted through air only. The patients informed the examiner when the volume became annoying. Sound level was increased by 5 dB at a time until patients felt annoyance. Pulsed mode (2.5 Hz/sec) was used with 1-2 beeps/freq.

Low Level Laser Therapy:

Laser light was administrated using three different probes:

- 904 nm, 120 mW, 5 Hz pulse, 7 minutes (50 J), administration over a circle area of 50 cm2 over the temporal lobe, the M. masseter, Proc. coronoideus, and the Lig. stylomandubulare.
- 808 nm, 500 mW, continuous light, administration via meatus for a minimum of 2 minutes (60 J) and a maximum of 15 minutes (450 J) in the beginning of the session. The laser probes were applied as close as possible to the tympani c membrane for the administration of as much laser light as possible to the inner ear. Contact mode with the tympanic membrane was not possible because of the size of the probe tip.
- 650 nm, 35 mW, continuous light, administration via meatus for 30 minutes (60 J), for the rest of the session. The laser probes were aimed towards the tympanic membrane and applied in contact mode between the outer regions of the meatus and the shell of the laser probe tip.

Pulsed Electromagnetic Field Therapy: BEMER 3000 system was used:

- Treatment session starts with the BEMER "bed" for 8 minutes using program "6".
- The BEMER 3000 standard electromagnetic intensive-applicator is used twice for 16 minutes during the laser treatment. It was applied behind the most afflicted ear of the patient suffering from hyperacusis and afterwards the intensive- applicator was moved to the same position of the other ear for another 16 minutes. Program "P3" was used for the intensive-applicator. The applicator was in contact mode with the mastoid bone behind the ear.

The BEMER 3000 system is a device approved for use in medical treatment in the EU, class 2A according to the ISO 9002 and DIN EN 46002.
Anti-oxidant Therapy - pharmacological drugs:

- Some patients took Gingko biloba tablets during the treatment period.
- Some patients took E-vitamin tablets during the treatment period.
- Some patients took multi vitamin tablets during the treatment period.
- Free Oxidative Radical Metabolites - measurement and control:

Reactive Oxygen Metabolites, dROMs, in the blood were analyzed in order to prescribe suitable doses of anti-oxidative tablets. A sample of 20 µl of capillary blood was analyzed spectrophotometrically with the Callegari CR2000 "FORM dROMs Free Oxygen Radicals Monitor".
Reactive Oxygen Metabolites were measured in U.Carr.

The normal interval for dROMs in the blood is 230-310 U.Carr. If the dROMs exceeded the upper limit 310 U.Carr, then anti-oxidants were prescribed in larger doses than the patients' actual intake.
The patients were treated twice a week, most of them for 6 weeks with an average total of 12 treatments with Low Level Laser Light, Pulsed Electromagnetic Field and in most cases a controlled amount of anti-oxidants. The time needed for a single treatment session is approximately 40 minutes. A couple of patients in this study underwent massage therapy during and/or immediately after the hyperacusis therapy in this study.

Results

THE FIRST GROUP - GROUP 1

From November 1999 to March 2004, laser treatment was performed and evaluated on all hyperacusis patients within the patient population treated at the clinic. The first 27 patients subjectively estimated their annoyance after the laser treatment in comparison with their annoyance before the start of the treatment.

In the first group of 27 hyperacusis patients evaluating their own hyperacusis annoyance subjectively after the treatment, the summary of the results reported by the patients is displayed in Table 2. Out of 27 hyperacusis patients (7 women, 20 men), 24 felt better (6 women, 18 men) after the treatment. The remaining 3 patients (I woman, 2 men) didn't get any changes in their hyperacusis.

Table 2 - Treatment results -subjective evaluation in group 1

Hyperacusis after treatment	Number of patients	Percentage
More annoyance	0	0%
No difference	3	11%
Less annoyance	24	89%
Total	27	100%

THE SECOND GROUP - GROUP 2

The results in the group of all 12 patients (2 women, l0 men), 24 ears (4 female, 20 male) with audiometrically measured hyperacusis are presented in Tables 3, 4, 5, 6, 7, 8 and 9. Table 3 displays audiometry levels in dB before treatment. Table 4 displays audiometry levels in dB after treatment. Table 5 displays the improvements in dB. Table 6 is a statistic analysis of each ear.

Table 7 is a statistic summary over every hyperacusis frequency improvement. Table 8 shows the improvement in intervals. Table 9 sums up the improvements of every difference between the observations made before and after therapy.

Table 3 - Audiometry levels in group 2 before therapy

Frequency	125	250	500	750	1000	1500	2000	3000	4000	6000	8000
Ear 1			(90)	(90)	(90)	(90)	80	80	80	85	75
Ear 2			(95)	(90)	(90)	(90)	85	85	80	75	70
Ear 3			(100)	(100)	(100)	(100)	(95)	(95)	(95)	(90)	75
Ear 4			(100)	(100)	(100)	(95)	(90)	(90)	85	80	80
Ear 5		80	75	75	70	75	70	70	70	70	70
Ear 6		80	80	80	80	85	70	70	70	65	65
Ear 7		(90)	(90)	(90)	(95)	75	75	80	85	80	
Ear 8		85	85	(90)	(90)	80	80	75	(90)	80	
Ear 9		80	85	85	80	75	75	70	65	60	55
Ear 10		80	85	85	85	85	75	75	70	70	65
Ear 11	35	35	40	40	40	55	65	65	70	65	60
Ear 12	50	50	50	45	50	50	65	65	70	55	55
Ear 13	80	85	85	85	85	80	75	75	65	60	
Ear 14	80	75	75	75	70	70	70	70	70	70	
Ear 15	75	80	80	80	85	80	80	80	80	80	

Ear 16	80	85	85	85	85	80	80	80	80	75	
Ear 17		(95)	(95)	(95)	(95)	85	85	85	75		
Ear 18							(95)	(100)	(95)	85	80
Ear 19			80	85	85	(90)	(90)	70	75	75	70
Ear 20			(95)	(95)	(95)	100)	(95)	85	(95)	80	80
Ear 21			(90)	(90)	85	85	85	80	75	70	70
Ear 22		80	85	85	80	80	80	70	70	65	65
Ear 23			(90)	85	85	85	75	70	85	(90)	
Ear 24			(90)	(95)	(95)	(90)	85	85	80		

"( )" around the values of the observations mean that they are not graded as hyperacusis and will not be used as statistical data for improvement and average.

Table 4 - Audiometry levels in group 2 after therapy

Frequency	125	250	500	750	1000	1500	2000	3000	4000	6000	8000
Ear 1			(>105)	(>105)	(>105)	(>105)	>105	>105	>105	95	>85
Ear 2			(>105)	(>105)	(>105)	(>105)	>105	>105	>105	>105	>85
Ear 3			(>105)	(>105)	(>105)	(>105)	(>105)	(>105)	(>105)	(>105)	>85
Ear 4			(>105)	(>105)	(>105)	(>105)	(>105)	(>105)	100	100	>85
Ear 5		80	75	75	75	80	80	75	75	75	70
Ear 6		80	80	80	80	85	75	70	70	70	65
Ear 7			(100)	(100)	(100)	(100)	90	85	85	100	>85
Ear 8			100	100	(95)	(100)	90	90	85	(100)	>85
Ear 9		>85	>105	100	100	95	90	90	80	75	70
Ear 10		>85	>105	>105	>105	105	100	100	100	90	80
Ear 11	40	40	50	50	50	65	70	65	75	70	70
Ear 12	50	55	55	55	50	55	65	65	75	70	65
Ear 13		>85	90	85	90	85	80	85	80	75	70
Ear 14		>85	90	90	90	90	90	85	80	80	75
Ear 15		>85	90	95	95	95	95	95	90	90	80
Ear 16		>85	95	95	100	100	95	95	90	90	80
Ear 17				(>105)	(>105)	(>105)	(>105)	>105	90	90	85
Ear 18							(>105)	(>105)	(>105)	>105	>85
Ear 19			>105	>105	>105	(>105)	(>105)	80	90	90	>85
Ear 20			(>105)	100	100	100	100	95	95	(90)	
Ear 21			(95)	(95)	90	90	90	90	90	90	>85
Ear 22		>85	90	90	85	85	85	85	85	80	80
Ear 23			(>105)	100	100	100	100	95	95	(90)	

					(100)	(>105)	(100)	(100)	100	95	90	
Ear 24												

">" means "the displayed value or even more".

">105" or "(>105)" means that the value was measured up to 100 dB but the patient didn't feel any annoyance at that level, therefore the level was registered as 105 dB. The parenthesis "( )" indicates that the observation measured before therapy was not regarded as hyperacusis. >85 means that the value was measured up to 80 dB but the patient didn't feel any annoyance at that level, therefore the level after treatment was set to 85 dB.

Table 5 - Audiometry level improvements between pre- and post treatment in group 2

Frequency	125	250	500	750	1000	1500	2000	3000	4000	6000	8000
Ear 1			(>15)	(>15)	(>15)	(>15)	>25	>25	>25	10	>10
Ear 2			(>10)	(>15)	(>15)	(>15)	20	20	25	30	15
Ear 3			(>5)	(>5)	(>5)	(>5)	(>10)	(>10)	(>10)	(>15)	>10
Ear 4			(>5)	(>5)	(>5)	(>10)	(>15)	(> 15)	15	20	>5
Ear 5			0	0	5	5	10	5	5	5	0
Ear 6			0	0	0	0	5	0	0	5	0
Ear 7			(10)	(10)	(10)	(5)	15	10	5	15	>5
Ear 8			15	15	(5)	(10)	10	10	10	(10)	>5
Ear 9		>5	>20	15	20	20	15	20	15	15	15
Ear 10		>5	>20	>20	>20	>20	25	25	30	20	15
Ear 11	5	5	10	10	10	10	5	0	5	5	10
Ear 12	0	5	5	10	0	5	0	0	5	15	10
Ear 13		>5	5	0	5	0	0	10	5	10	10
Ear 14		>5	15	15	15	20	20	15	10	10	5
Ear 15		>10	10	15	15	10	15	15	10	10	0
Ear 16		>5	10	10	15	15	15	15	10	10	5
Ear 17			(>10)	(>10)	(>10)	(>10)	>20	5	5	10	
Ear 18							(>10)	(>5)	(>10)	>20	>5
Ear 19			>25	20	20	(15)	(>15)	10	15	15	>15
Ear 20			(>10)	(>10)	(>10)	(>5)	(>10)	>20	(>10)	10	>5
Ear 21			(5)	(5)	5	5	5	10	15	20	>15
Ear 22		>5	5	5	5	5	5	15	15	15	15
Ear 23			(>15)	15	15	15	25	25	10	(0)	
Ear 24				(10)	(>10)	(5)	(10)	15	10	10	

The values are improvements in dB for every frequency in every ear after therapy. Blank spots were frequencies not measurable as annoying -not regarded as hyperacusis.

">" means "the displayed value or even more".

">105" or "(>105)" means that the value was measured up to 100 dB but the patient didn't fell any annoyance at that level, therefore the level was registered as 105 dB. The parenthesis"( )" indicates that the observation measured before therapy was not regarded as hyperacusis. >85 means that the value was measured up to 80 dB but the patient didn't feel any annoyance at that level, therefore the level after treatment was set to 85 dB.

Table 6 - Statistic hyperacusis analysis of every separate ear Frequency

	Total improvement (dB)	Number of observations	Average improvement (dB)
Ear 1	95	5	19.00
Ear2	110	5	22.00
Ear3	10	1	10.00
Ear4	40	3	13.33
Ears	35	10	3.50
Ear6	10	10	1.00
Ear7	50	5	10.00
Ear8	65	6	0.83
Ear 9	160	10	16.00
Ear 10	200	10	20.00
Ear 11	75	11	6.82
Ear 12	55	1I	5.00
Ear 13	50	10	5.00
Ear 14	130	10	13.00
Ear 15	110	10	11.00
Ear 16	110	10	11.00
Ear 17	40	4	10.00
Ear 18	25	2	12.50
Ear 19	120	7	17.14
Ear20	35	3	11.67
Ear21	75	7	10.71
Ear22	90	IO	9.00
Ear23	105	6	17.50
Ear24	35	3	11.67
Total	1830	169	10.83

Table 6 evidently shows that all patients in the trial improved their hyperacusis. In 18 years, the conditions were verified through audiometric test confirming an average improvement of 10dB or more for the frequencies graded as hyperacusis due to the sound levels before therapy.

Table 7 - Statistic foundation and average hyperacusis improvement in dB for all frequencies

Frequency (Hz)	125	250	500	750	1000	1500	2000	3000	4000	6000	8000
Before therapy	85	720	990	1075	1065	1000	1375	1585	1595	1535	1480
After therapy	90	765	1130	1225	1 215	1130	1610	1855	1840	1815	1655
Observations	2	10	13	14	15	13	18	21	21	21	21
Impr. (dB)	5	45	140	150	150	130	235	270	245	280	175
Aver. impr.(dB)	Feb 50	Apr 50	Oct 77	Oct 51	10.00	10.00	13. Jun	Dec 86	Nov 67	13.33	Aug 33

The statistic material for every frequency includes:
- First row: Frequency.
- Second row: Total sum in dB for patients suffering from hyperacusis before therapy.
- Third row: Total sum in dB for patients suffering from Hyperacusis after therapy.
- Fourth row: Number of patients suffering from Hyperacusis due to the specific frequency.
- Fifth row: Total improvement in dB among hyperacusis patients.
- Sixth row: Average improvement in dB among hyperacusis patients.

Table 8 - Statistic dB-groups of average improvement among the 24 ears in the group 2

Improvement range	Number of improved ears	Percentage of improved
Worse hyperacusis, < 0 dB	0	0%
0 - 4.99 dB	2	8%
5 - 9.99 dB	4	17%
10- 14.99 dB	12	50%
15-19.99 dB	4	17%
20-24.99 dB	2	8%
Total	24	100%

Table 9 - Statistic dB-groups of the number of improved frequencies graded as hyperacusis

Improvement	Number of observations
No improvement, 0 dB	0
Change for the worse	21
5dB	43
l0dB	36
15dB	38
20dB	20

25dB	9
30dB	2
Total	169

The patient with ears 5 and 6 in the table was noticed to have higher dROMs values (greater oxidative stress) than 310 U.Carr in his blood plasma throughout the whole treatment period. This patient made the least improvement in dB among all the patients in the second group.

One patient in the first group also had very high dROMs values, much higher than 310 U.Carr in blood plasma throughout the whole treatment period. That patient was one out of three in the first group who didn't notice any improvement.

One patient in the second group suffered from distortion. Sound started to be distorted at 60 dB before therapy. After therapy, distortion didn't appear until sound levels reached 90 dB.

Several patients suffered from otitis externa. This condition improved during the treatment period in almost all cases.

Many hyperacusis patients in this hyperacusis study also suffered from tinnitus. More than 55% of these patients permanently had less tinnitus after therapy.

Hearing capacity was improved among a great number of patients. The best improvement was 24.5 dB in average. The best improvement on a single frequency was 45 dB.

No damage was observed whatsoever in any patient in this study. No permanent side effects were noticed and none of the patients were harmed in any way by the mild, biostimulating low level lasers or by the pulsed electromagnetic field device.

Not a single patient obtained any observed, negative side-effect from Gingko biloba, E-vitamins, beta-carotene or any other anti-oxidant in the trial.

Side-effects noticed among patients in the study:

- A moderate and temporary increase of tinnitus symptoms, which were always reduced back to their original level or Jess. For two of the tinnitus patients the tinnitus symptoms totally disappeared.
- A moderate and most temporary enhancement of the hyperacusis, which diminished back to its original status or became even more diminished than before therapy,
- Tiredness was a quite common side-effect. Most patients who became tired found this side-effect to be a most "welcome" side-effect, as it contributed to the fact that they could sleep better at night.
- Balance was moderately affected in a negative way up to half an hour after treatment.
- Moderate pain was detected in the ear canal, probably due to anti- inflammatory processes.

Discussion

This study was performed with a combination of therapies. Of course one would want to know the results of every single monotherapy involved.

However the results in this study are positive and the treatment, which is mainly based upon the laser light therapy, definitely merit further attention and extended research.

Many patients with hyperacusis have been suffering from it for a long time - sometimes for many years. Among patients suffering from hyperacusis the average alteration during two months is expected to be very close to the "status quo" if the patients remain untreated. Some patients will develop worse hyperacusis, some will develop a milder form, a few may even be "cured" and some patients will remain just as hypersensitive to sound as they were at the beginning of the period. No great changes are expected during such a short period that lasts for two months (a little longer than the six weeks a normal treatment period takes). Therefore the results in this study are astonishing and at the same time very encouraging.

Some audiologists tend to advise their patients suffering from hyperacusis, to try to endure annoying or even painful sound volumes. It is well known that 81 dB is the most optimal sound level conveying a "training" effect for the hair cells of the inner ear because of the existence of actin-myosin proteins within the sound receptor cells. However, a lot of hyperacusis patients have painful experiences and experience severe hyperacusis, even after being exposed to sound levels not more powerful than 70 dB, if they are sensitive to sound volumes just as low and even lower than that. Often these hyperacusis patients also suffer from tinnitus and find their tinnitus to be more aggressive after being exposed to sound levels more powerful than what they can tolerate. Many patients also claim their tinnitus symptoms to be permanently worse after such exposure. Prescriptions to try to endure annoying or even painful sound levels could be disastrous for these patients.

The 40% limit of the possible share of patients obtaining positive "placebo effects" in tinnitus therapy could probably be applied to hyperacusis studies as well. But even if attention is paid to this, the results in this study surpass the 40% limit as much as possible among the patients in the second group. AJl patients in the second group had improved hyperacusis. This result is highly significant.

The results obtained are probably even better than the audiometrically measured results in the second group. This is probably the way it is because of the fact that sound levels higher than 100 dB could not be produced with the audiometry device. When patients got better, quite a lot of them didn't have any problems enduring sound levels of 100 dB. 22 measured observations could have had a higher level specified if another audiometry device would have been used. In the study measurement was stopped at l00 dB, and if the patient didn't feel any annoyance at that level, annoyance was specified to a level above, i.e. 105 dB. Sound level values of>l05 dB were actually 105 dB or more but 105 dB was the registration for that observation, forming the comparison material, even if the patient very well could have been able to tolerate a much higher level than 105 dB. Sound level values specified >85 dB were actually 85 dB or more, but 85 dB was the registered value.

After making a comparison between the two groups, it is obvious that most of the patients do detect and estimate the standard of their hyperacusis and its alteration over time quite well. This is probably also valid for patients suffering from tinnitus symptoms. The similarity between the two groups in this study asks the question as to whether the habituation process really is a major factor among the majority of the patients suffering from these two disorders. I do not think so. Tinnitus and hyperacusis symptoms could naturally be more annoying and the conditions experienced are worse if the patient focuses on them, but that doesn't mean that an active treatment should be avoided.

Patients suffering from these disorders also need to confirm their problems to themselves in order to be able to actively try to solve them and cope with the situation. Suppression is not a solution if there is a possibility to make the conditions better.

This hyperacusis and tinnitus treatment is similar. The positive effects of laser therapy on tinnitus symptoms are already very well known. Prochazka, Wilden, Hahn, Marti, Shiomi, Plath, Witt and many others have performed positive, scientific, medical studies in the field, often with laser therapy in combination with Gingko biloba and/or other therapies such as vertebral manipulation and the treatment of TMJ (tempooromandibular joint) or CMD (cranomandibular disorders). There is also a vast number of clinical reports supporting the positive effects of the scientific, medical studies on the treatment of tinnitus symptoms and other audiological and ENT-disorders. The positive effects on the amelioration of the inner ear are also well known from the work and studies of Lutz Wilden and the experiences of Ali Kolaylioglu, who once was an auscultator in my clinic.

One of the patients, treated for hyperacusis symptoms, was treated for two periods, each consisting of 15 and 14 treatments respectively, and the result after the second period was better compared to the result after the first one. This indicates that a good result can improve even more if therapy is performed repeatedly. This has also been observed among many tinnitus patients treated with the method. In the first group another one of the hyperacusis patients didn't experience any revolutionary effect after the first treatment period, but during the second period improvement was much greater. This indicates that patients might be more or less receptive to therapy during a certain period. But how do you optimize the receptiveness for hyperacusis treatment? This question requires further research before we can get closer to a satisfying answer.

A couple of patients underwent massage therapy during and immediately after this study. This excludes other therapeutic reasons for the improvement obtained in this study.

Does the result obtained have lasting effects and are they permanent? Well, permanence is a very difficult concept. But it is evident that the positive effects last for months and years.

The patient with ear 5 and 6 in the second group was the one who experienced minor improvement on hyperacusis levels. This patient had very high values of oxidative stress factors (dROMs) in blood plasma throughout the whole treatment period. The dROMs value was 852 U.Carr at the beginning - an absolutely extreme value that certainly depended on the use of estrogen pills (contraceptive tablets) well known to cause extremely high dROMs values, which of course contribute to the risk of developing severe diseases like many forms of cancer. Interesting about this issue is that the patient took so called "soft and gentle" contraceptives. The high dROMs values could partly depend on the fact that the patient didn't weigh much more than 40 kg, but there is no such thing as "soft and gentle" contraceptives. The patient was recommended to stop using contraceptives and so she did. After a week she said that she felt much better, a statement very common among women finishing their use of contraceptive tablets. Contraceptive tablets bring along great risks for "wear and tear" in tissue and cells, just like cytostatic medications, insulin and beta blockers do. After three weeks, the dROMs value was 634 U.Carr (better, but definitely not good at all), and three days before the end of the treatment period, the dROMs value had been adjusted in the right direction even further - down to 460 U.Carr (still a great oxidative stress value indicating great chemical stress in tissue and cells). Adjusting the dROMs value before treatment seems to be important, but the observations from a small amount of patients cannot be a determining factor whether this is of vital importance or not, but it seems like it is. There was also a female patient in the first group with a measured dROMs value of 822 U.Carr at the beginning of her treatment. Anti-oxidants were prescribed and less estrogen was part of the ordination to reduce oxidative stress, but the dROMs values didn't fall below 408 U.Carr during the treatment period. This female patient in the first group didn't experience any positive effects on hyperacusis levels after completing treatment. Maybe the estrogen played an important role for the result. Among other patients, treated for other hearing disorders there is a vast number of patients, hundreds of them, indicating that normal dROMs values in the interval 230-310 U.Carr could be beneficial to the outcome of the treatment. Extremely low values have also been seen, but seem to be more favorable to improvement than high dROMs values, but the best thing for a positive treatment result is probably to be within the normal interval.

Whatever anyone might criticize in or state against this study and clinical trial, the result speaks for itself and another study should be carried out without any problems and maybe in an even "more" controlled way, thereby confirming the results obtained therein. Nevertheless, this study is scientific, medical research. This is only the beginning of the exploration of this kind of combined therapy within this field. Of course there are always many parameters that could be discussed in any study. It would be preferable to carry out a randomized, double-blind, placebo-controlled study with a huge number of patients. But this would require solid funding and a Jot of dedicated people.
Hopefully this clinical trial Hyperacusis treatment with a combination of pulsed Electromagnetic Field - Bäckman awakens those who makes the decisions in funding medical research. My advice is to carry out similar trials on tinnitus symptoms, menieres disease, impaired hearing, balance disorders etc.

My intention is to perform an even larger study on tinnitus and/or hyperacusis and its treatment with Low Level Laser Therapy in combination with Pulsed Electromagnetic Field Therapy and Anti-oxidant Therapy to follow up this positive study. Some other interesting therapies lo combine the ones in this study with are negatively ionized oxygen and manipulation of the vertebral neck, jaw joints, jaw ligaments and jaw muscles, TMJ and CMD. There are also some interesting pharmaceutical therapies that could be worth trying in combination with these therapies.

Conclusions

- The combination of Low Level Laser Therapy & Pulsed Electromagnetic Field Therapy affects hyperacusis in a positive way and supports the hypothesis of this study. The positive results are clear and obvious. Low Level Laser Therapy in combination with Pulsed Electromagnetic Field Therapy and controlled anti-oxidant levels seem to be a beneficial treatment for raising the hyperacusis thresholds needed to avoid annoyance or pain for the patient.
- Reactive Oxygen Metabolites could play an important role having a repressing effect on biostimulation and anti-oxidants seem to have a beneficial effect on the result in hyperacusis treatment.
- Tinnitus symptoms were found to lessen and be eliminated with the therapy.
- Hearing thresholds were found to improve with the therapy.
- Distortion was found to improve with the therapy.
- Otitis externa was found to improve with the therapy.
- There were no major complications, neither severe nor permanent side- effects were observed from Low Level Laser Therapy in combination with Pulsed Electromagnetic Field Therapy and Anti-oxidant Therapy in this study.

Acknowledgements

I want to thank the surgeon and urologist Anders Larsson for introducing me to Low Level Laser Therapy in his private clinic in 1990. Ialso want to thank Lutz Wilden for introducing me to laser therapy for the treatment of inner ear diseases, disorders and dysfunctions. My sincere appreciation is addressed to Lutz Wilden, Miroslav Prochazka, Ali Kolaylioglu, Jan Tuner and Lars Hode for their dedication, scientific approach and limitless support. Without these people I would have been doing something completely different.

References

1. Demaree G.: http://hubel.sfasu.edu/courseinfo/SL98/www.hyperacusis.net.
2. Schwade, S.: Shedding light on supersensitive hearing: What to do when every small noise sounds like the big bang. Prevention, 1995; 47(8), 90-96.
3. Vernon J A, Oregon Health and Science University, USA.: Hyperacusis: Testing, Treatments and a Possible Mechanism. Audiology 24.2.2002; Volume 24, Number 2, Summary of Highlights From the 7th International Tinnitus Seminar.
4. Sanchez, L. & Stephens, D.: A tinnitus problem questionnaire in a clinic population. Ear & Hearing, 1997; 18, 210-217.
5. Goldstein, Shulman.: Tinnitus - Hyperacusis and the Loudness Discomfort Level Test - A Preliminary Report. International Tinnitus Journal 1996; 2:83-89
6. Anari, Axelsson, Eliasson, Magnusson: Hypersensitivity to sound- questionnaire data, audiometry, and classification. Scandinavian Audiology 1999; 28(4):219-230.
7. Kähari K, Zachau G, Ek.lof M, Sandsjo L, Möller C.: Department of Audiology, Goteborg University, Goteborg, National Institute for Working Life/West, Sweden. Assessment of hearing and hearing disorders in rock/jazz musicians. Int J Audiol. 2003 Jul; 42(5):279-88.
8. Kähari K.: The Influence of Music on Hearing. A Study in Classical and Rock/Jazz Musicians. Department of Otolaryngology, Faculty of Medicine, Goteborg University. 2002; ISBN 91-628-5339-2.
9. Katzenell U, Segal S.: Hyperacusis: review and clinical guidelines. Department of Otolaryngology, Otol. Neurotol. 2001 May; 22(3):321-6; discussion 326-7.
10. Schaaf-H, Klofat B, Hesse G: HNO. 2003 Dec; 51(12):1005-1I.11. Hyperacusis treatment with a combination of pulsed Electromagnetic Field - Bäckman
11. American Speech-Language Hearing Association. Hyperacusis. ASHA, 1995; 37, 53-54.
12. Rosen, M. R.: New treatment possibilities for hyperacusis--a painful, ultrasensitivity to normal sounds (letter to the editor). American Journal of Acupuncture, 1995; 23(1), 74- 76.
13. Hubacek J.: Experience with the Use of LLLT in ENT Medicine. Laser Partner 2000; No. 22.
14. Witt U, Felix C.: Selective photo-biochemo-therapy in the combination of laser and gingkoplant extracts acc. to the Witt method. 1989. Personal communication.
15. Olivier J, Plath P.: Combined low power laser therapy and extracts of Gingko biloba in a blind trial of treatment for tinnitus. Laser Therapy 1993; 5 (3): 137-139.
16. Plath P, Olivier J.: Results of combined low-power laser therapy and extracts of Gingko biloba in cases of sensorineural hearing loss and tinnitus. Adv Otorhinolaryngol. 1995; 49: 101-114.
17. Wilden L, Dindinger D.: Treatment of chronic diseases of the inner ear with low level laser therapy (LLLT). Laser Therapy, 1996; 8: 209-212.
18. Shiomi Y, Takahashi H, Honjo I, Kojima H, Naito Y, Fujiki N.: Efficacy of transmeatal low power laser irradiation on tinnitus: a preliminary report. Auris Nasus Larynx. 1997; 24(1): 39-42.
19. Wilden L.: The effect of low level laser light on inner ear diseases. In: Low Level Laser Therapy. Clinical Practice and Scientific Background. Eds. Jan Tuner, Lars Rode. Prima Books in Sweden AB (1999). ISBN 91-630-7616-0.
20. Wilden L, Ellerbrock D.: Amelioration of the hearing capacity by low- level-laser-light (LLLL). Lasermedizin. 1999; 14: 129-138.
21. Prochazka M, Tejnska R.: Noninvasive laser therapy of tinnitus: In: A window on the laser medicine world. Proc. SPIE. 1999. Vol. 4166: 223-223. Laser Partner, 2000; 4.
22. Hahn A, Senja I, Stolbova K, Cocek A.: Combined laser-EGb 761 tinnitus therapy. Acta Otolarngol Suppl. 2001; 545: 92-93.
23. Hahn A.: Combined tinnitus therapy with soft laser and EGb 761. Oral presentation at Barany Society Meeting, Seattle 2002.
24. Prochazka M, Hahn A.: Comprehensive laser rehabilitation therapy of tinnitus: long term double blind study in a group of 200 patients in three years. Laser Partner, 2002; 51.
25. Marti P.: Treatment through otolaser in combination with magnetic field therapy and oxygen-multistep-therapy. Cosmopolitan University & Universidad autonomo Gabriel Rene Moreno, Santa Cruz, Bolivia. 2001. Material published on the Internet.
26. Tauber S, Schorn K, Beyer W, Baumgartner R.: Transmeatal cochlear laser (TCL) treatment of cochlear dysfunction: A feasibility study for chronic tinnitus. Lasers Med Sci. 2003; 18(3): 154-61.
27. Beyer W, Baumgartner R, Tauber S.: Dosimetric analysis for low-level laser therapy (LLLT) of the inner ear at 593 nm and 633 nm. In: Effects of low-power light on biological systems IV. Eds. Bottiroli G, Karu T. Proc. SPIE. 1998; 3569: 13.
28. Tauber S, Baumgartner R, Schorn K, Beyer W.: Lightdosimetric quantitative analysis of the human petrosus bone: experimental study for laser irradiation of the cochlea. Lasers in Surgery and Medicine. 2001; 28: 18-26.
29. Nakashima
30. Beyer
31. Rogowski
32. Partheniadis-Stumpf

33. von Wedel
34. Walger
35. Shiomi Y et al.: Effect of low power laser irradiation on inner ear. Pract Otol (Kyoto). 1994; 87: 1135-1140.
36. Belkin M, Schwartz M.: Evidence for the existence of low-energy laser bioeffects on the nerv011s system. Nerosurg Rev. IR94; 11:7 17. - Hyperacusis treatment with a combination of pulsed Electromagnetic Field - Bäckman
37. Bashford J, Hallman H, Matsumoto J, Moyer S, Buss J, Baxter G.: Effects of 830 nm continuous wave laser diode irradiation on median nerve function in normal subjects. Lasers Surg Med. 1993; 13: 597-604.
38. Khullar S.: Reinnervation after nerve injury: the effects of low level laser treatment. In: Low Level Laser Therapy - Clinical Practice and Scientific Background. Eds Tuner- Hode. 1999; p 280-302. Prima Books in Sweden. ISBN 91-630-7616-0.
39. Khullar S et al.: The effects of low level laser treatment on recovery of nerve conduction and motor function after compression injury in rat sciatic nerve. Europ J Oral Sci. 1995; 103: 299-305.
40. Rochkind S et al.: Systemic effects of Low-Power Laser on the Peripheral and Central Nervous System, Cutaneous Wounds and Bums. Laser in surgery and Medicine. 1989; 9: 174-.
41. Rochkind S, Barrnea L, Razon N, Bartal A, Schwartz M.: Stimulatory effects of He-Ne low dose laser on injured sciatic nerve of rats. Neurosurgery. 1987; 20: 843-847.
42. Rochkind S, Nissan M, Alon M, Shamir M, Salame K.: Effects of laser irradiation on the spinal cord for the regeneration of crushed peripheral nerve in rats. Lasers Surg. 2001; 28: 216-219.
43. Rochkind S, Quaknine GE.: New trend in neuroscience: low power laser effect on peripheral and central nervous system (basic science, preclinical, and clinical studies). Neural Res 1992; 11: 2-11.
44. Rosner M, Caplan M, Cohen S, Duvdevani R, Solomon A, Assia E, Belkin M, Schwartz M.: Dose and temporal parameters in delaying injured optic nerve degeneration by low- energy laser irradiation. Lasers Surg Med Suppl. 1993; 13: 611-617.
45. Shamir M, Rochkind S, Sandbank J, Alon M.: Double-blind randomized study evaluating regeneration of the rat transected sciatic nerve after suturing and postoperative low-power laser treatment. Journal of Reconstructive Microsurgery. 2001; 17(2): 133-137.
46. Snyder-Mackler L, Bork C.: Effects of Helium-Neon laser irradiation on peripheral sensory nerve latency. Phys Ther. 1998; 86: 223-225.
47. Weintraub M.: Noninvasive laser neurolysis in carpal tunnel syndrome. Muscle Nerve.1997; 20 (8): 1029-1031.
48. Antipa C, Nacu M et al.: Clinical results of the low energy laser action on distal forearm posttraumatic nerve lesions. Laser Therapy. 1996; 1:36.
49. Khullar S et al.: Preliminary study of low-level laser for treatment of long- standing sensory aberrations in the inferior alveolar nerve. J Oral Maxillofac Surg. 1996; 54 (1) :2-7; discussion 7-8.
50. Rochkind S et al.: Double-blind Randomized Study Using Neurotube and Laser Therapy in the Treatment of Complete Sciatic Nerve Injury of Rats. Proc. 2nd Congr World Assoc. for Laser Therapy, Kansas City, 1998.
51. Snyder-Mackler L et al.: Effect of helium-neon laser irradiation on peripheral sensory nerve latency. Physical Therapy. 1988; 68: 223.
52. Walsh D et al:. The effect of low intensity laser irradiation upon conduction and skin temperature in the superficial radial nerve. Double- blind placebo controlled investigation using experimental ischaemic pain. Proc. Second Meeting of the Internat Laser Therapy Association. "London Laser". 1992.
53. Maier M, Haina D, Landthaler M.: Effect of Low Energy Laser on the Growth and Regeneration of Capillaries. Laser Therapy. 1993; 5 (2): 79-87.
54. Maegawa Y, Itoh T, Hosokawa T et al.: Effects of near-infrared low-level laser on microcirculation. Lasers Med Surg. 2000; 27: 427-437.
55. Petrischev N, Leontjeva N, Leotjeva T.: Influence of irradiation of helium-neon laser on microcirculation blood vessels. Proc. SPIE. 1996; Vol 2929: 198.
56. Wilden L, Karthein R.: Import of Radiation Phenomena of Electrons and Therapeutic Low-Level-Laser in Regard to the Mitochondrial Energy Transfer. Journal of Clinical Laser Medicine and Surgery. 1998; Vol. 16, No. 3, ISSN 1044-547 L. Hyperacusis treatment with a combination of pulsed Electromagnetic Field - Bäckman
57. Karu T.: Mechanisms of low-power laser light on cellular level. In: Lasers in Dentistry and Medicine. Ed: Simunovich Z. European Laser Medical Association. 2000. ISBN 953-6059-30-4.
58. Karu T.: "Low-power laser effects". In: Lasers in Medicine, Ed. by R. Waynant, Boca Raton,CRC Press. 2002;171-209, ISBN 0-8493-1146-2.
59. Karu T.: Photobiological Fundamentals of Low Power Laser Therapy. IEEE Journal of Quantum Electronics. 1987; 32 (IO): 1703-.
60. Karu T.: Photobiology of low-power laser effects. Health Physics. 1989; 56 (5): 691-704.
61. Karn T, Afanasyeva N et al.: Changes in absorbance of monolayer of living cells induced by laser irradiation at 633, 670 and 820 nm. IEEE J. Selected Topics in quantum Electronics. 2001; 7 (6): 982-988.
62. Karu T, Kolyakov S, Pyatibrat V et al.: Irradiation with a diode at 820 nm induces changes in circular dichroism spectra (270-780 nm) of living cells. IEEE J. Selected Topics in quantum Electronics. 2001; 7 (6): 976- 981.

63. Martin J, Migus A, Poyart C, Lecarpentier Y, Antonetti A.: Ultra-fast events in biological systems. Lab. d'optique Appliquée INSERM U275. Ecole Polytechnique- ANSTA, Palaiseau, Fr. p 218.
64. Derr V et al.: Free radical occurrence in some laser-irradiated biologic materials. Federal Proc. 1965; 24 (No I, Suppl 14): 99-103.
65. Klima H.: Effect of Weak Laser Light and Oxygen Activation in Open Biological Systems. LASER - Journ Eur Med Laser Ass. 1988; 1 (No 2): Tuner J, Hode L.: "Laser Therapy" - Clinical Practice and Scientific Background. Prima Books. 2002; ISBN 91-631-1344-9.
66. Fakuda, E.: Mechanical deformation and electrical polarisation in biological substances. Biorheology 5 (1968); 199-208.
67. Bassett, C. A. L.: Fundamental and practical aspects of therapeutic uses of pulsed electromagnetic fields, Critical Reviews in Biomedical Engineering, No 17, pp. 451-529 (1989).
68. Bassett C. A. L.: Beneficial effects of electromagnetic fields. Journ Cell. Bio-Chem. 5114 (1993): 387-393.
69. Becker, R. O.: Der Funke des Lebens, Piper, München. 1994.
70. Carpenter, D. O; Ayrapetan, S.: Biological Effects of Electric and Magnetic Fields: Sources and mechanism (Vol I); Beneficial and Harmful Effects (Vol2), Academic Press. 1994; ISBN: 0 12160262
71. Drexel H, Becker-Casademont R, Seichert N.: Physikalische Medizin: Licht und Elektrotherapie (Band 4), Hippokrates Verlag. 1988; ISBN: 3- 7773-0826.
72. Polk C, Postow E.: Handbook of Biological Effects of Electromagnetical Fields. CRC Press, 1996. ISBN: 0849306418.
73. Stemme 0.: Physiologie der Magnetfeldbehandlung: Grundlagen; Wirkungsweise; Anwendungen. Otto Stemme Verlag, München. 1992. ISBN: 3-9803094-01.
74. Warnake U: Survey of some working mechanisms of pulsing electromagnetic fields. Biochemistry and Bioenergetic. 1992.
75. Kafka, WA.: Emphyspace Literatur-Datenbank: Biologische Wirkung electromagnetischer Felder, 1999. Max-Planck-Institut für Verhaltensphysiologie, D- 82319 Seeweisen.
76. Kafka, WA.: Vasodilatorische Effekte durch speziell geformte electromagnetische Pulse niedrigster Energie. Emphyspace Report I, 1- 2, 1998.
77. Shore S, Vass Z, Wyss N, Altschuler R.: Trigeminal ganglion innervates the auditory brainstem. J. Comparative Neurology 2000; 419: 271-285.
78. Rubenstein B.: Tinnitus and cranomandibular disorders - is there a link? (thesis). Swed Dent J. Suppl. 1993; 95.
79. Bertolucci L, Grey T.: Clinical analysis of Mid-laser versus placebo treatment of arthralgic TMJ degenerative joints. J Cranomandib Practice. 1995; 13 (1): 26-29. Hyperacusis treatment with a combination of pulsed Electromagnetic Field - Bäckman
80. Bertolucci L, Grey T.: Clinical analysis of Mid-laser versus placebo treatment of arthralgic TMJ degenerative joints. J Cranomandib Practice. 1995; 13 (1): 26-29.
81. Bjorne A.: Tinnitus aureum as an effect of increased tension in the lateral pterygoid muscle (letter). Otolaryngol Head Neck Surg. 1993; 109: 969.
82. Bjorne A.: Cranomandibular Disorders in Patients with Meniere 's Disease: A Controlled Study. Journal of Orofacial Pain. 1996; Vol 10, No. I p 29-37.
83. Cho KA. Park JS, Ko MY.: The effect of low level laser therapy on pressure threshold in patients with temporomandibular disorders. A double blind study. J of Korean Academy of Oral Medicine. 1999; 24 (3): 281-300.
84. Conti PC.: Low-level laser therapy in the treatment of temporomandibular disorders (TMD): a double-blind pilot study. Cranio. 1997; 15 (2): 144-149.
85. Ibanez J, Medico R.: Laser therapy in temporomandibular dysfunction. Rev Fac Odont Univ Nae (C6rdoba). 1989; 17 (1-2): 21-30.
86. Kim S, Park J.: The effect of low level laser therapy at trigger points in masseter and other muscles. J Korean Acad Med. 1996; 21 (1): 3.
87. Sattayut S.: A study on the influence of low intensity laser therapy on painful temporomandibular disorders. 1999. University of London PhD thesis.
88. Application of low power laser therapy in closed lock temporomandibular joint dysfunction. Lasers in Surgery and Medicine. 1992; Suppl 4: 84.

Sources

89. Prochazka, M.: 2002-2004. Personal communication.
90. Kolaylioglu, A.: 2001-2004. Personal communication.
91. Wilden, L.: 1998-2004.Personal communication.

My Experiences with the BEMER Therapy in Patients with Tinnitus

Dr. Szilágyi Imre, chief physician, head of department
"Dr. Bugyi István" Hospital, Szentes, Otorhinolaryngology Department

Tinnitus is a symptom that has been observed with increasing frequency in our patients during recent years and decades. According to international figures (based on British and Swedish surveys), this condition causes long-term problems in 8-10% of the population. The number of patients with tinnitus has increased in recent years in Hungary, as well. This symptom can be caused by many diseases, and therefore patients with tinnitus must undergo a thorough examination.

Tinnitus can be either objective, when it can also be heard by the physician observing the patient (very seldom), or subjective, when the symptoms are observed only by the patient.

After the examinations, in case of the majority of the patients the cause of tinnitus cannot be determined. Treatment of this patient group has always been a great challenge for otorhinolaryngology specialists.

Over time, many different medicines and treatment methods were used in an attempt to treat tinnitus patients. The table below summarizes the most important medicines and treatment methods used at present:

Medicinal products	Vasodilators, agents to improve brain microcirculation, blood viscosity reducing agents, anxiolytics, tranquilizers, Lidocain, serotonin antagonists, etc.
Different treatment methods	Tinnitus retraining therapy, hyperbaric oxygen therapy, various physiotherapies
Different stimulation techniques applied around the ears	Electric stimulation, high frequency ultrasound stimulation, electromagnetic stimulation

Intravenous administration of brain circulation and microcirculation improving agents (pyracetam, pentoxyphyllin, vinpocetine) comprise the most widely used therapies in Hungary. This is also the therapy applied in case of tinnitus patients at our department for years.

About 4 years ago, we started to use BEMER therapy in addition to the above described therapy, as a result of which significant improvement of the therapeutic outcome was observed.

In order to scientifically confirm the positive effects of the BEMER therapy in the treatment of tinnitus, we have conducted a randomized, double-blind, placebo-controlled clinical study.

Patients admitted to our department with tinnitus, who had been previously examined, were divided into two groups. Patients who were given odd and even numbers at admission were included into Group I and Group II, respectively. A number of 108 and 106 patients were included in the first and the second group, respectively. Patients in Group I were administered 200 mg pentoxyphyllin in infusion and 2 x 1200 mg piracetam orally. In addition, 1 session of BEMER therapy was administered using BEMER 3000 Signal Plus device. The program used was as follows: mat P2 and intensive applicator P4 placed on the temporal region of the skull. This treatment was continued for 8 days.

Patients in Group II received the same medicines as those in Group I. However, in their case we used placebo BEMER therapy, i.e. during a simulated BEMER treatment session the device was not activated. Each patient treated with real BEMER therapy was followed by a patient treated with placebo BEMER therapy. These sessions were performed by a qualified assistant and the physician assessing the results received the data only after the completion of the treatment.

The study results are summarized in the table below:

Results of Patient Group I (n=108): (receiving real BEMER therapy)			Results of Patient Group II (n=106): (receiving placebo treatment)		
Tinnitus resolved	24	22.20%	Tinnitus resolved	9	8.50%
Tinnitus improved	51	47.30%	Tinnitus improved	39	36.76%
Tinnitus unchanged	33	30.50%	Tinnitus unchanged	57	53.80%
Tinnitus worsened	0	0.00%	Tinnitus worsened	1	0.94%

When comparing the data in the table, it can be determined that a significantly higher number of patients reported that the tinnitus was resolved or had improved in the group receiving real BEMER therapy (Group I) than in the placebo group. The results were evaluated using statistical analyses. The statistical significance of the difference in the distribution of the status change in the two patient groups was checked using the $\chi 2$ test showing a value of $p=0.001$. Based on that, it can be stated that the difference between the results of these two groups is statistically highly significant.

These statistical analyses therefore confirmed that the BEMER therapy significantly improved the results obtained using medicines only. Our study confirmed our previous clinical experiences that BEMER therapy can be successfully administered in patients with tinnitus.

BEMER Therapy Applied in Endocrinology

Dr. Balogh Imre, Debrecen, Dentofit 2000, professional manager

Classic endocrine syndromes (hormonal hypostimulation or hyperstimulation) cause changes in the internal balance of the body that are usually associated with visible bodily changes (weight gain, intense growth of body hair, bulging eyes and hair loss). It is the responsibility of the endocrinologist to restore the hormonal balance and, by doing so, to ameliorate and eliminate the patients' complaints. Among the treatments using physical agents, the BEMER device using lower energy pulsating electromagnetic radiation plays an increasing role (affecting motor disorders and vascular syndromes). The following section describes some less known BEMER effects observed in my endocrinology practice.

In addition to its effects that can be used in everyday medical practice, the BEMER therapy has some promising "hot points" as well, which allow for future therapeutic or preventive interventions. It is a common feature of the syndromes concerned that they can be considered "epidemics" as regards their incidence.

I. Hypothyroidism

The vast majority of hypothyroidism cases result from the underactivity of the thyroid gland. This may have two main causes: thyroxin and triiodinetironin deficiency developed as a result of autoimmune chronic thyroiditis (Hashimoto-thyroiditis) and the underactivity caused by the so-called ablative therapeutic interventions (surgery of the thyroid gland, radioactive iodine therapy).

This syndrome occurs mainly in women. Over 40, 5-10% of the women suffer from hypothyroidism.

The proportion of elderly women (above 65) suffering from hypothyroidism is 13%. The most common symptoms include fatigue, progressive weight gain, hair loss, negative mood and infertility and miscarriage in women of childbearing potential. As regards routine laboratory results, a major warning sign can be a high cholesterol level.

In establishing the diagnosis, TSH and FT4 values may be indicative. The anti- TPO antibody value, which is indicative of the inflammatory activity of the autoimmune thyroid process, may be used to determine whether it is an active or an inactive disease that is already "burnt out" from an immunological point of view.

BEMER therapy was used in an adjuvant setting in patients previously undergone hormone-replacement therapy, in whom certain complaints (mainly fatigue) still remained despite the permanent euthyreosis (normal TSH level). Naturally, the dose of the hormone treatment was not adjusted during, and for three months after, the BEMER therapy.

The quantitative evaluation of the results was performed using the Rand Vitality Questionnaire (higher scores indicate higher vitality). Our patients filled out this questionnaire before, immediately after and 3 month after the 1-month BEMER therapy. A large proportion of the patients (92%) reported a significant increase of vitality, and a decrease in, or elimination of, fatigue. In the control group (lying on BEMER mats but not receiving effective therapy) the vitality scores showed no or only a limited increase. The scores obtained in the questionnaires, repeatedly filled out three months after the treatment was completed, did not show a significant decrease compared to the results obtained immediately at the end of the treatment. Three months after the BEMER therapy was completed, the anti-TPO antibody, which shows a good correlation with the immune activity, decreased or remained at a level similar to that measured at baseline.

The evaluation of the results showed that in the patient group treated with BEMER therapy subjective fatigue significantly decreased, and the mood of the patients and therapy compliance (positive attitude towards the hormone treatment) improved. The decrease in the serum anti-TPO levels raises the issue whether the BEMER signal (as an immune-modulating physical agent) can be used in the autoimmune conditions of the thyroid.

However, the possibility of influencing immune processes requires further detailed investigations. The fact that during the treatment using a BEMER device TSH level showed no remarkable changes emphasizes the effects on small arteries, skeletal muscles and the immune system in addition to leaving the metabolism and hormonal status unchanged.

II. Post-partum thyroiditis (PPT)

Post-partum thyroiditis is a less known condition, which however, should be addressed due to its high incidence after birth (affecting 1 in every 15 mothers) and repeated occurrence (relapse).

Autoimmune thyroiditis usually cause transient underactivity of the thyroid ("tired-mother syndrome"); however, cases of transition to hypo-thyreosis requiring a lifelong treatment are not uncommon (25-50%).

Women with normal thyroid function before pregnancy, showing high anti-TPO titer, are at increased risk of developing this disease, just like women with type 1 diabetes. Women with a history of PPT are also predisposed to the recurrence of this disease after birth. The anti-TPO level lowering effect of the BEMER therapy, described above, suggested the possibility of administering this treatment in addition to selenium supplementation (the BEMER therapy may be safely administered during pregnancy). The development or recurrence of PPT was observed in none of our 7 patients (healthy women, but with high anti-TPO titer and with a history of PPT after an earlier pregnancy).

The administration of BEMER therapy in both primary and secondary prevention may play an important role in the reduction of the incidence of this disease. Follow-up studies of several years may clarify whether the BEMER therapy is capable of reducing the risk of transitioning to long-term underactivity in women who had already suffered from PPT.

III. Graves-Basedow Syndrome (GB) and associated endocrine orbitopathy (EOP)

As regards hyperthyroidism (overactive thyroid), Graves-Basedow syndrome with immunological origin is also an especially important and common disorder. When the immune system is abnormally overactive, specific antibodies are formed which force the thyroid cells to continuously produce hormones (TSHR -Ab or TRA K) at an enhanced rate and independently from feedback regulation.

However, autoimmune inflammation causes changes not only in the thyroid tissue, but also in the connective tissue and the eye muscles in the (so-called retro-bulbar) region behind the eyes.

The typical clinical image of the EOP, associated with the GB syndrome in 10- 30% of the cases, is created by the accumulation of substances (pro- inflammatory cytokines: TNF -α, IL -2 and IFN -γ) causing inflammation through local paracrine mechanisms: "bulbous" eyes, stabbing-pushing feeling and "foreign body" feeling in the eyes, lacrimation, photosensitivity and double vision.

The usefulness of BEMER therapy in this syndrome lies in the anti- inflammatory effect of the Bemer-signal that inhibits TNF-α (similarly to pentoxyphyllin used in the treatment of EOP). Therefore, the use of a BEMER device is expected to produce results only in the active, inflammatory phase of the disease. In mild cases of EOP (CAS<3) the efficacy of BEMER therapy is similar to that obtained with pentoxyphyllin infusion therapy. In addition to a significant amelioration of subjective complaints, the orbit MRI and DTPA-SPECT evaluations also confirmed the amelioration of the inflammatory activity affecting the orbit configuration.

In the treatment of the EOP BEMER therapy constitutes a very useful supplementary option to reduce the injuries caused by the autoimmune inflammation (secondary prevention).

IV. Diabetes mellitus (DM) and insulin resistance

Tissue insulin resistance plays a crucial role in the development of type 2 DM associated with the malfunctioning of insulin secreting β-cells. One of the main factors in the development of this disease is the so-called abdominal obesity, i.e. the accumulation of the abdominal fat tissue. One of the parameters that can be used to describe insulin resistance in clinical conditions is the HOMA- index (calculated using the values of plasma glucose and e.g. insulin determination).

During the BEMER therapy of five patients with known insulin resistance, but still not suffering from diabetes (i.e. pre-diabetes, a condition preceding diabetes) the HOMA-index significantly decreased after one month into the therapy, following which it usually returned to the pre-treatment level in some 60-90 days. A similar decrease of the HOMA-index was not observed in the control group. No significant difference was detected in the physical status of the patients, thus no substantial changes were observed regarding body weight and body fat determined using the DEXA method. Further analysis of this phenomenon may provide a theoretical option to influence the tissue insulin resistance which plays a determinant role in the development of type 2 DM.

V. Polycystic ovary syndrome or disease (PCOS or PCOD)

Based on the so-called "Rotterdam criteria" approved in 2003, the incidence of the PCOS is 26%, affecting, half a million (!) women in Hungary. The absence of ovulation renders family planning more difficult (menstruation disorders and fertility), while esthetic problems (enhanced hair growth, obesity etc.) cause grave psychological burden to the patients. Due to associated comorbidities (metabolic syndrome, DM, hypertension and cardiovascular diseases), morbidity and mortality rates are expected to show a substantial increase.

One of the characteristics of this disease is insulin resistance (similarly to type- 2 diabetes).

In our ambulatory care facility, BEMER therapy was administered to eight patients who showed no ovulation despite a metformin therapy of at least six- months. Upon the completion of the therapy, 3 patients showed ovulation cycles and one woman had a full-term pregnancy. Two of the five PCOS patients, who had undergone no treatment besides BEMER therapy, also had a successful pregnancy. The observations showed that BEMER therapy, based on a mechanism of action unknown so far, can be used as a therapeutic option to help women with PCOS to get pregnant.

VI. Erectile Dysfunction (impotence)

Erectile dysfunction can be caused by endocrinological (testosterone deficiency, high prolactin level), neurogenic (neuropathy caused by alcohol and diabetes or sclerosis multiplex), vascular (diabetes, atherosclerosis and hypertension), urological (congenital abnormalities and injuries), adverse reactions to drugs (blood lowering agents, drugs used in psychiatry) and psychological factors.

Being aware of the positive effects on blood vessels (small vessels and capillaries) of the BEMER therapy, it is not surprising that this therapy should have its place among the currently known therapeutic options. In combination with medicines and psychotherapy or as a stand-alone therapy, the physiological impact of the BEMER-signal shows substantial efficacy.

We used this therapy mainly in desperate patients who fell in the trap of therapeutic nihilism when surgical and hormonal therapy could not be used after proper urological and hormonal examination, and the standard phosphodiesterase-inhibitor drug therapy was not feasible (it was either medically contra-indicated or the patient refused the drug therapy).

BEMER therapy had positive results in 16 out of 19 patients (IIEF > 22 points). The results obtained at the end of the treatment were usually maintained by the patients for 3-4 months, after which the majority of them required a new cycle of BEMER therapy of at least 1 month.

VII. Osteoporosis (OP)

The number of patients with osteoporosis shows an increasing tendency worldwide (at least 1 million patients in Hungary). The cost of treatment represents a continuously increasing financial burden, also due to new therapeutic procedures (intermittent parathormone – teriparatid, monoclonal antibody against RAN KL – denosumab). In terms of its etiology, osteoporosis can be primary (post-menopausal and senile osteoporosis) or secondary (osteoporosis due to other diseases: hormonal, hematopoietic disorders and adverse effects). In addition to the estrogen deficiency, the accumulation of cytokines with local actions (TNF α, interleukines, RANK ligands) also plays a role in postmenopausal osteoporosis. Senile osteoporosis is mainly associated with the decrease in the activity of the osteoblasts, as well as calcium and vitamin D deficiency.

In addition to the excellent pain relief activity (fractures) of the BEMER therapy in the everyday practice, due to the inhibition of TNF α and increase of the osteoblast activity, which theoretically can be used, this therapy can become an important supplementary therapeutic option. In patients treated with a widely used, so-called antiresorptive (bisphosphonate) therapy and BEMER therapeutic system, the increase in the bone density is slightly above that measured in the control group; however, another measure of the efficiency of the therapy is the decrease in the fracture risk currently cannot yet be evaluated because of the short follow-up period. In case of vertebral fractures, the pain relief effect was markedly higher compared with the control group.

In addition to this therapy, we should find a place for the BEMER therapy in the prevention of the osteoporosis together with calcium and vitamin D supplementation, and appropriate physical exercises. Groups at particularly high risk should be identified (positive family history, durable physical exercises, conditions associated with sex hormone deficiency and long-term drug treatment: corticosteroids, heparin and warfarin). In these groups, long-term BEMER therapy may reduce the incidence of diseases associated with substantial burden to both the individual and society.

BEMER Therapy Applied in Internal Medicine

Influence of the Pulsed BEMER Magnetic Field on the Biopolymers Produced by the Pseudomonas Aeruginosa Bacterium

Kesserü P, Kiss I; Institute for Biotechnology at the Zoltán Bay Foundation for Applied Research Budapest

SUMMARY: *The extremely low-frequency BEMER magnetic field is capable of exerting a physical effect and breaking down the structure of generated biopolymers without affecting the quantity and viability of the bacteria responsible for the synthesis. The effect which destroys the investigated structure is not permanent.*

[SUMMARY from the February 01, 2010 Lecture at Budapest Congress 03.26.2011: In further in vitro tests, we demonstrated that the weak BEMER electromagnetic field is not able to modify the sensitivity of the investigated pseudomonas aeruginosa bacteria to Ciprofloxacin antibiotics. The biopolymer investigation, however, showed that the applied electromagnetic field improved the antibiotic's access to the target cells significantly by breaking up the biopolymer structure.]

Introduction
Cystic fibrosis (CF, mucoviscidosis) is a recessively inherited autosomal disease and is one of the most common congenital metabolic diseases. Its frequency is different in different populations. In the Caucasian (white) population, it occurs with a frequency of 1:3.000. In Hungary, one in 25 people carries at least one copy of the defective allele.

Molecular background
In cystic fibrosis, the TfR gene mutates. The CFTR gene is one of the largest genes in the human genome for which more than 500 mutations have now been described. The CFTR gene is located in region 31.1-31.2 of the longer arm on chromosome 7. The most common mutation is the loss of the phenyl aniline at position 508.

The product of the CFTR genes is the regulator protein for transmembrane conductance of the cystic fibrosis, located in the epithelia of the drainage channels of the glands. In a healthy organism, it supports production of sweat, various digestion enzymes and mucus. The disease can occur at different level of severity and coincides with thickening of the secretions for all endocrine and holocrine glands. Under normal conditions and following the applicable signal (in healthy function) at the drain protein of the CFTR, chloride ions then sodium ions and water flow into the lumen of the glands, thereby adjusting the normal viscosity of the glandular secretion. As a result of the mutation, however, the protein does not occur or occurs defectively, so that it cannot perform this function. Water and ions are not transported into the lumen and, as a result, the secretion thickens, its viscosity increases, and the viscous mucus for a rich breeding ground for a large range of bacterial secondary infections.

Clinical symptoms of cystic fibrosis
The defective function of the CFTR protein can be observed most clearly in the following organs:
- In the pancreas: The lack of this gland causes digestion problems.
- In the epididymis: Blocking of the canals of the epididymis means that 95% of male patients are sterile.

- The thickened mucus blocks the exit drains of the holocrine glands and is reflected in the change in mucus production.
- In babies, mecinium ileus, i.e. obstruction as a result of thickening of the intestinal contents, indicates the presence of the disease.
- The symptoms occur in diseased children gradually, depending on the severity of the cystic fibrosis.
- Body height and weight remain underdeveloped.
- Protein deficiency
- Deficiency symptoms for fat-soluble vitamins (E, D, K, A)
- Hammer toes
- Typical attendant phenomenon: inflammatory changes in almost all glands
- In the respiratory system: chronic and sudden attacks of coughing, returning and chronic pneumonia. Breathing difficulties, depositing of viscous secretion in the airways so that insufficient oxygen is supplied to the lung and it gradually dies.

The most serious difficulties in the lung are caused primarily by colonization of the bacteria that typically occur in the airways. Such bacteria include various klebsiella strains, staphylococcus aureus, haemophilus influanzeae and pseudomonas aeruginosa. A total of 80% to 95% of cystic fibrosis patients die from bacterial infections originating in respiratory passages at the age of between 20 and 30. In 67% of the cases, the pseudomonas aeruginosa bacterium is responsible for the pathological inflammation of the lung tissue or the degeneration of the cell structure. Pseudomonas aeruginosa is a gram-negative bacterium that can be identified in almost all environmental samples. It is an extremely adaptable bacterium with a broad range of tolerance which causes patients as well as clinical practitioners a lot of problems because of its polyresistance to antibiotics. It has a very large number of pathogenesis factors, including endotoxins, proteases and pyocyanin, as well as mucus biopolymers as secondary metabolism products, with the aid of which the bacterium can colonize over the long term on the applicable carriers or even in the alveoli of the lungs. Under this mechanical protective cover, the bacterium is even harder to reach for a range of antibiotics than in free cell form.

The symptomatic treatment of cystic fibrosis is extremely complex because the problem affects the entire organism. Treatment is frequently limited to longer or shorter retention of quality of life. On the other hand, long-term healing and treatment of chronic and recurring illnesses in the respiratory system is of vital importance to patients suffering from this disease. Both chemotherapeutic (antibiotics etc.) and physiotherapeutic procedures are known for the treatment of the catarrh condition caused by the inflammatory processes in response to the bacterium and the viscous mucus that is collected in the respiratory system.

In addition to oral use of Fluimucil, ACC, salt solution in various concentrations (0.9, 2, 3, 4%), Mucopront and Paxirasol, inhalation of "Salvus" branded spa water is also a common means of clearing the thickened mucus. Tobramicin (as an inhalable aerosol) and Ciprofloxacin (oral or intravenous) are used most frequently as antibiotic therapy to repress the pseudomonas aeruginosa bacterium spreading in the alveoli of the lungs and responsible for the inflammatory processes. There are also now inhalation preparations available that prevent or alleviate inflammatory processes via steroid ingredients (Pulmicort) or Pulmozyme with recombinant DNAse, which is able to reduce the population of bacteria that has already died in the mucus of the lungs and causes further thickening. In the USA, inhalation preparations with mixed components are used successfully both to dissolve the mucus and to kill off existing bacteria (preparation with Tobramicin, concentrated NaCl and recombinant DNAse). Bronchodilating medicans (Berodual, Berotec, Salbutamol, Ventolin, Spiropent, Bricanyl) also have a role in treating cystic fibrosis to guide mucus-dissolving and inhaled antibiotics better to their target.

Physiotherapy, breathing technique or sale pipe cure, which contribute to clearing the mucus collected in the lungs, are an essential part of pulmotherapy after mucus has been successfully dissolved.

Physiotherapy methods and procedures have also been established to support highly viscous or already mobilized, less viscous lung fluid.

High-frequency chest wall oscillation (HFCWO)
Devices used to oscillate the chest wall at high frequency (HFCWO: High Frequency Chest Wall Oscillation) are primarily used in the USA. The chest wall is set in motion with variable force and frequency using a compressor. The advantage is that the device is simple for patients to use and set up and contributes to distributing aerosol preparations. It must be assumed that more effective coughing is the result of interaction between the mucus and the airflow and/or the result of reduction in the adhesion of the mucus. Compared to traditional chest wall physiotherapy, this method has been shown to be useful and effective and, in terms of clearing mucus, even more efficient. The Hayek Oscillator is a variant of the HFCWO, which is not however as efficient in terms of clearing mucus.

The disadvantages include the relatively high price, even for Americans (at USD 16,780) and the necessity of permanent installation.

Intrapulmonary percussive ventilation (IPV)
IPV is a device that also contributes to mobilizing the mucus. It generates oscillation as does the HFCWO. However, it does not function via the chest wall, but orally using a ventilator with compressor. The air quantity as well as the pulsation frequency can be adjusted and there are also versions with continuous vibration (both when breathing in and out) and vibration only when breathing in (the latter allows for passive breathing out). The efficiency in terms of mucus removal has been demonstrated in multiple investigations. In tests, the efficiency of two chest wall oscillators and two oral devices was compared in terms of mucus removal and oxygen saturation and no significant differences were identified. These devices are generally expensive. However, as treatment can be performed autonomously, they are cost efficient.

Flexible chest compression strap
Straps with Velcro fasteners that hold the chest down after a long exhaled breath are common and therefore also available in Hungary. The strap does hinder expansion of the chest when breathing in, but is flexible enough to allow inhalation, and it contributes significantly to breathing out.

In Hungary (with approx. 10 million inhabitants at present), there are currently 540 registered patients known to have cystic fibrosis, including both adult and child patients. However, the number of persons actually affected is higher. In the USA, there are more than 30.000 patients with cystic fibrosis.

In the future health policy of the EU, support for the treatment of rare diseases will play a role. However, it is essential that countries that require financial support identify the exact number of persons affected.

Research task and objective
In our investigations, we considered the question of whether extremely weak electromagnetic fields generated by the BEMER signal plus electromagnetic therapy device, made by Innomed AG, are capable of exerting physical effects on the structure of the biopolymers produced by the pseudomonas aeruginosa that regularly cause problems in cystic fibrosis. The positive physiological effects of the use of the BEMER therapy system are generally known and demonstrated. However, there is no or at least no publicly available data regarding how the generated magnetic field affects bacterial systems. The treatment may facilitate clearance of lung mucus and the bacteria protected by the polymer may be

more susceptible to selected antibiotics if the special BEMER signal breaks down the structure of the biopolymer.

Materials and methods

Bacteria used Pseudomonas aeruginosa bacteria from the environment (not of clinical origin) were used in the experiments. Previous work had established that, in suitable nutrient solution, these bacteria are capable of producing viscous and elastic biopolymers.

Biopolymer production

The nutrient solution for polymer production was inoculated with a pseudomonas aeruginosa bacterial culture enriched for 24 hours in rich nutrient solution. These systems were then treated in incubators at 37°C for 72, 48 and 24 hours to allow the applicable polymer to be synthesized. During the experiments, 95 ml of biopolymers were created for each case.

Rheological measurements

The change in the flow characteristics of the untreated polymer samples and the samples treated with the magnetic field was determined using a programmable Brookfield DV-II rotation viscometer. During measurement, the rotor is submerged into the sample on the sampling cup and rotated by the unit via a calibrated spring. The viscous resistance of the fluid against the rotor can be measured from the movement of the spring. The spring movements are measured by a rotary transducer.

The flow diagram of the fluid can be obtained from the measurement and the value of the apparent viscosity can be calculated from the flow curve. This measure of calculation is outlined in Figure 1. The polymer generated by the bacteria has no homogeneous structure, but behaves like a highly viscous gel or a fluid, depending on the concentration. Qualitative evaluation of the rheological measurement curves is only possible in such cases by taking into account all the individual measurement points, as the quality and viscosity of the biopolymer changes almost constantly.
The quotient of the measurement results is formed when determining the apparent viscosity. The apparent viscosity for the individual measurement point is given by the quotient from the rotary velocity of the measurement head (shear rate) and the shear stress defined by the measurement device and associated with this speed.

During measurement, a sample of 2x16 ml was taken from each biopolymer solution from the lower phase (the lower range in the polymer), as shown in Figure 2. The first sample (16 ml) was used as an untreated control for the applicable system, where the second sample (16 ml) was taken immediately after magnetic field treatment (as verum). The flow characteristics were then determined.

The rheological measurements were performed at 37 °C, the temperature of polymer production.

Effect of the magnetic field

The intensive application (IA) unit of the BEMER signal plus device was used to apply the magnetic field. The magnetic field strength was applied at 100 µT (level 10, 8 minutes), 50 µT (level 5, 8 minutes) and with continuous transition of 60-100 µT (P4, 20 minutes). For some of the treatments with magnetic field, the glass wall of the container (0.1-0.2 cm thick) was the only physical distance between the IA and the biopolymer to be treated. In the other cases, the IA was placed at a distance of 5 cm from the biopolymer.

In the first series of tests, the biopolymer was treated a total of 6 times after inoculation with the bacterium (100 µT, level 10, 8 minutes, distance: 0.1-0.2 cm), 3 times daily, with 3 hours between applications. After the 6th treatment, the rheological characteristics of the biopolymer over the 48 hours were investigated, then treatment was repeated as described and the flow characteristics of the biopolymer were determined again after the second round of treatment. The biopolymer used as control for the experiment was left untreated for 48 hours (without applied magnetic field) and, after the incubation period of 48 hours, a sample was taken and the flow characteristics were determined. The control biopolymer was then subject to magnetic field treatment identical to the treatment applied to the verum system and the rheological curve of this biopolymer was then also determined.

In the subsequent experiments, the biopolymers of different ages (24, 48 and 72 hours) were only treated once with magnetic field and the rheological curve was immediately recorded in the samples taken therefore (treated sample).

The sample taken from the biopolymer solutions prior to treatment was used as control measurement. All measurements and magnetic field treatments were performed in multiple, entirely independent systems. The number of systems is given in the presentation of the test results.

Results
Investigations of the inhomogeneity of the biopolymer and description of the aspects of evaluation
The composition of the biopolymer is inhomogeneous as a result of its biological origin. In the upper range of the nutrient solution, an almost gel-like viscous material is synthesized at high oxygen concentrations, whereas the polymer structure becomes increasingly weak (viscous fluid) in the direction of the lower oxygen partial pressures.

Fortunately, the determined values for the apparent viscosity in sample 1 (hereafter referred to as the untreated control sample) do not deviate significantly from sample 2 (the latter sample is hereafter referred to as the treated sample, as these samples did undergo magnetic field treatment after the control values were measured). The data from the two sequential measurements can therefore be compared with regard to whether the magnetic field had or did not have an effect that weakened the structure. It is important to take into account the inhomogeneity of the biopolymers when evaluating the measurement results, as, in many cases, the values for the apparent viscosity of the verum samples were almost identical to or exceeded the values for the untreated control sample after treatment (see Figures 18.25.31.79.80. in the Appendix). The physical effects of the magnetic field rule out the possibility that it may contribute in any way to strengthening the biopolymer structure, so that the greater structural strengths measured in the samples after treatment are clearly the result of the inhomogeneity of the biopolymer. This thesis is also support by the phenomenon shown in Figure 4, i.e. that the biopolymer has only become more homogeneous during continuous treatment, but its structure has not been strengthened.

The samples already had higher viscosities in sample 3, so that it could easily have been the case that fractions from the upper biopolymer with stronger structure entered into sample 2 (the sample taken after magnetic field treatment). Cases in which the structure of the biopolymer samples was stronger after treatment than the control samples before treatment were evaluated in this case in the same way as if the magnetic field treatment had been without effect, so that the adjective "unchanged" has been applied in these cases.

The structure-destroying effect of the magnetic field can be clearly observed from most rheological curves (e.g. Figures 4, 7 in the Appendix). In these cases it was also possible to determine that the biopolymer structure has become thinner after treatment without stating the apparent viscosity value. However, the situation was not this unambiguous in all cases (e.g. Figures 23, 27). Deviations between the untreated control sample and the treated samples only occurred at higher shear rate values for the flow curves reproduced in Figure 23 of the Appendix and the calculated apparent viscosity values. We also assessed the effect of the magnetic field as positive in these cases, as it reduced the structural stability of the biopolymer to a definite extent, though not drastically – the treated sample could withstand greater mechanical stress (at higher shear rate values the measurement cylinder of the rheometer rotates faster in the sample), the sample less stress.

The fact that the rheological curve for the untreated samples shows that the shear stress value suddenly falls as the shear rate increases and then rises again or remains the same can be explained by the exceptionally strong structure of the biopolymer. In such cases (the effect is also described as a slip effect), the investigated material – in this case the biopolymer – is simply coiled around the rod of the measuring head and thereby moves in a significant quantity out of the measurement volume (the cylindrical volume between the cylinder of the sample holder and the measuring head). As the material thereby no longer affects the rotating body in full quantity, the measurement device returns a weaker signal in these cases, as if the structure suddenly became weaker. This phenomenon, therefore, is typically of strongly structured viscous fluids that still retain elastic properties.

In materials with similar substances, it is also typical at which shear rate values this slip effect begins to occur. If the structure is weakened, this effect does not occur or start only at explicitly higher shear rate values. In samples in which this effect was significant before treatment with magnetic field and the slip effect was not identified or only identified at higher shear rate values after treatment, the effect of the magnetic field was assessed as positive, i.e. as destroying the structure.

Advance test
Advance tests were performed to investigate whether the biopolymer synthesis of the pseudomonas aeruginosa bacteria can be prevented by regular application of the BEMER magnetic field.
Change in the flow curves of biopolymers after 48 hours following 100 µT

The viscoelastic biopolymer

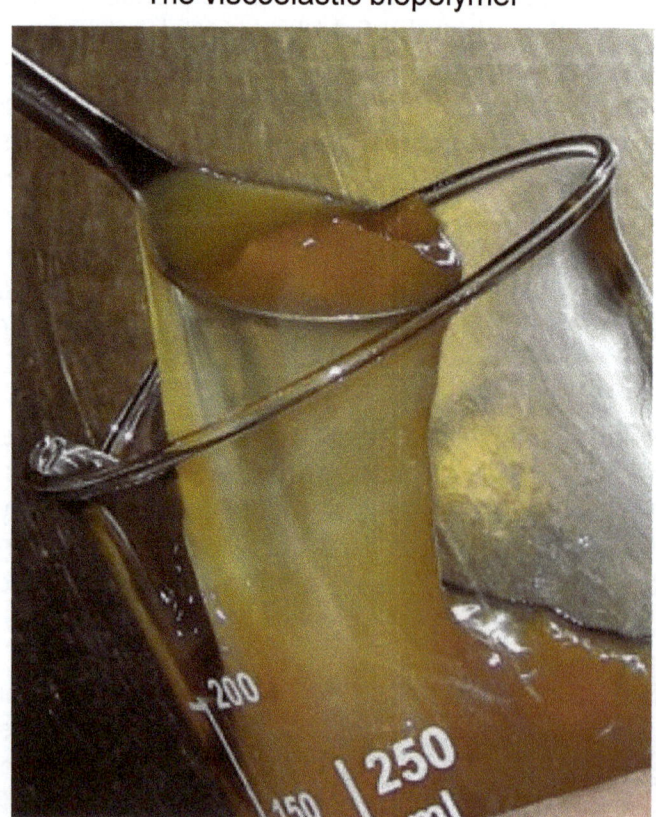

Effect of 60 to 100 µT on biopolymers 24 to 48 hours old with direct treatment and at a distance of 5 cm

The BEMER signal plus therapy device programs also make it possible to select a treatment in which the field strength of the magnetic field continuously increases. Program P4 is typically recommended to treat deep-lying problem areas. This program provides a magnetic field continuously increasing from 60 to 100 µT over 20 minutes when using the IA.

It was therefore relevant to investigate the influence of the longer-lasting magnetic field with varying field strength of biopolymers 24 hours old in the case of direct magnetic field treatment.

Table 5: Qualitative change in 24-hour-old biopolymers in response to magnetic field influence of 60-100 µT from immediate proximity

Biopolymer structure	Number of samples (units)	Percentage distribution (%)
Weakened	6	35.3
Unchanged	11	64.7
Total	17	100

The results in Table 5 demonstrate an unexpected effect. Up until this point, the magnetic field therapy was never as ineffective in any single case. In only 35.3% of the investigated samples (17 units) was it possible to demonstrate unambiguously that the biopolymer structure was weakened after treatment.

However, during treatment it was observed that the top phase of the biopolymer frothed up during treatment and that the almost cartilage-like solid gel structure explicitly typical on the top layer of the biopolymer disintegrated. This effect certainly influenced the measurement/effectiveness.

Biopolymers with stronger structure (48 hours old) were then investigated using the same treatment program and the source of the magnetic field was also placed 5 cm away from the biopolymer.

This demonstrates what is for practical purposes the highest possible positive result, whereby it has been possible unambiguously in all investigated systems (9 units) to weaken the structure of the biopolymers using the continuously rising pulsed magnetic field.

Similarly in this case, it was observed that the systems frothed up and therefore the structure of the top, gel-like viscous biopolymer fraction was destroyed and that it was partially mixed with lower phases.

SUMMARY: On the basis of the evaluation of the presented results of the experiment, the following findings have been made in connection with the effect of the BEMER signal magnetic field on the structure of the biopolymer produced by the pseudomonas aeruginosa bacterium:

- The extremely low-frequency BEMER magnetic field is capable of exerting a physical effect and breaking down the structure of generated biopolymers without affecting the quantity and viability of the bacteria responsible for the synthesis. The effect which destroys the investigated structure is not permanent. The biopolymer strands are able to re-organize themselves and thereby develop a more homogeneous biopolymer structure. At the current stage of research, it remains unexplained whether this process would also occur if there were no living bacteria left in the system and only the chemical processes between the macromolecules could occur.

- Deviating results were obtained with regard to the destructive effect of the magnetic fields of varying strength. The positive effect, in our opinion, was less dependent on the strength of the magnetic field and the distance at which treatment was applied than on the quality of the treated biopolymer, which modified autonomously in systems of similar age owing to its biological origin.

- The quality therefore proved decisive with regard to the modifiability of the biopolymers. No results could be obtained for highly structured materials (72 hours old). However, the measurement results indicate that the magnetic field was not sufficiently effective when working with biopolymers that were "too thin" (there were a number of such cases among biopolymers 24 hours old). Irrespective of the type of magnetic field treatment, the best results were achieved in 48-hour-old biopolymers.

- Weakening of the structure of the markedly gel-like parts was observed over the course of 20 minutes of magnetic field treatment at several field strengths. In 24-hours-old samples (after magnetic field treatment), this reduced the inhomogeneity otherwise typical of the system and reduced the mixture of the biopolymer on sampling, which in turn lead to seemingly low effectiveness. The phenomenon was observed again during similar treatment of 48-hour-old samples, but did not cause similar problems.

- A total of 135 biopolymers were treated with the BEMER magnetic field in the series of experiments. Irrespective of the type and nature of treatment, the biopolymer structure was weakened by the magnetic field in a total of 62.9% of the samples.

On the basis of the presented results, the BEMER therapy may exert a positive effect for targeted treatment of patients suffering from cystic fibrosis in the form of short-term reduction of the viscosity of lung fluid, that may contribute the clearing the fluid. The weakening and subsequent potential re-ordering of the biopolymer structure may also make the bacteria responsible for polymer production accessible and therefore susceptible to antibiotics. However, this conclusion needs to be verified by further investigation.

BEMER Therapy Applied in Pain Therapy

Experiences Regarding the Effectiveness of Electromagnetic Treatment for Various Rheumatological Diseases

Rheumatology: Lecture at Budapest Congress 03.27.2011

Dr. Gomez Roberto, Dr. Izabella Gomez

SUMMARY: The VAS and WOMAC summary score results from patients with osteoarthritis of the knee demonstrate the effectiveness of the therapy. The VAS and ROM results from patients with shoulder inflammation and regression of bursitis are also evidence of the anti-inflammatory effect of the therapy. Researchers have been studying the effect of pulsed electromagnetic fields on living organisms for a long time. Technical development has recently made it possible to obtain greater insight into their mechanism of action. Numerous reports on this subject have been published, but the results provided are not unambiguous and are disputable.

In Hungary, treatment with magnetic energy is a recognized and frequently applied therapeutic procedure. It is being increasingly applied at more points and with extended indication. Diseases of the musculoskeletal system with inflammation are among the best known and most important indications for the treatment.

We here report our findings with magnetic therapy in three disease groups: osteoarthritis of the knee, adhesive capsulitis of the shoulder associated with diabetes mellitus and bursitis. Before starting pulsed magnetic treatment and in the course of treatment, the patients were not permitted to take anti-inflammatory medication or other anti-inflammatory physiotherapy treatment. The VAS and WOMAC summary score results from patients with osteoarthritis of the knee demonstrate the effectiveness of the therapy. The VAS and ROM results from patients with shoulder inflammation and regression of bursitis are also evidence of the anti-inflammatory effect of the therapy.

Authors: Dr. Roberto Gomez, Dr. Izabella Gome.

Pain Relief with BEMER Treatment in Neurology

Polyneuropathy Lecture at Budapest Congress 03/27/2011

Dr. Eva Csecsei - Neurologist, Psychiatrist, Practice Medical Director, Budapest, Lipötväros City Center Health Service

SUMMARY: The BEMER pain therapy, adjuvant drug therapy and psychotherapy together make it possible to alleviate and/or end pain.

Pain is one of the most common complaints patients bring to their doctors. Every third person on Earth experiences some form of recurring or persistent pain. In Hungary, the large proportion of patients affected by this problem is well shown by the fact that, for example, the life-time prevalence of lower back pain is 60-70%, that is, about 1,000,000 patients. The number of patients with migraine and tension headache is similar. Alleviation and removal of chronic pain is the major challenge for pain therapy, alongside alleviation of acute pain and mitigation of pain after operations.

Among the different types of pain, the least comprehensible pain in patients is pain caused by primary damage to the nervous system. We have processed 6 years' material from using the BEMER therapy at our neurological practice in the center of Budapest and have organized the experience we have gained from treating pain in our own protocol answered for 165 patients. In addition to experience of BEMER treatment with 43 different patients with peripheral neuropathic pain (painful polyneuropathy, postherpetic neuralgia and trigeminal neuralgia), we also report findings from therapy for 24 patients treated for pain in the central nervous system (migraines, multiple sclerosis and post stroke pain), as well as improvement and healing in 82 of our patients treated for sacroiliac pain of varying etiology. The picture is rounded off by pain associated with several rare diseases and various traumas to the central nervous system.

In pain relief, the potential effects of the BEMER therapy on pain are as follows:
- dilates blood vessels and improves blood supply by stimulating the nitrogen-monoxide system in the body,
- improves microcirculation in damaged tissues and facilitates the excretion of acids and metabolic waste products,
- transports more macrophages, lymphocytes and antibodies to the pain center,
- reduces swelling and facilitates the optimal regeneration of damaged tissues by activating the anti-inflammatory enzymes,
- helps cells to have access to more oxygen by improving microcirculation.

Among the different types of pain, neuropathic pain induced by the primary damage of the nervous system causes the most senseless suffering to our patients. We have processed the data collected over 6 years using the BEMER therapy in our neurology practice in the centre of Budapest. These data were processed retrospectively. In our presentation, we systematized the experiences collected in 165 patients during the treatment of pain according to the protocol configured by us. 85% of the patients suffered of different pain which cannot be sufficiently relieved by drug therapy. Our patients were administered BEMER therapy for sessions of 25-30 minutes, which were financed by the NHF at the neurology outpatient department and could be settled as "magnetotherapy". These sessions were administered over a period of 2.5 weeks. Treatment was administered using BEMER mat applicator P1 + BEMER 3000 MFA (Multifunctional Applicator) or pillow applicator P4.

We used the Bemer 3000 Signal Plus devices.

Mean age of the patients was 43 years (22-80 years); the proportion of men and women was 32% and 68%, respectively.

In addition to the experiences of 43 patients with different peripheral neuropathic pain (painful polyneuropathy, postherpetic neuralgia, trigeminus neuralgia), we also present the results obtained in 24 patients treated for neurogenic pain of the central nervous system (migraine, SM and post-stroke pain), as well as the improvement and treatment of 82 patients treated for lower back pain of different etiology.

Most laymen and, unfortunately, most physicians believe that pain always has a physical origin and frequently request and perform many unnecessary tests to find a logical explanation. The dominant view is "There has to be something" which leads to erroneous diagnoses and unnecessary drug treatments. The experience of pain and reaction to pain largely depend on the current psychological and physical state, education and pain-related beliefs of the patient.

Excluding the above, as a "simple operator" we cannot achieve long-term results in the treatment of patients suffering from pain. It can be established that in the treatment of pain caused by neurogenic neuropathies, somatization disorders and depression, well-known analgesics (aspirin, NSAIDs and paracetamol) are insufficient, and sometimes severe adverse reactions or drug addictions can occur.

In 30-45% of the patients suffering from pain an improvement is observed after they were given placebo. The treating physician proceeds correctly if he or she tries to make use of the placebo effect and takes into account the recommendations of evidence-based medicine. The most efficient placebo is the competence and reassuring and positive radiance of a good physician.

The "nocebo effect" (the effect of an incompetent, anxious, flustered and frustrated physician) can render ineffective the best agents and methods with confirmed efficacy in the treatment of pain. About 10-15% of the patients have such an encounter. The same can happen when an incompetent colleague disqualifies a well initiated BEMER therapy administered for pain relief purposes, and hinders or completely interrupts the treatment.

Pain cannot be objectively measured; however, we try to quantify it using different scales. The intensity of pain may be measured using verbal, numerical or visual scales. On such a visual scale (VAS), we observed a decrease in the mean scores of 61% after 2 to 5 weeks of treatment using a BEMER device.

In addition, our patients reported the improvement of the motor performance (25%), elimination of somatic complaints (5%), psychological complaints and the elimination of the associated depression (32%) and a significant improvement in the quality of life (75%).

This therapy resolved tissue damages, trauma-related complaints and pain in 100% of the cases (2 patients with spine trauma). Acute pain should be promptly and effectively reduced. 3 patients with acute lumbago were locally treated with the BEMER therapy 5-7 times a day. After 2 days, the patients reported a reduction in pain of 60% which allowed for further corrective- gymnastic therapy and supplementary physical therapy.

Pain is a complex phenomenon. Depression, emotional liability and adoption of the "patient role" frequently associated with chronic pain disorder require a complex treatment plan.

The combination of the BEMER pain therapy, the adjuvant pharmacotherapy and psychotherapy allows the reduction and/or relief of the pain.

Utilizing the BEMER Therapy in Neurosurgical Diseases

Neurosurgery at Budapest Congress 03.27.2011

Dr. Zoltän Nemeti, Specialist for Neurosurgery, BEMER specialist advisor (Kenezy Hospital, Department for Accident and Hand Surgery, Neurosurgery)

SUMMARY: I became acquainted with the options offered by BEMER by integrating this type of treatment into my work. I now assess the possible benefits of its application for each patient and am therefore able to provide more and more patients with operation-free improvement and more effective healing after injury.

The majority of diseases in the central nervous system are not surgical diseases. A proportion of cases that fall under neurosurgery require an operation, depending on type, and the timing also varies within wide limits. For example, 70-80% of slipped discs are not operated on or an operation can be put off for years, whereas traumatic bleeding hemorrhaging in the skull requires operation immediately. Non-surgical healing methods and complex rehabilitation are most applicable before and after intervention or instead of intervention.

Patients and methods: During my work, I mainly encountered patients to whom I was not able to recommended neurosurgical intervention or for whom before or after operation there was no suitable, effective medication or methods, or the degree of residual symptoms and complaints made a return of the patient to a normal way of life impossible. I therefore began to engage with the BEMER magnetic therapy to my own great satisfaction and that of my patients.

Over 3 years more than 200 patients (232) received BEMER therapy. At total of 50% had neck and lumbar spine disease and 10% of those underwent an operation either as primary treatment or subsequently because conservative treatment had been unsuccessful. Those suffering injury after accidents (14%) and patients with nervous system complications following an illness (12%) made up a significant group. Some patients had lost their faith in traditional medical treatment entirely. They had experienced no improvement from such medicine for a long time and they believed their chances of recovery were hopeless. I can inform you, with great pride, that we saw improvement in quality of life even in these cases by using BEMER. These examples form part of this lecture. We will also present a number of cases where we did not achieve any objective success (8%). Results: Proper medical examination and necessary care were not neglected in any of the cases. The recommended magnetic therapy treatment was applied autonomously or as part of complex treatment. We based the degree of change in symptoms and complaints on our own opinion and the opinion of the patients, as well as by tracking objective symptoms, and we documented change using the popular Visual Analog Scale, i.e. VAS values, which measures the degree of initial pain, symptoms and the improvement achieved on a 10-point scale.

For practical reasons, we have established 4 success groups. At the start of treatment, the VAS value was higher than 7 in each case. The proportion of symptom-free/healed patients reached 40%. A total of 36% reported residual complaints regarding their future life of a significant extent after treatment. The symptoms in 16% of cases fell by at least half, which meant, inter alia, a reduction in necessary medication, better treatability, more lasting strength and less sickness benefits for our patients. In 10 cases (8%), we did not achieve any improvement. The medical history in these cases was mainly sacroiliac arthritis, spondylolisthesis or multiple serious spine operations, where magnetic therapy would not be expected to reduce the serious mechanical damage. We observed an interesting effect in 2 cases. After myocarditis had reduced in response to the treatment, tachycardia became apparent. In another patient, itchy rashes appeared over the entire body, so that the otherwise effective treatment had to be stopped.

Conclusion: I became acquainted with the options offered by BEMER by integrating this type of treatment into my work. I now assess the possible benefits of its application for each patient and am therefore able to provide more and more patients with operation-free improvement and more effective healing after injury.

Effect of BEMER Magnetic Field Therapy on the Level of Fatigue in Patients with Multiple Sclerosis: A Randomized, Placebo-Controlled Double-Blind Study

Piatkowski J; Kern S.; Ziemssen T; J alternative and complementary medicine; Vol15; 5; 2009; 507-511

SUMMARY: In this pilot study, we were able to demonstrate a beneficial effect of the BEMER therapy on MS fatigue. Although we recognized a placebo effect, there was a statistically significant benefit for treated patients after 12 weeks. From our personal experience, MS patients suffering from MS fatigue can benefit from electromagnetic field therapy.

The Journal of Alternative and Complementary Medicine, Volume 15, Number 5, 2009, pp. 507–511[a]
Mary Ann Liebert, Inc. DOI: 10.1 089=acm.2008.0501

Abstract

Objectives: Electromagnetic field therapy has been reported to be beneficial in patients with multiple sclerosis (MS) with significant fatigue. This study was designed to evaluate the long-term effects of Bio-Electro-Magnetic - Energy- Regulation (BEMER) on MS-related fatigue.

Design: This was a monocenter, patient- and rater-blinded, placebo-controlled trial.

Patients: There were 37 relapsing-remitting patients with MS with significant fatigue in the study. Interventions: The intervention consisted of BEMER magnetic field treatment for 8 minutes twice daily in comparison to placebo for 12 weeks.

Outcome measures: The primary outcome criterion was change in the Modified Fatigue Impact Scale (MFIS) between baseline and 12weeks. The secondary outcome criteria were changes of the Fatigue Severity Scale (FSS), a depression scale (ADS-L), Multiple Sclerosis Functional Scale (MSFC), and the Expanded Disability Status Scale (EDSS).

Results: There was evidence of a significant difference of MFIS value (primary outcome criterion) after 12 weeks in favor of the verum group (26.84 versus 36.67; $p = 0.024$). In addition, FSS values were significantly lower in the verum group after 12 weeks (3.5 versus 4.7; $p = 0.016$). After 6-week follow-up, the verum and the placebo groups did not differ in experienced fatigue (MFIS, FSS). Regarding the subscales of the MFIS, there was a significant decrease in physical ($p=0.018$) and cognitive ($p = 0.041$), but not in psychologic subscales only in the verum group regarding the timepoints baseline and 12 weeks. BEMER therapy was well tolerated.

Discussion: In this pilot study, we were able to demonstrate a beneficial effect of BEMER intervention on MS fatigue. As this was only a pilot study, trials with more patients and longer duration are mandatory to describe long-term effects.

Introduction

FATIGUE is among the most common symptoms of multiple sclerosis (MS), affecting at least 75% of patients [1], for many of whom it constitutes one of the worst and most dis- tressing features [2]. Fatigue is reported in all clinical pheno- types of MS and affects patients of all ages [3]. This symptom is an integral part of the disease process that is usually present at the time of diagnosis and in some cases represents one of the reasons for which patients originally consult a neurologist. Fatigue is not closely related to physical signs of disability or with magnetic resonance imaging markers of disease activity,although it does seem to increase when the patient experiences relapses [2, 4]. Fatigue is a major cause of unemployment in patients with MS.s..7 The etiology and pathophysiology of MS-related fatigue remain unknown. Studies have failed to demonstrate an association between MS-related fatigue and the level of disability, clinical disease subtype, or gender.8 Imaging studies using positron emission tomography suggest that fatigue in MS is related to hypometabolism of specific brain areas, including the frontal and subcortical circuits.9 Different components of fatigue have been described such as motor and cognitive fatigue and lassitude. Management strategies include medications, exercise, and behavioral therapy [10]. There have been reports on the positive effects of immunomodulatory drugs on fatigue [11]. However, the efficacy of the treatment remains quite disappointing [10]. In addition to pharmacological interventions, non- pharmacological treatments including yoga, aerobic exer-cises, cooling therapy, and energy conservation techniques have been used successfully. A recent meta-analysis summarized promising data on electromagnetic field devices [12] Richards et al. and Lappin et al. demonstrated a positive effect of low-level pulsed, electromagnetic field devices worn by the patients [13, 14]. Unfortunately, there were no long-term data available. Although Mostert and Kesselring showed disappointing data on pulsed magnetic field therapy as an additional effect of a multimodal neurological rehabilitation program on fatigue [15], Sandyk documented improved physical and cognitive fatigue in case studies of patients with MS after a course of treatment [16, 17]. It is only hypothetical why there is a positive impact of magnetic field therapy on MS fatigue. Factors such as energy metabolism, oxygen supply, and microcirculation are discussed [12]. The tendency for positive results warrants further investigation using a double- blinded, controlled protocol. There are different patterns of pulsed magnetic field therapies available. Bio-Electro- Magnetic-Energy-Regulation (BEMER, Innomed International AG, Lichtenstein) therapy uses broadband, extremely weak, low frequent pulsed electromagnetic fields induced by flexible, flat electric coils [18]. Although there have been several anecdotal positive reports with this device, no placebo-controlled, double-blinded study is currently available in the literature.

Our study was designed to evaluate the long-term effect of BEMER therapy in patients with MS with significant fatigue in a typical outpatient setting: Patients with relapsing-remitting MS and significant fatigue were randomized to BEMER or placebo treatment and were evaluated after 6 and 12 weeks using different fatigue scales. We hypothesize that patients with relapsing-remitting MS who use the BEMER for 8 minutes twice a day for 12 weeks will experience improvement in fatigue, compared to patients who use a placebo device.

Methods
The present study was a randomized, patient and rater- blinded, placebo- controlled trial conducted in a neurological outpatient center in Dresden. The study lasted 3 months and was performed between 2006 and 2007. The study protocol was approved by the international ethical committee in Freiburg, Germany (EC 02/TS/06). It was conducted according to the Declaration of Helsinki (Hong Kong Amendment) and pertinent national legal and regulatory requirements. Prior to study entry, each patient provided written, informed consent and was free to withdraw from the study at any time for any reason without consequences on the care provided.

Forty-one (41) ambulatory patients with clinically definite, relapsing-remitting MS were randomly assigned to treatment with BEMER or to sham therapy twice a day over 3 months. The sample size was calculated before using the software nQuery Advisor 6.0 (Statistical Solutions, Cork, Ireland) with a power of 97% (two-sided test, α=0.05). A total of 4 patients were lost to follow-up (2 verum, 2 placebo); all 4 had no time left for the two applications per day. Data analysis was therefore restricted to the remaining 37 patients with complete data sets because no follow-up data were available for the last 4 patients.

Female and male patients between 18 and 65 years were enrolled in the study when they (1) had relapsing-remitting MS as defined by Poser et al. [19], (2) accepted the informed consent, and (3) had sig- nificant fatigue as reported by the patient. Reasons to refuse were (1) previous therapy with pulsed electromagnetic fields, (2) acute relapse of MS within the last month as we were interested in the effect of magnetic field therapy on chronic fatigue that can be interfered with by an acute relapse, (3) psychiatric or neurological disorders other than multiple sclerosis, (4) actual treatment with amantadine, aminopyridine, or modafinil as drug therapy for fatigue to avoid interference of anti-fatigue effects of drugs and magnetic field therapy or (5) pregnancy.

Randomization to the verum and the placebo group was performed by block randomization. Patients and physician/statistician were blinded. All patients were told in the informed consent document that there was a 50% chance to receive placebo and verum treatment. All devices looked identical and were numbered. The placebo-verum coding was only used for the final analysis. The success of blinding was not evaluated, and patients were unblinded after the end of the study.

The BEMER therapy was used to stimulate by extremely weak, low-frequency pulsed electromagnetic fields (with mean of 14μT) induced by flexible, flat electric coils. The BEMER signal consists of a series of half-wave-shaped sinusoidal intensity variations. Starting out with low values, the intensity initially increases slowly and then drops again to a value that, however, is located at a higher level within the impulse than the initial value. This sequence keeps repeating itself, while the intensity variations gets denser and the drift from the zero line gradually increases. Correspondingly, the ups and downs keep getting steeper. The intensity process repeats itself 33.3 times per second.

After 2 minutes, the magnetic field changes its polarity. The duration of the signal sequences was set empirically via a control device to a period of 8 minutes. In this way, the magnetic field of the BEMER 3000 systems is, in the first approximation, a typical pulsing constant electromagnetic direct current field that is asymmetrical to the zero line. The BEMER device includes a control device that produces the patented BEMER signal and that could be turned on/off by the patient. It is connected with an all-metal mat that is hooked up to the control device via a connecting cable and rolled out.

For this study, patients with MS were asked to lie down on the mattress for 8 minutes twice every day in their private home. Compliance of the patient was controlled by a special diary. In the treatment group (verum), the BEMER mattress was activated whereas in the control group (placebo), no magnetic field was generated although there was the typical BEMER sound.

TABLE 1. DEMOGRAPHIC CHARACTERISTICS OF THE MULTIPLE SCLEROSIS PATIENTS IN THE VERUM AND THE PLACEBO GROUP

	Verum	Placebo
N	19	18
Age	44±8.3	47.5±8.6
% Female	89.5%	72%
Duration of disease (years)	10.5±9.8	6.8±5.8
EDSS	3.7±2.2	3.1±1.3
MSFC	-0.7±1.8	-0.4±0.8
% Patients on immunomodulation	53%	89%
% Patients on GA	16%	33%
% Patients on IFN	37%	56%

Patients were evaluated at inclusion and after 6 and 12 weeks of treatment at the same time of day (10 AM). At each visit, patients underwent a full neurologic assessment, any relapses occurring since the previous visit were ascertained, and disability was assessed with the Expanded Disability Status Scale (EDSS) [20]. Multiple Sclerosis Functional Composite (MSFC) was performed each time. Fatigue was assessed by the patient using the fatigue severity scale (FSS), a visual analogue scale scored from 0 (no fatigue) to 10 (maximum possible fatigue), and with the Modified Fatigue Impact Scale (MFIS) [21] in its validated German translation.

Data are presented as mean±standard deviation. EDSS, expanded disability status scale; MSFC, Multiple Sclerosis Functional Scale; GA, glatiramer acetate; IFN, interferon-β.

This is a 21-item questionnaire that yields a total score ranging from 0 (no impact of fatigue) to 84 points (maximum impact of fatigue), as well as three subscales representing the physical (score range 0-36), cognitive (score range 0-40), and psychosocial (score range 0-8) dimensions of fatigue. Depression was evaluated by the long German version of the Center for Epidemiologic Studies Depression Scale (CES-D).

Group differences in MFIS, FSS, MSFC, EDSS, and ADS-L scores between the verum and the placebo groups were evaluated at the different timepoints by Student's t-test for independent samples. Changes in fatigue scores over time were statistically assessed by paired t-tests for the placebo and the verum group, respectively. Differences in gender group composition were assessed with a x^2-test. All comparisons were two-tailed and a p value of <0.05 was taken as being statistically significant.

The BEMER devices were kindly supplied by Innomed International AG, Liechtenstein. No additional support was provided.

Results

Study population and baseline characteristics Baseline demographic characteristics are presented in Table 1. The verum and the placebo groups did not statistically differ in terms of age or gender group composition.

At baseline, both groups did not differ in terms of EDSS (Student's test: t = 1.21; not significant (n.s.)), MSFC (Stu- dent's t-test: t = 0.7; n.s.), duration of disease (Student's t-test: t = 1.10; n.s.) and ADS-L (Student's t-test: t = -1.23; n.s.).

Fatigue scores (MFIS, FSS) were slightly higher in the placebo group compared to the verum group, but this effect did not reach statistical significance. (Student's t-test: MFIS: t = -1.36; n.s.; FSS: t = -1.15; n.s.) (Table 2).

Primary outcome criterion: MFIS baseline versus 12-weeks treatment Regarding the primary endpoint of our study, there was evidence of a significant difference of MFIS value after 12

After 6-week treatment, the verum and the placebo groups did not differ in experiencing fatigue (Student's t-test for independent samples; MFIS 6weeks: t= -1.38; n.s.; FSS6weeks:t= -2.03; n.s.) (Table 2). However, looking at changes in fatigue over time, there was a decrease in fatigue measured by the FSS in the verum but not the placebo group after 6 weeks compared to baseline (paired t-test: FSS6week/verum; t = 2.68; p =0.015; FSS 6weeks/placebo: t = 0.98; n.s.) (Table 3). No differences for the MFIS or MFIS subscales (physical, cognitive, psychologic) were observed over time for either group (paired t-test: MFIS 6weeks/verum: t = 1.14; n.s .; MFIS 6weeks/placebo: t = 0.98; n.s.).

Self-rated depressive symptoms by the CE5-D did not differ between groups after 6 weeks' treatment (Student's t-test for independent samples: ADS- L6weeks: t = -0.76; n.s.). There was also no change in depressive symptom expression over tin1e in either group (paired t-test: ADS-L6weeks/verum: t = 0.33; / ADS-L6weeks/placebo: t = 0.45; n.s.).

Secondary outcome criteria: Baseline versus 12-week treatment

In addition to significant different fatigue ratings by MFIS between the verum and the placebo group, there was evidence for a significant difference of FSS value after 12 weeks in favor of the verum group (26.84 versus 36.67; Student's t-test for independent samples: MFIS 12 weeks: t =-2.36; p=0.024) treatment in favor of the verum group (Student's t-test for independent samples: FSS 12 weeks: f = -2.53; p = 0.016). In the verum group but not in the placebo group, there was a significant decrease in perceived fatigue over this 12-week period (paired t-test; FSS 12 weeks/verum: 3.87; p =0.001; MFIS 12 weeks/verum: t =3.12; p =0.006; FSS 12 weeks/placebo: 1.50; p =n.s.; MFIS 12 weeks/placebo: t =0.53; p =n.s.). Regarding the subscales of the MFIS, there was a significant decrease in physical (paired t-test: MFIS/- phys 12 weeks/verum: t = 2.6; p =0.018; MFIS/phys 12 weeks/placebo: t =0; n.s.) and cognitive (paired t-test: MFIS/cog 12 weeks/verum : t =2.2; p =0.041; MFIS/cog 12 week/placebo: t =0.43; p =n.s.) but not in psychologic subscales (paired t-test: MFIS/psy12-psy 12 weeks/verum: t =1.83; n.s.; MFIS/psy12weeks/placebo: t = 1.44; n.s.) only in the verum group regarding the timepoints base-line and 12 weeks of treatment.

Table 2. Changes of Modified Fatigue Impact Scale (MFIS) Overall Score as Well as Physical, Cognitive, and Psychological Subscores in the VErum and Placebo Groups at Baseline, 6 Weeks, and 12 Weeks

	Baseline				6 Weeks				12 Weeks			
	Verum		Placebo		Verum		Placebo		Verum		Placebo	
	Mean	SD	Mean	SD	Mean	SD	Mean	SD	Mean	SD	Mean	SD
MFIS	31.68	13.24	37.83	14.26	29.21	14.85	36.06	15.25	26.84	12.061	36.67	13.253
Physical	17.21	6.78	17.72	7.84	14.58	6.70	17,5	7.91	14.11	5.801	17,72	6.47
Cognitive	12.26	7.15	16.33	6.23	11.95	8.84	15.06	6.86	10.37	6.825	15,83	6.373
Psychologic	2.74	2.38	3.78	2.42	2.68	1.64	3.50	2.07	2	1.563	3.11	1.568

Changes of MFIS overall score. Data are presented as mean± standard deviation (SD).

Table 3. Changes of MSFC, EDSS, MFIS, FSS, and ADS-L in the Verum and the Placebo Group at Baseline, 6 Weeks, and 12 Weeks

	Baseline				6 Weeks				12 Weeks			
	Verum		Placebo		Verum		Placebo		Verum		Placebo	
	Mean	SD	Mean	SD	Mean	SD	Mean	SD	Mean	SD	Mean	SD
MSFC	-0.7	1.8	-0.4	0.8	-0.5	19	-0.2	0.8	-0.3	1.8	0.0	-0.8
EDSS	3.8	2.1	3.1	1.3	3.8	2.1	3.1	13	3.8	2.1	3.1	1.3
FSS	4.5	1.2	5.0	1.4	3.8	1.4	4.8	1.6	3.5	1.3	4.7	1.6
ADS-L	13.7	7.5	16.8	8.05	13.2	11.3	15.8	9.6	11.1	8.1	14.8	8.7

Data are presented as mean± standard deviation (SD).
MSFC, Multiple Sclerosis Functional Scale; EDSS, Expanded Disability Status Scale; MFIS, Modified Fatigue Impact Scale; FSS, Fatigue Severity Scale; ADS-L,.

Self-rated depressive symptoms by CES-D did not differ between groups after 12 weeks of treatment (Student's t-test for independent samples: ADS-L 12 weeks: t= 1.35; n.s.). There was a tendency for decreased depressive symptoms compared to baseline in the verum group, but this effect did not reach statistical significance (paired t-test: ADS-L 12 weeks/verum: t = 2.03; (0.058/n.s.)/ADS-L 12 weeks/placebo: t = 0.89; n.s.).

There were no significant side-effects during verum and placebo application.

Discussion

Our study was focused on the effects of the new type of pulsed low-frequency electromagnetic fields of the BEMER 3000 device on MS fatigue after 6 weeks and 12 weeks. The patients were evaluated by a panel of different questionnaires (MFIS, FSS, ADS-L) in addition to MSFC and EDSS testing.

Using a randomized placebo-controlled protocol, we were able to demonstrate a modest, but statistically significant advantage for the verum treatment group concerning an effect on the MFIS and FSS over a 3-month period. Although both groups showed a decrease in fatigue over the intervention time, MFIS score was significantly lower in the verum than in the placebo group 3 months later, which reflects a statistical advantage of the BEMER treatment ac- cording the predefined primary outcome criteria.

There is growing evidence in the literature of a beneficial effect of magnetic field therapy on different MS symptoms such as fatigue, bladder control, spasticity, and quality of life. Nielsen and Sinkjaer reported a reduction of spasticity by magnetic stimulation over the thoracic myelon [23]. while Sandyk reported cases of prompter recovery from fatigue following physical activity by an extracranially applied electromagnetic field [17, 24]. A recent meta-analysis summarized the beneficial effects of electromagnetic fields on MS fatigue, but recommended long-term studies [12].

Other experiments have already investigated the effect of electromagnetic fields on MS fatigue so far. Lappin et al. demonstrated a reduction of MS fatigue by 0.5 points on a modified five-item scale out of the MS Quality of Life Inventory by wearing a small portable pulsing electromagnetic device next to the skin over the brachial plexus 24 hours a day for 4 weeks [14]. Expressed in relative terms, this was a decrement of fatigue by roughly 20%. The placebo effect of the sham intervention in their study was 0.36 points (about 14%). A preliminary study of the same study group with 30 patients with the same device used 24 hours per day over a 2-month period also demonstrated a beneficial effect of pulsed magnetic field therapy on a combined performance scale rating for bladder control, cognitive function, fatigue level, mobility, spasticity, and vision [13].

In contrast, Mostert and Kesselring used a device (magnetic cell regeneration system by Santerra) that was comparable to the BEMER system as it was applied for 16 minutes twice daily. They were not able to demonstrate a beneficial effect of pulse electromagnetic field therapy as an additional component to a multimodal neurologic rehabilitation program on fatigue [15]. In comparison to our study, the level of fatigue was slightly higher as measured by the FSS (5.5). Unfortunately, other studies could not be compared regarding the baseline fatigue level because they used other scales. Because Mostert and Kesselring described a wide variability of measurements using the visual analogue scale, we decided to focus our evaluation of MS fatigue only on FSS and MFIS scales. In contrast to this study, we measured fatigue level not directly after the application of electro- magnetic field therapy, but in the study center always at 10 AM. Our patients were not enrolled in a specific rehabilitation program, which may have additional positive effects on MS fatigue that may be confounded in their study. Mostert and Kesselring have already described that a special rehabilitation program with short-time exercise treatment was able to reduce MS fatigue in a significant way [24]. Of course, there are statistical limitations to this study.

Although this study was a randomized, placebo-controlled trial, the number of participants was limited, with only 19/18 only Lappin et al. interventions for fatigue in adults with multiple sclerosis, investigated more than 55 patients per group, but only for 4 weeks [14]. Larger trials on this issue are needed in order to confirm the findings from this pilot study. Again, it is not possible to compare the different devices, as the physiology of magnetic field therapy is not well known. Magnetic field therapy is used in a lot of clinical settings. Unfortunately, scientific data on mechanism and so on are still missing. We are beginning to investigate physiologic changes induced by magnetic field therapy.

Conclusions

In this pilot study, we were able to demonstrate a beneficial effect of BEMER therapy on MS fatigue. Although we recognized a placebo effect, there was a statistically significant benefit for treated patients after 12 weeks. From our personal experience, MS patients suffering from MS fatigue can benefit from electromagnetic field therapy. Because devices for pulsed electromagnetic therapy like BEMER are quite expensive, we recommend individual tests for several weeks to see whether there is an individual benefit for the MS patient with significant fatigue.

Disclosure

No competing financial interests exist.

References

1. Freal JE, Kraft GH, Coryell JK. Symptomatic fatigue in multiple sclerosis. Arch Phys Med Rehabil 1984;65:135-138.
2. Fisk JD, Pontefract A, Ritvo PG, et al. The impact of fatigue on patients with multiple sclerosis. Can J Neurol Sci 1994; 21:9-14.
3. Ziemssen T. Multiple sclerosis beyond EDSS: Fatigue and depression. J Neurol Sci 2008;273:S32-S35.
4. Vercoulen JH, et al. The measurement of fatigue in patients with multiple sclerosis: A multidimensional comparison with patients with chronic fatigue syndrome and healthy subjects. Arch Neurol 1996;53:642-649.
5. Smith MM, Arnett PA. Factors related to employment status changes in individuals with multiple sclerosis. Multiple Sclerosis 2005;11:602- 609.
6. Krupp LB. Fatigue in multiple sclerosis: Definition, pathophysiology and treatment. CNS Drugs 2003;17:225-234.
7. Jackson MF, Quaal C, Reeves MA. Effects of multiple sclerosis on occupational and career patterns. Axone 1991;13:16-17, 20-12.
8. Bakshi R. Fatigue associated with multiple sclerosis: Diagnosis, impact and management. Multiple Sclerosis 2003;9:219-227.
9. Filippi M, Rocca MA . Toward a definition of structural and functional MRI substrates of fatigue in multiple sclerosis. J Neurol Sci 2007;263:1-2.
10. Lee D, Newell R, Ziegler L, Topping A . Treatment of fatigue in multiple sclerosis: A systematic review of the literature. Int J Nurs Pract 2008;14:81-93.
11. Ziemssen T, Hoffmann J, Apfel R, Kem S. Effects of glatiramer acetate on fatigue and days of absence from work in first-time treated relapsing-remitting multiple sclerosis. Health Quality Life Outcomes 2008;6:67. rheumatoid arthritis, or systemic lupus erythematosus: A systematic review. J Adv Nurs 2006;56:617-635.
12. Richards TL, et al. Double-blind study of pulsing magnetic field effects on multiple sclerosis. J Altern Complement Med 1997;3:21- 29.
13. Lappin MS, Lawrie FW, Richards TL, Kramer ED. Effects of a pulsed electromagnetic therapy on multiple sclerosis fatigue and quality of life: A double-blind, placebo controlled trial. Altern Ther Health Med 2003;9:38-48.
14. Mostert S, Kesselring J. Effect of pulsed magnetic field therapy on the level of fatigue in patients with multiple sclerosis: A randomized controlled trial. Multiple Sclerosis 2005;11: 302-305.
15. Sandyk R. Treatment with weak electromagnetic fields im- proves fatigue associated with multiple sclerosis. Int J Neu- rosci 1996;84:177-186.
16. Sandyk R. Immediate recovery of cognitive functions and resolution of fatigue by treatment with weak electromag- netic fields in a patient with multiple sclerosis. Int J Neurosci 1997;90:59-74.

17. Walther M, Mayer F, Kafka W, Scl1utze N. Effects of weak, low- frequency pulsed electromagnetic fields (BEMER type) on gene expression of human mesenchymal stem cells and chondrocytes: An in vitro study. Electromagnetic Biol Med 2007;26:179-190.
18. Poser CM. Clinical diagnostic criteria in epidemiological studies of multiple sclerosis. Ann NY Acad Sci 1965;122:506- 519.
19. Kurtzke JF. Rating neurologic impairment in multiple sclerosis: An expanded disability status scale (EDSS). Neurology 1983;33:1444- 1452.
20. Multiple Sclerosis Council for Clinical Practice Guidelines. Fatigue and Multiple Sclerosis: Evidence-Based Management Strategies for Fatigue in Multiple Sclerosis. Washington, DC: Paralyzed Veterans of America, 1998:1-33.
21. Hautzinger M. Die CES-D Skala. Ein Depressionsmessinstrument für Untersuchungen in der Allgemeinbevölkerung. Diagnostika 1988;34:167-173.
22. Nielsen JF, Sinkjaer T. Long-lasting depression of soleus motoneurons excitability following repetitive magnetic stimuli of the spinal cord in multiple sclerosis patients. Multiple Sclerosis 1997;3:18-30.
23. Sandyk R. Resolution of sleep paralysis by weak electromagnetic fields in a patient with multiple sclerosis. Int J Neurosci 1997;90:145- 157.
24. Mostert S, Kesselring J. Effects of a short-term exercise training program on aerobic fitness, fatigue, health perception and activity level of subjects with multiple sclerosis. Multiple Sclerosis 2002;8:161-168.

Long-Term Effects of BEMER Electromagnetic Field Therapy on the Level of Fatigue in Patients with Multiple Sclerosis: An Open-Label Follow-Up Study

Piatkowski J; Haase R; Ziemssen T; Journal of Alternative and Complementary Medicine; Vol 17, 2011
Joachim Piatkowski (1), Rocco Haase (2), Tjalf Ziemssen (2)

(1) Neurological Practice, Reichenbachstrasse, Dresden, Germany and (2) MS Center Dresden, Clinic and Polyclinic for Neurology, University of Technology, Dresden, Germany.

SUMMARY: This long-term open-label study demonstrated the beneficial effects of long-term BEMER therapy on MS-related fatigue. Electromagnetic field therapy may be a useful complementary treatment for MS patients with severe fatigue. Long-term effects of the BEMER electromagnetic field therapy on fatigue in patients with multiple sclerosis – open-label follow-up study.

Short title: **Long-Term Electromagnetic Field Therapy in MS Fatigue**

Corresponding author: Dr. Tjalf Ziemssen, MS Center Dresden, Clinic and Polyclinic for Neurology, Carl Gustav Carus University Hospital, University of Technology Dresden, Fetscherstr. 74, 01307 Dresden, Germany.

Abstract

Background: A number of studies have shown that electromagnetic field therapy has beneficial effects on fatigue in multiple sclerosis (MS) patients.

Primary study objective: To evaluate the long-term effects of BEMER (Bio-Electro-Magnetic-Energy-Regulation) therapy on MS-related fatigue, we designed a crossover control trial of a previously performed randomized controlled trial and a long-term open-label follow-up trial. Study design and setting: Monocentric, crossover and open-label follow-up trial at a single neurological practice.

Participants: 37 patients with relapsing-remitting MS with severe fatigue.

Intervention: After 12 weeks' randomized exposure to low-frequency pulsed magnetic fields for 8 minutes twice daily or to placebo treatment, a crossover trial (from control group to verum and vice versa) was performed for another twelve weeks, followed by a 3-year open-label follow-up trial.

Primary outcome measures: The most important outcome criteria were changes in the Modified Fatigue Impact Scale (MFIS) and the Fatigue Severity Scale (FSS) between the end of the first double-blind trial and the follow-up trial/end of the crossover trial (12 weeks). Secondary outcome criteria were changes on the general depression scale – long version (ADS-L), the Multiple Sclerosis Functional Scale (MSFC), and the Expanded Disability Status Scale (EDSS).

Results: The MFIS and FSS scores were significantly lower in the open-label group than in the control group after follow-up (MFIS: 16.78 compared to 42.54; $p = 0.00$; FSS: 2.35 compared to 5.16; $p = 0.00$). Participation in the open-label treatment was the strongest predictor of low fatigue outcome after follow-up (ANCOVA MFIS 3 years: $p = 0.00$, $\eta^2 = 0.597$) Patients who had previously received the placebo treatment demonstrated a significant regression of fatigue after verum treatment (MFIS: 33.23 to 22.42, $p = 0.006$; FSS: 4.13 to 3.04, $p = 0.005$). BEMER therapy was well tolerated.

Conclusions: This long-term open-label study demonstrated the beneficial effects of long-term BEMER therapy on MS-related fatigue. Electromagnetic field therapy may be a useful complementary treatment for MS patients with severe fatigue.

Introduction

Fatigue affects more than 75% of multiple sclerosis (MS) patients and is therefore one of the most common symptoms of the disease. [1] For the majority of patients, it is one of the worst and most oppressive impairments. [2] Fatigue is reported in all clinical phenotypes of MS and affects patients of all ages. [3] The symptom is an integral part of the disease process. It is usually present at the time of diagnosis and in many cases is the reason for examination by a neurologist.

Fatigue is not closely related to physical disability or MRT markers that indicate disease activity. However, it appears to be increased when the patient experiences a relapse. [2,4] The etiology and pathophysiology of MS fatigue are not known. Studies have not been able to demonstrate connections between MS fatigue, degree of disability, clinical sub-type of the disease or gender. [5]

Management strategies include medication, physical activity and behavioral therapy. [6] Positive effects of immunomodulating mediation on MS fatigue are reported. [7] The efficacy of treatment, however, remains disappointing. [6]

The potential benefit of non-pharmacological electromagnetic field therapy, reported recently in a meta-analysis [8], required further investigation, even if the modulating mechanisms of MS fatigue are still far from being explained. [8] We therefore initially conducted a randomized controlled double-blind trial [9] (RCT) on the effects of BEMER (Bio-Electro-Magnetic-Energy-Regulation) electromagnetic field therapy (BEMER, Innomed International AG, Liechtenstein). In the trial, patients with relapsing-remitting MS and associated severe fatigue were treated in a typical practice environment with extremely weak, low-frequency pulsed broadband electromagnetic fields. [10] The results showed that, after 12 weeks of treatment, the participants in the verum group had a significantly lower level of fatigue on the various fatigue scales than the participants in the placebo group (t3). [9]

The study protocol was supplemented by a single crossover control study and an open long-term follow-up study to follow up these results.

In our hypothesis, we assumed that regular BEMER therapy over a period of three years will reduce the fatigue in MS patients compared to patients who do not receive the therapy. We also expected that patients who move from the placebo to BEMER treatment in the crossover phase would show a gradual reduction of fatigue compared to the end of the placebo trial.

Materials and methods

This trial is a monocentric, open-label crossover and follow-up trial, performed in a neurological practice in Dresden, Germany. The crossover trial lasted twelve weeks (t3 to t5) and was performed between 2006 and 2007. The open-label long-term trial was performed in 2009, three years after completion of the crossover trial. The study protocol was approved by the international ethical committee in Freiburg, Germany. It was conducted according to the Declaration of Helsinki (Hong Kong Amendment) and pertinent national legal and regulatory requirements. Prior to start of the study, each patient provided written, informed consent.

The participants were free to withdraw from the study at any time for any reason without consequences on the care provided.

The study protocol has been described elsewhere. 9 In summary: Thirty-seven (37) ambulant patients between 18 and 65 years of age with clinically diagnosed, relapsing-remitting MS were evaluated over a period of three months (t1 to t3). They underwent bio-electromagnetic energy regulation therapy (BEMER therapy, BEMER, Innomed international AG, Liechtenstein) or a placebo intervention. Patients and study physicians/evaluators were blind. The patients were unblinded after the end of the first study.

During BEMER therapy, extremely weak, low-frequency pulsed electromagnetic fields (average field strength: 14 µT) are generated by flexible, flat electrical coils. A detailed description has been published elsewhere. 9 As in the first study, MS patients were asked to lie down on the mattress in their home twice per day for 8 minutes each time. Patient compliance was monitored by a special diary where patients recorded their correct use of the BEMER device.

Of the 18 patients in the placebo group, 13 took part in the follow-up crossover study. One patient had to be excluded from the analysis, as the time intervals for data acquisition were not met. The crossover patients were evaluated at inclusion (t3) and after 6 weeks (t4) and 12 weeks (t5) of treatment at the same time of day (10 am).

After the crossover study, all 37 patients were asked whether they would like to participate in an open-label, long-term follow-up study with continuing BEMER therapy. A total of 9 patients agreed to further treatment (open-label group). All patients were re-evaluated after three years (t6).

At each visit (t1 to t6), the patients underwent a full neurological examination. Relapses that occurred between appointments were documented and disability was assessed at each visit using the Expanded Disability Status Scale (EDSS). [11] The Multiple Sclerosis Functional Composite (MSFC) was also performed at each appointment. Fatigue was recorded using the Fatigue Severity Scale (FSS) and the Modified Fatigue Impact Scale (MFIS) in its validated German translation. [12] The FSS values are between 0 (no fatigue) and 7 (maximum possible fatigue). The 21 items on the MFIS yield a total score from 0 (no impact of fatigue) to 84 points (maximum impact of fatigue). Depression was determined using the German long version of the Center for Epidemiologic Studies Depression Scale (CES-D) and the general depression scale – long version (ADS-L). [13] Group differences in the MFIS, FSS, MSFC, EDSS and ADS-L scores between the open-label and the control groups at the different points in time were determined using the Student's t-test for independent samples. Changes in fatigue values over time were determined in the open-label and control groups using paired t-tests and, in the crossover study, using the Wilcoxon signed-rank test. Differences in the gender composition of the groups were determined using an χ^2 test. The effects of treatment on fatigue at the end of the open-label study were evaluated by analysis of covariance (ANCOVA), whereby the two treatments were applied as factor variable and the initial values at t1 and t3 as adjustments. All comparisons were bilateral and a p-value of <0.05 was taken as statistically significant. All statistical calculations were performed using SPSS 17.0 (SPSS Inc., Chicago, IL, USA).

Results
Study population and baseline characteristics
The demographic baseline characteristics (t1) of the verum group (N=19) and the placebo group (N=18) do not differ in terms of age, gender composition of the group and the test values described above. Comparison of the baseline characteristics (t1) of the open-label (N=9) and the non-open-label control group (N=28) identified no differences in terms of age, gender composition of the group, EDSS value (Student's t-test: tt1 = 0.48; n.s.), MSFC value (Student's t-test: tt3 = -0.36; n.s.) or ADS-L value (Student's t-test: tt1 = 0.98; n.s.). Fatigue values (MFIS and FSS) tended to be higher in the control group than in the open-label group. However the differences were not statistically significant (Student's t-test: MFIS tt1 = 1.70; n.s.; FSS tt1 = 1.40; n.s.) (Table 1).

Primary objective, open-label trial: MFIS & FSS values after RCT (t3) and follow-up (t6)

The MFIS and FSS values were significantly lower in the open-label group than in the control group after three-year follow-up (t6) (MFIS 16.78 compared to 42.54; Student's t-test for independent samples: MFIS 3 years (t6) = 6.31; p = 0.00; FSS t6 = 5.85; p = 0.00). At the start of the open-label trial (t3), the MFIS values did not differ between the groups (MFIS 25.11 compared to 33.71; Student's t-test for independent samples: MFIS t3 t = 1.72; n.s.).

However, the FSS values of the groups did differ significantly at the start of the open-label phase, though only to a limited extent (Student's t-test for independent samples: FSS t3 t= 2.82; p = 0.008) (Table 1).

Evaluation of the changes in fatigue over time identified an insignificant trend to lower FSS values in the open-label group after three years (paired t-test: FSS t3 t6 t = 1.10; n.s.), whereas fatigue had increased in the control group (paired t-test: FSS t3 t6 t = -4.32; p = 0.00). The MFIS values similarly fell in the open-label group (paired t-test: MFIS t3 t6 t = 2.67; p = 0.028), but increased in the control group (paired t-test: FSS t3 t6 t = -5.06; p = 0.00) (Table 1).

ANCOVAs were applied to the last MFIS and FSS values (t6) ANCOVA MFIS t6: $\eta2$= 0.804; FSS t6: $\eta2$= 0.812) to be able to distinguish the effects of open- label treatment from the original RCT intervention. 9 Participation in the open- label group was the best predictor for a lower fatigue value after the follow-up trial (ANCOVA study t6: F= 45.927; p = 0.00; $\eta2$= 0.597; power = 1.00; ANCOVA FSS t6: F= 31.901; p= 0.00; $\eta2$= 0.507; Power= 1.00). Allocation to the verum or placebo group for first intervention did not prove a significant factor with regard to the fatigue values at the end of the follow-up trial (ANCOVA MFIS t6: F= 1.047; p= 0.31; $\eta2$= 0.033; Power= 0.171; ANCOVA FSS t6: F= 3.774; p= 0.061; $\eta2$ = 0.109; Power= 0.469). The differences in adjusted means on the MFI, open-label versus control group (20.60 versus 41.23; ANCOVA: MFIS t6 p = 0.00) and FSS open-label versus control group (2.90 versus 4.96; ANCOVA: FSS t6 p = 0.00) at t6 underlines the benefit in the open-label group. No interactive effects were identified between the open- label and the RCT phase (ANCOVA: MFIS t6 F= 0.006; n.s.; FSS t6 F= 0.231; n.s.). Accordingly, the differences in fatigue values between the verum and placebo group identified at t39 disappeared after the three-year follow-up (t6) (MFIS t6 33.58 versus 39.11; Student's t-test for independent samples: MFIS t6 t= -1.099; n.s.; FSS 4.27 versus 4.70; Student's t-test for independent samples: FSS t6 t= -0.743; n.s).

Secondary objective, open-label trial. RCT (t3) compared to the follow-up study (t6)
There were no differences in the self-assessed depression symptoms on the CES-D between the groups at the end of the follow-up study (t6) (Student's t- test for independent samples: ADS-L t6 t = 1.38; n.s.). There was a tendency towards higher MSFC values in the open-label group (Student's t- test for independent samples: MSFC t6 t = 1.85; n.s.). There were no changes in MS disability according to EDSS.

Primary outcome of the crossover study: MFIS & FSS values after RCT (t3) and crossover (t6)
During the crossover trial (t3 to t5), the MFIS and FSS values fells significantly from 33.23 to 22.42 (Wilcoxon MFIS t3 t5: Z = -2.764; p = 0.006) and from to 3.04 (Wilcoxon FSS t3 t5: Z = -2.803; p = 0.005) respectively.

Secondary outcome of the crossover study: RCT (t3) compared to the crossover study (t5)
The MSFC value increased during crossover treatment (from 0.26 to 0.54, Wilcoxon MSFC t3 t5: Z = -2.936; p = 0,003), whereas the values on the depression scale continuously improved, as already identified during the RCT 9 (ADS-L: from 11.42 to 7.25, Wilcoxon ADS-L t3 t5: Z= -2.255; p= 0.024).

Discussion

The aim of this study was to identify the long-term effects of magnetic field therapy (pulsed low-frequency electrocmagnetic fields) on MS fatigue. The patients were evaluated with regard to fatigue, disability, severity of disease and depression using various tests and questionnaires (MFIS, FSS, ADS-L, MSFC and EDSS). Alleviation of MS fatigue after continuous treatment with pulsed low-frequency electromagnetic fields (open-label treatment group) was demonstrated on the basis of an open-label test protocol, whereas the severity of the disease remained constant. The results of this study solidify the results of the original RCT 9, which had already demonstrated positive impacts of the pulsed low-frequency electromagnetic fields.

There is increasing evidence of the positive effects of electromagnetic field therapy on various MS symptoms, such as fatigue, bladder control and spasticity, as well as quality of life. Nielsen and Sinkjaer have demonstrated a reduction in spasticity following local magnetic stimulation of the thoracic medula. [14] Sandyk reports cases of prompter recovery from fatigue caused by physical exertion thanks to treatment with electromagnetic fields. [15,16] A meta-analysis has summarized the positive effects of electromagnetic field therapy on MS fatigue, but there is no evidence from long-term studies. [8] In a different study, Lappin et al. demonstrated a reduction in MS fatigue by 20% after four weeks of continuous treatment of the brachial plexus with pulsed electromagnetic fields. [17] However, the fatigue of the placebo group also fell by 14% in the study. The same researchers demonstrated an improvement in bladder control, cognitive functions, fatigue, mobility, spasticity and vision on a combined improvement scale used to evaluate 30 MS patients, who carried a portable device at all times for a period of two months to generate pulsed electromagnetic fields. [18] Although a similar device to the BEMER system was used, i.e. the magnetic cell regeneration system from Santerra, no improvement in fatigue was demonstrated during treatment with pulsed electromagnetic fields (twice daily for 16 minutes) as part of a multimodal neurological rehabilitation program. [19] In contract to this study, the patients in that study demonstrated a higher fatigue value (FSS: 5.5) when the fatigue values were determined directly after magnetic field treatment. In addition, the patients in the present study did not take part in a special rehabilitation program, which might have hidden positive effects on MS fatigue. Mostert and Kesselring also describe reduction of MS fatigue by a special rehabilitation program with short physical exercises. [20] The comparability of the results is further hindered by the use of different scales to determine the severity of fatigue and by the fact that the period of magnetic field treatment selected was different in each case. As the visual analog scale used by Mostert and Kesselring showed significantly variable results, we decided to use the FSS and MFIS to evaluate MS fatigue in this study.

There are statistical limits that must be observed. The participants in the open- label and crossover study were recruited without restriction or randomization, so that bias may have occurred. The small size of the open-label group (N=9) may have limited the ability to demonstrate treatment effects, even though other studies reporting positive effects have been performed with a similar number of patients. [18,19] Studies with larger patient groups are definitely necessary to conform the results in this study. A further disadvantage was the fact that the crossover study could not be performed in full.

Conclusions

This long-term study demonstrated the beneficial effects of regular BEMER therapy on MS fatigue, lasting up to three years. From our experience, electromagnetic field therapy may be a useful therapeutic treatment in MS fatigue. As the purchase costs are high, we recommend individual efficacy analyses over a number of weeks to filter out patients that do not respond to the treatment.

Conflicts of interest

There are no financial conflicts of interest.

Table 1. Changes in the fatigue, disability and depression values in the open-label group (N=9) and the control group (N=28) at inclusion (baseline), after RCT and after follow-up

The data are means +/- standard deviation (SD). * p< 0.01

	Baseline (t1)		Ende RCT (t3)		offene Follow-up-Studie (t15)	
	Offen Mean SD	Kontrolle Mean SD	offen Mean SD	Kontrolle Mean SD	offen Mean SD	Kontrolle Mean SD
MFIS	28,00 13,88	36,82 13,45	25,11 11,83	33,71 13,44	16,78* 8,76	42,54* 11,15
FSS	4,23 1,34	4,93 1,29	2,91* 1,45	4,44* 146	2,35 1,13	5,16 1,29
MSFC	-0,38 2,09	-0,58 1,13	-0,11 2,03	-0,20 1,18	0,45 0,85	-0,21 096
EDSS	3,17 2,15	3,50 1,69	3,17 2,15	3,50 1,69	3,22 2,12	4,07 1,76
ADSL	13,00 6,50	15,93 8,20	8,22 6,26	14,43 8,63	12,56 9,07	17,11 8,48

MFIS, Modified Fatigue Impact Scale; FSS, Fatigue Severity Scale; MSFC, Multiple Sclerosis Functional Scale; EDSS, Expanded Disability Status Scale; ADS-L, general depression scale – long version.

References

1. Freal JE, Kraft GH, Coryell JK. Symptomatic fatigue in multiple sclerosis. Arch Phys Med Rehabil 1984;65:135-138,
2. Fisk JD, Pontefract A, Ritvo PG, et al. The impact of fatigue on patients with multiple sclerosis. Can J Neurol Sci 1994;21:9-14.
3. Ziemssen T, Multiple sclerosis beyond EDSS: Fatigue and depression. J Neurol Sci 2008;273:S32-S35.
4. Vercoulen JH, et al. The measurement of fatigue in patients with multiple sclerosis: A multidimensional comparison with patients with chronic fatigue syndrome and healthy subjects. Arch Neurol 1996;53:642-649.
5. Bakshi R. Fatigue associated with multiple sclerosis: Diagnosis, impact and management, Multiple Sclerosis 2003,9:219-227.
6. Lee D, Newell R, Ziegler L, Topping A. Treatment of fatigue in multiple sclerosis: A systematic review of the literature. Int J Nurs Pract 2008;14:81—93.
7. Ziemssen T, Hoffmann J, Apfel R, Kern S. Effects of glatiramer acetate on fatigue and days of absence from work in first-time treated relapsing- remitting multiple sclerosis. Health Quality Life Outcomes 2008;6:67.
8. Neill J, Belan I, Ried K. Effectiveness of non-pharmacological interventions for fatigue in adults with multiple sclerosis, rheumatoid arthritis, or systemic lupus erythematosus: A systematic review. J Adv Nurs 2006;56:617-635.
9. Piatkowski J, Kern S, Ziemssen T. Effect of BEMER Magnetic Field Therapy on the Level of Fatigue in Patients with Multiple Sclerosis: A Randomized, Double-Blind Controlled Trial. J Altern Complement Med, 2009 May;15(5):507-11.
10. Walther M, Mayer F, Kafka W, Schutze N. Effects of weak, low- frequency pulsed electromagnetic fields (BEMER type) on gene expression of human mesenchymal stem cells and chondrocytes: An in vitro study. Electromagnetic Biol Med 2007;26:179-190.
11. Kurtzke JF. Rating neurologic impairment in multiple sclerosis: An expanded disability status scale (EDSS). Neurology 1983;33:1444-1452,
12. Multiple Sclerosis Council for Clinical Practice Guidelines. Fatigue and Multiple Sclerosis: Evidence-Based Management Strategies for Fatigue in Multiple Sclerosis. Washington, DC: Paralyzed Veterans of America, 1998:1-33.

13. Hautzinger M. Die CES-D Skala: A depression scale for evaluation of general populations [in German]. Diagnostika 1988;34:167-173.
14. Nielsen JF, Sinkjaer T, Long-lasting depression of soleus motoneurons excitability following repetitive magnetic stimuli of the spinal cord in multiple sclerosis patients, Multiple Sclerosis 1997;3:18-30.
15. Sandyk R. Immediate recovery of cognitive functions and resolution of fatigue by treatment with weak electromagnetic fields in a patient with multiple sclerosis. Int J Neurosci 1997;90:59-74.
16. Sandyk R. Resolution of sleep paralysis by weak electromagnetic fields in a patient with multiple sclerosis, Int J Neurosci 1997;90:145-1 57.
17. Lappin MS, Lawrie FW, Richards TL, Kramer ED, Effects of a pulsed electromagnetic therapy on multiple sclerosis fatigue and quality of life: A double-blind, placebo controlled trial. Altern Ther Health Med 2003;9:38-48.
18. Richards TL, et al. Double-blind study of pulsing magnetic field effects on multiple sclerosis. J Altern Complement Med 1997;3:21-29,
19. Mostert S, Kesselring J. Effect of pulsed magnetic field therapy on the level of fatigue in patients with multiple sclerosis: A randomized controlled trial. Multiple Sclerosis 2005;11:302-305.
20. Mostert S, Kesselring J. Effects of a short-term exercise training program on aerobic fitness, fatigue, health perception and activity level of subjects with multiple sclerosis, Multiple Sclerosis 2002;8:161-168.

Effect of BEMER Therapy on the Strength of Tensor Fascia Lata Muscle in Sclerosis Multiples

Dr. Duray Péter, internist, motor rehabilitation specialist, sport physician, medical economist

In the treatment of sclerosis multiplex, magnetic therapies have always been the most efficient procedures in physiotherapy. This study aimed at measuring the effect of the BEMER therapy on the strength of lower limb extensor muscles in sclerosis multiplex. In the study, 20 patients underwent a physical examination, the EDSS (disease-specific disability test), the FIM (Functional Independence Measurement) to evaluate the disability, and Multicont II computer dynamometric test to measure muscle strength and a video recording to present motor coordination at timepoint 0, regardless of the patients' age, gender, SM type and disease stage. The lower limb muscle strength test was isometrically illustrated by measuring the maximum voluntary torque. Subsequently, we administered the BEMER therapy over 6 weeks, and then the above measurements and tests were repeated. During these 6 weeks, no adjustments were made in the drug therapy, life style and frequency of physical therapy. The results were compared with the baseline and the opinion of the patients. The beneficial effects of the BEMER therapy can be inferred from the changes in the lower limb muscle strength.

Results

Overall, according to the objectivized and measured values, all 20 patients showed improvement in muscle strength. On average, compared with the baseline, an increase in muscle strength of 75% and 32% was measured on the weaker and the stronger lower limb, respectively. The difference between the muscle strength of the two lower limbs decreased that lead to the improvement of the walking pattern, balance and coordination. The patients were administered a disease-specific scale, the EDSS, which ranges from 10 (full disability) to 0 (walking without aid).

This test evaluates the relation between the use of aids and walking distance, and their common presence, where an improvement was observed in both measures. Walking distance increased, while the use of aids decreased. On average, the EDSS scores improved from 4.0 to 3.5. The Functional Independence Measurement (FIM) was also used, which illustrates independent activities, including grooming, clothing and use of toilette. This measure also improved. FIM scores increased from 117 to 122. Therefore, the values correlated with the clinical experiences and the opinion of the patients.

The clear improvement of the clinical symptoms that were not measured included incontinency, fatigue and mood.

BEMER Therapy Combined with Physiotherapy in Patients with Musculoskeletal Diseases: A Randomised, Controlled Double Blind Follow-Up Pilot Study

Franciska Gyulai, Katalin Rába, Ildikó Baranyai, Eniky Berkes, and Tamás Bender

Hospitaller Brothers of St. John of God, ´Arp´ad fejedelem ´utja 7, Budapest 1023, Hungary

Received 12 March 2015; Revised 5 May 2015; Accepted 5 May 2015
Academic Editor: Antonella Fioravanti

Background.
This study evaluates the effect of adjuvant BEMER therapy in patients with knee arthrosis and chronic low back pain in a randomized double blind design. Methods. A total of 50 patients with chronic low back pain and 50 patients with osteoarthritis of knee took part in this study and were randomized into 4 groups. Hospitalized patients received a standardized physiotherapy package for 3 weeks followed by BEMER therapy or placebo. Results. In patients with low back pain, the comparison of the results obtained at the first and second visit showed a significant improvement in restingVAS scores and Fatigue Scale scores.TheOswestry scores and Quality of Life Scale scores showed no change. In patients with knee arthrosis, the comparison of the first and second measurements showed no significant improvement in the abovementioned parameters, while the comparison of the first and third scores revealed a significant improvement in the Fatigue Scale scores and in the vitality test on the Quality of Life Scale. Conclusions. Our study showed that BEMER physical vascular therapy reduced pain and fatigue in the short term in patients with chronic low back pain, while long-term therapy appears to be beneficial in patients with osteoarthritis of knee.

1. Introduction

Electromagnetic field has been used in healing for centuries and has a medical literature of many decades, as well [1]. During the 1960s, Bassett confirmed that this therapy has a stimulating effect on callus formation and thus one aim of the studywas to evaluate the effect of pulsed electromagnetic field on osteoblastic activity both in vitro and in vivo [2]. There are only a few areas of physiotherapy that are so controversial in the medical community as this therapy. Many people refer to it only as an alternative therapy, while others see it as a treatment for a number of conditions. One reason for this is that prominent medical journals publish articles expressing completely opposed positions on the effects of magnetic therapy used in a specific indication. (Pulsed electromagnetic field generators use different signal formats, so they produce different effects. Identical impulse format is for this therapy what identical active substance is for medicines.) There are many data available for both ultrasound and TENS as conventional physical therapies; however, these evidences are not convincing [3, 4]. As regards electromagnetic therapies, pulsed magnetic therapy is widely used, unlike therapy in static magnetic fields. In the case of pulsed electromagnetic field (PEMF), a number of different frequency ranges can be used. One of the assumed mechanisms of action of the electromagnetic field is the ion cyclotron resonance effect, through the modulation of ion bindings, an effect on free radicals, and an effect on heat shock proteins.The beneficial effect on angiogenesis may play a role in the facilitation of callus formation [5]. PST (Pulsed Signal Therapy) is different from PEMF as PST is an extended version of PEMF, whose beneficial effects on human chondrocytes were confirmed by in vitro studies [6]. Moreover, PEMF also has a chondroprotective effect [7]. BEMER (Bio-Electro-Magnetic-Energy-Regulation) devices operate with special parameters, and the "weak" magnetic field is only a vehicle and a special pulsed signal was developed to this end (BEMERsignal), the primary effect of which is an improvement in tissue microcirculation.

In contrast to the known magnetic field wave patterns that can easily be described by mathematical formulae, the BEMER therapy developed by J. Klopp essentially applies the specifically developed

BEMER signal patterns. As a result, a significant increase in the vasomotion of microvessels, arteriovenous pO2 difference, number of open capillaries, arteriolar and venular flow volume, and flow rate of red blood cells is observed in a specific microcirculatory area. This change in the microcirculation status was demonstrated by combining high-resolution intravital microscopy, computer image processing, and measurement of microflow rate using laser reflection spectroscopy [8, 9]. BEMER devices generate a maximum magnetic induction of 100–150 µT; for comparison, the magnetic field of Earth in Budapest is approximately 47-48 µT.

Treatment time is usually 20 minutes a day (depending on the applicator) for 3-4 weeks depending on the diagnosis. Improvement of microcirculation and reducing fatigue are the clinical applications that have so far been confirmed.

Aim of the study was to evaluate the effect of adjuvant BEMERtherapy on pain, fatigue, and quality of life in patients with knee arthrosis and chronic low back pain. The primary outcomes were to assess the effect of BEMER therapy on knee and low back pain caused by degenerative changes. The secondary outcomes were to evaluate the adverse effects and to record the changes in fatigue and to investigate the effect on quality of life.

2. Materials and Methods

2.1. Study Design. This is a single-centre, randomized, placebo-controlled, double blind follow-up study. A total of 50 patients with chronic low back pain and 50 patients with knee arthrosis were enrolled in this study who had been hospitalized for 3 weeks at the Rheumatologic Rehabilitation Department of the Hospitaller Brothers of St. John of God.

2.1.1. Ethics. The patients signed an Informed Consent Form before the study. The study was approved by the Ethics Committee.

2.1.2. Procedure. In addition to complex standard physiotherapy, half of the patients also received additional BEMER therapy, while the other half received additional placebo BEMER therapy; patients could not tell the placebo treatment from the real treatment. Randomisation was conducted by an independent person (by means of drawing lots). During this study, neither the study doctor nor patients or study assistants knew the treatment given. Unblinding took place only after study completion.

2.1.3. Participations. Demographics: average age was 67.29 years ± 5.44 years (males) and 66.7 years ± 7.73 years (females) in patients with chronic low back pain and 67.11 years ± 8.8 years (males) and 65.3 years ± 7.46 years (females) in patients with osteoarthritis of knee; with 2 and 3 exceptions, all patients with chronic lower back pain and with osteoarthritis of knee, respectively, were females. There were no differences in gender and age between the treatment and placebo group.

Inclusion Criteria for Patients with Low Back Pain. These include
  i. patients with chronic nonspecific low back pain with nonseverely reduced mobility;
  ii. males and females of 20 to 80 years of age;
  iii. nonspecific low back pain for at least 12 weeks;
  iv. palpable tenderness of the paravertebral muscles and/or painful limited mobility of the lumbar spine;
  v. low back pain VAS (visual analogue scale) score of at least 30mmon a 100mmvisual analogue scale during exercise;
  vi. the patients have not received systemic or local steroid therapy or physical therapy or balneotherapy, within 2 months prior to the study; physiotherapywas allowed.

Exclusion Criteria for Patients with Low Back Pain. These include

i. acute low back pain;
ii. organic neurological deficit associated with lower back pain;
iii. the underlying cause is likely to be vertebral compression fracture caused by osteoporosis or other factors;
iv. underlying malignancy;
v. pain caused by inflammatory spine conditions;
vi. spondylolisthesis (grade 2 or higher);
vii. pregnancy.

Inclusion Criteria for Patients with Osteoarthritis of Knee. These include
i. males and females of 30 to 80 years of age with mild or moderate knee arthrosis reporting knee pain characteristic of arthrosis for at least 3 months;
ii. diagnosis of knee arthrosis confirmed by imaging meeting ACR (American College of Rheumatology) criteria [10].

Exclusion Criteria for Patients with Osteoarthritis of Knee. These include
i. inflammatory rheumatic conditions;
ii. palpable effusion in the knee;
iii. knee injury within 6 months prior to the study;
iv. intra-articular steroid within 1 month prior to the study;
v. intra-articular hyaluronic acid within 6 months prior to the study;
vi. patients with femoral neuralgia or radiculopathy;
vii. NSAID (nonsteroidal anti-inflammatory drug) therapy or chondroprotective therapy modified within 1 month prior to the treatment;
viii. knee surgery within 6 months;
ix. pregnancy.

Intervention. All patients were administered a standardized physiotherapy package during the study (individual and group exercises (30 minutes): underwater whirlpool massage (10 minutes), TENS therapy on the low back or knee (15 minutes every day), and aquagym (30 minutes every other day)).

In addition to the standard complex physical therapy 50% of the patients received BEMER therapy, whereas 50% received placebo BEMER therapy

Each BEMER session lasted 20 minutes; parameters were using mattress applicator (B. Body Pro): 7–35 microTesla, intensive applicator (B. PAD): 60–100 microTesla, or mattress applicator (B. Body Pro) intensity levels 2-3-4–10, intensive applicator (B. PAD) intensity levels 6-7-8-9-10 and using vascular motion signal configuration (BEMER signal). The device was a BEMER International AG (Liechtenstein) product. Accessories were mattress with therapy unit (B. Body), flexible, intensive, small surface unit (B. PAD) and B. SPOT (intensive point-like unit), and B. LIGHT unit as needed (may be connected to light therapy unit). The B. BOX Professional control units have 10 different levels of intensity and 3 predefined programmes. The intensity levels are applied during the general full body surface treatment according to the basic programme, while programmes P1– P3 are used gradually to achieve the "deep effect" during targeted treatments. Patients in both groups were treated in supine position while receiving B. BODY mattress applicator treatment. Low back pain patients received B. PAD therapy placed in the low back region at the same time as the full body treatment. Knee pain patients had the B. PADapplicator placed on their knees at the same time as the full body treatment. Therapy sessions lasted 20 minutes each with the B. BODY and B. PAD applicator, respectively:

parameters evaluated: pain intensity on a visual analogue scale (VAS) of 10 cm;
General Quality of Life Questionnaire SF 36 [11, 12];
Facit Fatigue Scale (fatigue intensity ranged from 1 to 50) [13];

Oswestry Index for patients with low back pain [14, 15];
WOMAC Index for patients with knee pain [16, 17].

We used the data from only those patients who received at least 12 sessions of treatment (each patient completed 15 sessions).

Study Procedure.

(1) Before starting the therapy, the physician takes a detailed history, performs a physical examination,

(2) At the end of the therapy sessions, the physician examines the patient, administers the abovementioned questionnaires, and asks about the adverse effects.

(3) Follow-up period after 15 weeks (the patient has returned the self-administered WOMAC, Oswestry, and SF36 questionnaires).

2.2. Statistical Analysis. The analyses focused on pairwise comparisons among the two selected study arms based on the intention-to-treat (ITT) principle. The One-Sample Kolmogorov-Smirnov Test was applied for testing normality. Analysis of covariance (ANCOVA) was used with the analgesic as a covariate to measure effectiveness by comparing study arms.Thesignificance level was set at alpha = 0.05 (twotailed). All analyses were carried out using the R-software version 2.9.1 (R Development Core Team, 2009).

3. Results

3.1. Low Back Pain. Of the 25 patients with low back pain, 4 patients (2 cases with acute fever and 2 older patients have misunderstood how to fill out the questionnaires) and 6 patients (2 cases with acute fever and 4 patients had poor compliance) were excluded from the placebo group and the treatment group, respectively, after the second measurement. Of the patients with knee arthrosis, 2 patients (because of gastroenteritis) and 6 patients (2 cases with acute fever and 4 patients whose questionnaires could not be evaluated) were excluded from the placebo group and the treatment group, respectively. No adverse effects were seen. In the group with low back pain, the comparison of the results from the first and second visit showed a significant improvement in resting VAS scores and Fatigue Scale scores and the exercise VAS scores were close to the level of significance, while no changes were found in the Oswestry scores and Quality of Life (see Table 1). Based on the comparison between the first and third measurements, there was no significant change in either value (see Table 2).

3.2. Knee Osteoarthritis. As regards knee complaints, the comparison of the results of the first and second measurements showed no significant improvement in either parameter (moreover, VAS scores were better in the placebo arm) (see Table 3). Based on the comparison of the first and third measurements, scores on the Fatigue Scale improved significantly, just as the vitality score on the Quality of Life scale (see Table 4).There were no changes in medication.

4. Discussion

Preliminary data suggest that BEMER therapy may have a pain-relieving and fatigue-reducing effect in the treatment of chronic low back pain, even in the short term (studies conducted on large patient populations are required to confirm this). However, for long-term improvement, the therapy should be applied for a long period of time (but to prove this, also further examinations are required.). There was no short-term beneficial effect during knee therapy, probably due to the fact that Program P2 should be used instead of Program P3 (as the deep effect is not that pronounced, however, this is only a hypothesis and needs further studies to be demonstrated), although it was effective in the long term. In this study, we used BEMER therapy not as monotherapy but as adjuvant physiotherapy for inpatients. Many studies with pulse electromagnetic field (PEMF) in patients with locomotor diseases have been published. In patients with osteoarthritis of knee, PEMF was administered as adjuvant therapy in a total of 483 patients in 9 studies, which showed an improvement in the total clinical score [18]. Based on 14

TABLE 1: Comparison of values before and after treatment of low back pain.

Dependent variable	Therapy	Descriptive statistics		N	p values of ANCOVA
		Mean	Std. deviation		
Resting VAS diff. Tests 1 and 2	Physio + BEMER	26.84	13.68	19	0.0229
	Physio + placebo	15.00	15.23	21	
Resting VAS rel. Tests 1 and 2	Physio + BEMER	0.55	0.28	18	0.0620
	Physio + placebo	0.35	0.44	18	
Exercise VAS val. diff. Tests 1 and 2	Physio + BEMER	29.79	15.11	19	0.0547
	Physio + placebo	21.33	17.06	21	
Exercise VAS val. rel. Tests 1 and 2	Physio + BEMER	0.44	0.23	18	0.0179
	Physio + placebo	0.30	0.28	20	
Oswestry diff. Tests 1 and 2	Physio + BEMER	9.80	8.16	19	0.6872
	Physio + placebo	9.27	11.72	21	
Oswestry rel. Tests 1 and 2	Physio + BEMER	0.24	0.18	18	0.8190
	Physio + placebo	0.21	0.28	20	
Fatigue GFI diff. Tests 1 and 2	Physio + BEMER	12.40	9.53	9	0.0218
	Physio + placebo	6.71	9.22	9	
Fatigue GFI rel. Tests 1 and 2	Physio + BEMER	0.32	0.28	8	0.0153
	Physio + placebo	0.22	0.23	7	
Physical functioning nbs diff. Tests 1 and 2	Physio + BEMER	−3.45	3.17	15	0.4952
	Physio + placebo	−3.15	6.95	14	
Physical functioning nbs rel. Tests 1 and 2	Physio + BEMER	−0.10	0.10	14	0.5188
	Physio + placebo	−0.09	0.22	13	
Role physical nbs diff. Tests 1 and 2	Physio + BEMER	−13.17	14.35	15	0.7722
	Physio + placebo	−8.42	14.84	16	
Role physical nbs rel. Tests 1 and 2	Physio + BEMER	−0.49	0.63	14	0.8037
	Physio + placebo	−0.37	0.59	15	
Bodily pain nbs diff. Tests 1 and 2	Physio + BEMER	−14.57	9.75	15	0.1431
	Physio + placebo	−7.68	8.05	19	
Bodily pain nbs rel. Tests 1 and 2	Physio + BEMER	−0.44	0.36	14	0.2485
	Physio + placebo	−0.24	0.25	18	
General Heath nbs diff. Tests 1 and 2	Physio + BEMER	−2.81	8.23	12	0.9361
	Physio + placebo	−2.74	6.06	17	
General Heath nbs rel. Tests 1 and 2	Physio + BEMER	−0.09	0.27	11	0.9707
	Physio + placebo	−0.10	0.20	16	
Vitality nbs diff. Tests 1 and 2	Physio + BEMER	−7.92	6.86	12	0.6338
	Physio + placebo	−5.01	5.05	16	
Vitality nbs rel. Tests 1 and 2	Physio + BEMER	−0.20	0.20	11	0.6240
	Physio + placebo	−0.12	0.13	15	
Social functioning nbs. diff. Tests 1 and 2	Physio + BEMER	−7.33	8.59	13	0.7860
	Physio + placebo	−4.75	9.37	19	
Social functioning nbs. rel. Tests 1 and 2	Physio + BEMER	−0.23	0.28	13	0.8866
	Physio + placebo	−0.17	0.34	18	
Role emotional nbs diff. Tests 1 and 2	Physio + BEMER	−12.93	17.67	14	0.3680
	Physio + placebo	−7.84	14.36	16	
Role emotional nbs rel. Tests 1 and 2	Physio + BEMER	−0.62	1.07	13	0.4572
	Physio + placebo	−0.41	0.89	15	
Mental health nbs diff. Tests 1 and 2	Physio + BEMER	−8.28	8.77	12	0.5300
	Physio + placebo	−6.05	8.85	16	
Mental health nbs rel. Tests 1 and 2	Physio + BEMER	−0.22	0.28	11	0.9709
	Physio + placebo	−0.17	0.31	15	
Physical component summary diff. Tests 1 and 2	Physio + BEMER	−4.99	4.45	7	0.1974
	Physio + placebo	−6.04	9.23	12	
Physical component summary rel. Tests 1 and 2	Physio + BEMER	−0.14	0.13	7	0.1514
	Physio + placebo	−0.22	0.34	11	
Mental component summary diff. Tests 1 and 2	Physio + BEMER	−7.82	11.09	7	0.6788
	Physio + placebo	−5.38	8.76	12	
Mental component summary rel. Tests 1 and 2	Physio + BEMER	−0.26	0.42	7	0.6899
	Physio + placebo	−0.16	0.27	11	

TABLE 2: Comparison of values before and 3 months after treatment of low back pain.

Dependent variable	Therapy	Mean	Std. deviation	N	p values of ANCOVA
Resting VAS diff. Tests 1 and 3	Physio + BEMER	15.94	22.98	18	0.7766
	Physio + placebo	8.74	17.38	19	
Exercise VAS val. diff. Tests 1 and 3	Physio + BEMER	15.44	22.67	18	0.6571
	Physio + placebo	11.26	20.90	19	
Oswestry diff. Tests 1 and 3	Physio + BEMER	5.87	9.91	18	0.9773
	Physio + placebo	4.68	14.74	18	
Fatigue GFI diff. Tests 1 and 3	Physio + BEMER	5.04	9.84	13	0.5316
	Physio + placebo	2.80	7.96	12	
Physical functioning nbs diff. Tests 1 and 3	Physio + BEMER	−1.18	5.66	13	0.4034
	Physio + placebo	−1.03	4.11	13	
Role physical nbs diff. Tests 1 and 3	Physio + BEMER	−4.49	11.55	14	0.4105
	Physio + placebo	0.64	10.25	14	
Bodily pain nbs diff. Tests 1 and 3	Physio + BEMER	−6.45	6.28	15	0.1099
	Physio + placebo	−2.44	7.93	18	
General heath nbs diff. Tests 1 and 3	Physio + BEMER	−3.57	4.24	12	0.9441
	Physio + placebo	−2.17	5.57	14	
Vitality nbs diff. Tests 1 and 3	Physio + BEMER	−5.35	6.54	10	0.7085
	Physio + placebo	0.25	6.64	12	
Social functioning nbs. diff. Tests 1 and 3	Physio + BEMER	−1.54	10.11	13	0.6081
	Physio + placebo	−0.56	10.30	18	
Role emotional nbs diff. Tests 1 and 3	Physio + BEMER	−5.36	19.31	13	0.2712
	Physio + placebo	−1.86	14.76	15	
Mental health nbs diff. Tests 1 and 3	Physio + BEMER	−4.36	7.28	9	0.9854
	Physio + placebo	−3.84	7.84	15	
Physical component summary diff. Tests 1 and 3	Physio + BEMER	−2.99	5.57	6	0.9299
	Physio + placebo	−2.06	5.05	10	
Mental component summary diff. Tests 1 and 3	Physio + BEMER	−9.97	2.68	6	0.4874
	Physio + placebo	−1.31	10.13	10	

studies included in another review article, significant improvement in knee arthritis was seen after 8 weeks as compared to patients receiving placebo [19]. Turkish authors administered PEMF therapy in addition to ultrasound treatment and physiotherapy, but there was no difference between the two groups (thosewho received PEMF as adjuvant therapy and those who received no additional PEMF therapy) [20]. In patients with osteoarthritis of knee, a static magnetic knee protector with a field of 35mT was used for 12 weeks (placebo-controlled study). There were no differences between the two groups in the outcome parameters [21]. In a double blind controlled study conducted in patients with fibromyalgia, although the number of cases was limited, a significant pain-relieving effect was confirmed following treatment with a weak electromagnetic field [22]. Hungarian authors studied thirty patients with obliterative vascular disease of the lower limb.They measured pain-free and maximum walking distance using a treadmill. After the placebo period, the patients were administered 8 sessions of BEMER physical vascular therapy, then i.v. pentoxiphylline therapy. Pain-free and maximum walking distance was measured after each session of therapy. As a result of BEMER physical vascular therapy, pain-free and maximum walking distance increased by 57.4%. Combined therapy (BEMER physical vascular therapy + rheological therapy) increased the measured values by 81.9% and 84.0%, respectively. Combined therapy led to a significant improvement in the walking distance as compared to the pretherapy level [23]. According to a double blind controlled study, BEMER therapy (2 × 8 minutes for 12 weeks) alleviated fatigue in patients with multiple sclerosis; subsequently, a 3-year open-label trial confirmed the long-term effect [24, 25]. A double blind study involving musculoskeletal patients was first published in 2009 [26].

TABLE 3: Comparison of values before and after treatment of knee osteoarthritis.

Dependent variable	Therapy	Descriptive statistics			p values of ANCOVA
		Mean	Std. deviation	N	
Resting VAS diff. Tests 1 and 2	Physio + BEMER	15.94	15.67	18	0.9901
	Physio + placebo	20.58	26.68	24	
Exercise VAS val. diff. Tests 1 and 2	Physio + BEMER	18.22	17.17	18	0.3630
	Physio + placebo	25.79	21.55	24	
Fatigue GFI diff. Tests 1 and 2	Physio + BEMER	6.03	6.08	10	0.4270
	Physio + placebo	4.96	9.57	7	
Physical functioning nbs diff. Tests 1 and 2	Physio + BEMER	−2.76	5.25	9	0.6392
	Physio + placebo	−3.83	6.20	17	
Role physical nbs diff. Tests 1 and 2	Physio + BEMER	−13.47	13.53	14	0.7978
	Physio + placebo	−9.48	15.85	18	
Bodily pain nbs diff. Tests 1 and 2	Physio + BEMER	−6.97	6.35	17	0.7382
	Physio + placebo	−6.59	6.04	17	
General heath nbs diff. Tests 1 and 2	Physio + BEMER	−2.96	4.19	13	0.2222
	Physio + placebo	−0.95	3.36	13	
Vitality nbs diff. Tests 1 and 2	Physio + BEMER	−7.64	11.28	14	0.0788
	Physio + placebo	−2.38	9.81	20	
Social functioning nbs diff. Tests 1 and 2	Physio + BEMER	−8.15	10.50	16	0.2459
	Physio + placebo	−5.90	11.92	17	
Role emotional nbs diff. Tests 1 and 2	Physio + BEMER	−13.93	19.70	15	0.8289
	Physio + placebo	−7.96	19.48	14	
Mental health nbs diff. Tests 1 and 2	Physio + BEMER	−5.45	11.67	12	0.9227
	Physio + placebo	−3.72	8.51	19	
Physical component summary diff. Tests 1 and 2	Physio + BEMER	−2.65	4.30	6	0.8054
	Physio + placebo	−5.86	7.68	7	
Mental component summary diff. Tests 1 and 2	Physio + BEMER	−11.58	18.21	6	0.4531
	Physio + placebo	−4.96	7.78	7	
WOMAC "A" diff. 1-2	Physio + BEMER	20.11	19.26	17	0.9221
	Physio + placebo	17.81	17.51	24	
WOMAC "B" diff. 1-2	Physio + BEMER	15.78	18.41	16	0.7126
	Physio + placebo	14.21	20.91	24	
WOMAC "C" diff. 1-2	Physio + BEMER	10.87	15.48	17	0.9848
	Physio + placebo	15.16	14.94	24	
WOMAC total diff. 1-2	Physio + BEMER	13.46	15.10	17	0.8817
	Physio + placebo	15.00	13.83	24	

4.1. Limitations of the Study. This is a pilot study. Unfortunately, many of the patients failed to return or misunderstood how to fill out the questionnaires during the three-month period for returning them, which led to a decrease in the number of cases. Furthermore, the Fatigue Scale includes many questions that are uncharacteristic of inpatients and can be evaluated only in outpatients: if, for example, a patient fails to answer Questions 2, 3, and 4, the entire questionnaire will be unevaluable (the software will ignore it). Some patients failed to completely fill out the SF 36 and the Fatigue Scale because they did not perform a specific physical activity during hospitalization. In the case of SF 36, patients failed to answer 1 or 2 questions in a number of item groups. They either did not understand the questions or were not allowed to perform a specific activity. Unfortunately, these cases also led to worse results because more significant improvements would have been possible in many cases in a larger study population.

TABLE 4: Comparison of values before and 3 months after treatment of knee osteoarthritis.

Dependent variable	Therapy	Descriptive statistics			p values of ANCOVA
		Mean	Std. deviation	N	
Resting VAS diff. Tests 1 and 3	Physio + BEMER	13.03	25.03	20	0.6565
	Physio + placebo	12.2	24.99	20	
Exercise VAS val. diff. Tests 1 and 3	Physio + BEMER	14.85	19.81	20	0.6760
	Physio + placebo	13.30	24.59	20	
Fatigue GFI diff. Tests 1 and 3	Physio + BEMER	4.22	8.54	16	0.0235
	Physio + placebo	−3.30	8.52	11	
Physical functioning nbs diff. Tests 1 and 3	Physio + BEMER	−2.27	6.49	16	0.8051
	Physio + placebo	−3.68	6.96	13	
Role physical nbs diff. Tests 1 and 3	Physio + BEMER	−1.89	13.91	19	0.8724
	Physio + placebo	−5.28	13.50	17	
Bodily pain nbs diff. Tests 1 and 3	Physio + BEMER	−6.41	8.90	18	0.3015
	Physio + placebo	−3.38	6.08	18	
General heath nbs diff. Tests 1 and 3	Physio + BEMER	−5.12	8.08	18	0.4666
	Physio + placebo	−1.43	3.69	12	
Vitality nbs diff. Tests 1 and 3	Physio + BEMER	−5.78	8.61	18	0.0079
	Physio + placebo	2.55	6.98	14	
Social functioning nbs. diff. Tests 1 and 3	Physio + BEMER	−1.47	10.45	17	0.5787
	Physio + placebo	−0.30	11.14	17	
Role emotional nbs diff. Tests 1 and 3	Physio + BEMER	−6.55	13.14	17	0.0371
	Physio + placebo	−1.74	15.98	16	
Mental health nbs diff. Tests 1 and 3	Physio + BEMER	−3.76	12.16	16	0.1842
	Physio + placebo	5.67	8.63	12	
Physical component summary diff. Tests 1 and 3	Physio + BEMER	−4.50	12.57	12	0.6942
	Physio + placebo	−3.20	4.22	5	
Mental component summary diff. Tests 1 and 3	Physio + BEMER	−6.41	11.74	12	0.1940
	Physio + placebo	2.47	11.81	5	
WOMAC "A" diff. 1-3	Physio + BEMER	11.55	18.26	20	0.7254
	Physio + placebo	12.53	21.92	18	
WOMAC "B" diff. 1-3	Physio + BEMER	9.60	21.21	20	0.3888
	Physio + placebo	13.44	31.24	18	
WOMAC "C" diff. 1-3	Physio + BEMER	8.98	20.77	20	0.7020
	Physio + placebo	8.51	21.09	18	
WOMAC total diff. 1-3	Physio + BEMER	8.45	17.92	20	0.4711
	Physio + placebo	10.15	18.97	18	

5. Conclusions

Our study suggests the possibility that BEMER therapy administered in combination with traditional physiotherapy procedures reduces chronic lower back pain in the short term and may be effective in the long-term treatment of patients with osteoarthritis of knee. However, well-performed studies with a larger sample size are required for a more exact evaluation of the abovementioned effects.

Abbreviations

PEMF: Pulsed electromagnetic field
BEMER: Physical vascular therapy
WOMAC: TheWestern Ontario and McMaster Universities Arthritis Index
VAS: Visual analogue scale

ACR: American College of Rheumatology.

Conflict of Interests

Devices were made available by BEMER Medical Technic Ltd. for the completion of the study which subsequently were donated to the hospital. Neither the hospital nor the study doctors received any other support in relation to this study.

Authors' Contribution

Each author contributed to the conception and design of the study.

Acknowledgment

The authors thank Lajos Katona for performing the statistical analysis.

References

[1] M. S. Markov, "Expanding use of pulsed electromagnetic field therapies," Electromagnetic Biology & Medicine, vol. 26, no. 3, pp. 257–274, 2007.

[2] C. A. Bassett, "The development and application of pulsed electromagnetic fields (PEMFs) for ununited fractures and arthrodeses," Orthopedic Clinics of North America, vol. 15, no. 1, pp. 61–87, 1984.

[3] S. Ebadi, N. Henschke, N. Nakhostin Ansari, E. Fallah, and M. W. van Tulder, "Therapeutic ultrasound for chronic low-back pain," Cochrane Database of Systematic Reviews, vol. 3, Article ID CD009169, 2014.

[4] T. E. McAlindon, R. R. Bannuru, M. C. Sullivan et al., "OARSI guidelines for the non-surgical management of knee osteoarthritis," Osteoarthritis and Cartilage, vol. 22, no. 3, pp. 363–388, 2014.

[5] S. D. Monache, A. Angelucci, P. Sanit`a et al., "Inhibition of angiogenesis mediated by extremely low-frequency magnetic fields (ELF-MFs)," PLoS ONE, vol. 8, no. 11, Article ID e79309, 2013.

[6] A. Fioravanti, F. Nerucci, G. Collodel, R. Markoll, and R. Marcolongo, "Biochemical and morphological study of human articular chondrocytes cultivated in the presence of pulsed signal therapy," Annals of the Rheumatic Diseases, vol. 61, no. 11, pp. 1032–1033, 2002.

[7] A. Ongaro, A. Pellati, F. F. Masieri et al., "Chondroprotective effects of pulsed electromagnetic fields on human cartilage explants," Bioelectromagnetics, vol. 32, no. 7, pp. 543–551, 2011.

[8] R. C. Klopp, W. Niemer, and W. Schmidt, "Effects of various physical treatment methods on arteriolar vasomotion and microhemodynamic functional characteristics in case of deficient regulation of organ blood flow. Results of a placebocontrolled, double-blind study," Journal of Complementary & Integrative Medicine, vol. 10, pp. S39–S41, 2013.

[9] R. C. Klopp, W. Niemer, and J. Schulz, "Complementarytherapeutic stimulation of deficient autorhythmic arteriolar vasomotion by means of a biorhythmically physical stimulus on the microcirculation and the immune system in 50-year-old rehabilitation patients," Journal of Complementary & Integrative Medicine, vol. 10, pp. S29–S37, 2013.

[10] R. D. Altman, M. C. Hochberg, R. W. Moskowitz, and T. J. Schnitzer, "Recommendations for the medical management of osteoarthritis of the hip and knee: 2000 update," Arthritis & Rheumatism, vol. 43, no. 9, pp. 1905–1915, 2000.

[11] J. E. Ware Jr. and C. D. Sherbourne, "The MOS 36-item shortform health survey (SF-36). I. Conceptual framework and item selection," Medical Care, vol. 30, no. 6, pp. 473–483, 1992.

[12] A. Czimbalmos, Z. Nagy, and Z. Varga, "P´aciens megel´egedetts ´egi vizsg´alataz SF-36 k´erd˝o´ıvvel, a magyarorsz´agi norm´al´ert ´ekek meghat´aroz´asa," N´epeg´eszs´eg¨ugy, vol. 4, no. 1, pp. 4–19, 1999.

[13] D. Cella and C. J. Nowinski, "Measuring quality of life in chronic illness: the functional assessment of chronic illness therapy measurement system," Archives of Physical Medicine and Rehabilitation, vol. 83, no. 12, supplement, pp. S10–S17, 2002.

[14] B.W. Koes, M. W. van Tulder, and S.Thomas, "Diagnosis and treatment of lowback pain," BritishMedical Journal, vol. 332, no. 7555, pp. 1430–1434, 2006.

[15] G. Ormos, ´A. Czimbalmos, J. Csiki, P. Huszt´ak, and C. S. Szab´o, "K´et der´ekf´aj´asspecifikus ´allapot felm´er˝os index hazai valid´al´asa," Rehabilit´aci´o, vol. 24, no. 2-3, pp. 65–68, 2014.

[16] N. Bellamy, W. W. Buchanan, C. H. Goldsmith, J. Campbell, and L. W. Stitt, "Validation study of WOMAC: a health status instrument for measuring clinically important patient relevant outcomes to antirheumatic drug therapy in patients with osteoarthritis of the hip or knee," Journal of Rheumatology, vol. 15, no. 12, pp. 1833–1840, 1988.

[17] P. M´arta, G. Gy¨orgy, P. Attil´an´e, and R. Istv´an, "A WOMAC VA3.0 index magyar verzi´oj´anak vizsg´alata t´erd- ´es cs´ıp˝oarthrosisos betegeken," Magyar Reumatol´ogia, vol. 40, pp. 94–97, 1999.

[18] P.Vavken, F. Arrich, O. Schuhfried, and R. Dorotka, "Effectiveness of pulsed electromagnetic field therapy in themanagement of osteoarthritis of the knee: a meta-analysis of randomized controlled trials," Journal of Rehabilitation Medicine, vol. 41, no. 6, pp. 406–411, 2009.

[19] S. R. We, Y. H. Koog, K.-I. Jeong, and H. Wi, "Effects of pulsed electromagnetic field on knee osteoarthritis: a systematic review," Rheumatology, vol. 52, no. 5, pp. 815–824, 2013.

[20] E. Ozgüclü, A. Cetin, M. Cetin, and E. Calp, "Additional effect of pulsed electromagnetic field therapy on knee osteoarthritis treatment: a randomized, placebo-controlled study," Clinical Rheumatology, vol. 29, no. 8, pp. 927–931, 2010.

[21] C.-Y. Chen, T.-C. Fu, C.-F.Hu, C.-C.Hsu, C.-L. Chen, and C.-K. Chen, "Influence of magnetic knee wraps on joint proprioception in individuals with osteoarthritis: a randomized controlled pilot trial," Clinical Rehabilitation, vol. 25, no. 3, pp. 228–237, 2011.

[22] A. W. Thomas, K. Graham, F. S. Prato et al., "A randomized, double-blind, placebo-controlled clinical trial using a lowfrequency magnetic field in the treatment of musculoskeletal chronic pain," Pain Research andManagement, vol. 12, no. 4, pp. 249–258, 2007.

[23] S. I. Bern'at, "Effectiveness of pentoxifylline and of bioelectromagnetic therapy in lower limb obliterative arterial disease," Orvosi Hetilap, vol. 154, no. 42, pp. 1674–1679, 2013.

[24] J. Piatkowski, S. Kern, and T. J. Ziemssen, "Effect of BEMER magnetic field therapy on the level of fatigue in patients with multiple sclerosis: a randomized, double-blind controlled trial," Journal of Alternative and ComplementaryMedicine, vol. 15, no. 5, pp. 507–511, 2009.

[25] J. Piatkowski, R. Haase, and T. Ziemssen, "Long-term effects of Bio-electromagnetic-energyregulation therapy on fatigue in patients withmultiple sclerosis," AlternativeTherapies in Health and Medicine, vol. 17, no. 6, pp. 22–28, 2011.

[26] G. Bernatzky, W. Kullich, F. Aglas et al., "Elektro-magnetische Felder bei Patienten mit chronischen R¨uckenschmerzen (lowback pain): Eine doppelblinde randomisierte Duo-Center- Studie," Schweizerische Zeitschrift f¨ur Ganzheitsmedizin, vol. 21, no. 3, pp. 149–156, 2009.

BEMER Therapy Applied in Neurology

Treatment of Stroke and Motor Neurone Disease with BEMER Therapy

Dr. Terezia Szemerszki, Specialist for Neurology

SUMMARY: The efficacy of traditional therapy can be improved to a significant extent by applying the BEMER treatment. Applied in the acute phase, the treatment promotes the reduction in secondary damage caused by intracranial pressure by optimizing metabolism in the nerve cells and reducing the temporary diffuse or circumscribed edema caused by the disease.

Stroke is the third most common cause of death globally, including in developed countries, and the major cause of disabilities. In 90% of cases, the brain mass is damaged by vasospasm and hemorrhaging occurs in 10% of cases. When a strokes occurs, the entire area of the brain where deficits occur does not die immediately, but the functionality of "penumbral" or "sleeping" areas can still be saved by applying relevant methods. The efficacy of traditional therapy can be improved to a significant extent by applying the BEMER treatment. Applied in the acute phase, the treatment promotes the reduction in secondary damage caused by intracranial pressure by optimizing metabolism in the nerve cells and reducing the temporary diffuse or circumscribed edema caused by the disease.

As neurologist and a physician performing Carotid ultrasound, I see many acute and chronic patients. I learned of the BEMER therapy 4 years ago and since then I have been using it successfully and with conviction to treat my patients. I would like to present some cases.

A.D. The 15-year-old boy was intubated by emergency services after a night out and brought in to traumatology with a peripheral venous catheter after collapsing at home in a state of shock. Consumption of illegal drugs could not be confirmed or ruled out. He had no external cuts and his pupils were constricted. His left limbs were lame and there was only a sluggish reaction to pain stimulus in his right limbs. The urgent cranial CT identified no issues other than the cerebral edema, so he was taken to the neurology toxicology department. In the evening, brain stem symptoms were identified (partial vertical nystagmus). The control cranial CT the next day found extensive malacia in the brain stem (pons) and 10 mm malacia in the cerebellum carotid without UH deviation. Cranial MR and MR angiography, in addition to the previous deviation, confirmed closure of an 8 mm section in front of the basilar origin. On day 3 of treatment, the patient's mother visited and requested BEMER therapy, which we started the next day with the BEMER 3000 PLUS device, 3 times per day (mat 3.10 and PI thereafter, cushion P4 under the head). He initially became more awake, opened his eyes spontaneously and on request, then began to move independently, first the upper right and then the lower left body. The breathing and feeding tubes were removed at the end of week 4. Swallowing improved gradually. The patient developed good comprehension even in the presence of motor aphasia.

S.C. The 46-year-old man was brought into the neurology department having suffered from severe headaches for 1 week that were not responding to aspirin and with vomiting caused by impaired vision. On admission, he had no neurological signs of focal abnormality. The urgent cranial CT indicated no deviation, but the blood content of the liquor taken from a lumbar puncture indicated subarachnoid hemorrhage. Cranial MR and MR angiography showed two small aneurysms in the anterior communicating artery. The change was treated with the endovascular procedure in the neurosurgery department. Thereafter, worsening clouded awareness developed in addition to the rear head binding and the response to pain stimulus was only sluggish in the limbs. The cranial CT did not detect hemorrhage and the two anterior cerebral arteries indicated local circulatory disturbance. An MRSA infection worsened the patient's condition further and bedsores developed. After improvement following rehabilitation treatment, he was discharged home, though he was not able to move his lower limbs or control feces/urine. Treatment with BEMER Classic started in month 7 after the onset of his illness (mat 3 and P1 in week 1, then mat 3 and P1 from week 2, mat 4 and P1 from week 3, and cushion P3 for shoulder pain). In week 2 of treatment, he was able to control feces/urine during the day and, in week 3, he was able to bend his legs well. In week 4 he was able to raise his legs from the hip.

Amyotrophic lateral sclerosis (ALS), which is caused by the death of the central motor neurons, is a rare progressive disease that currently has no known cure. The symptoms are atrophy and weakening of the musculature, first in typical areas, then over the entire body, as well as involuntary muscle twitching, followed by difficulty swallowing and breathing.

L.Z. A 55-year-old male patient treated since early childhood for schizophrenia and Parkinson's disease. His mother noticed around a year ago that he was holding his pen and spoon strangely. She did not consider the change to be significant because of his underlying illness. For several months thereafter, however, he increasingly asked for help doing up his shirt and tying his shoelaces.

Observation status: Soft musculature over entire body. Loss of muscle on both sides between the 1st and 2nd finger of each hand and in the pectoral girdles. Small, frequent muscle twitching in the pectoral girdle muscles. Clutching and holding ability of the hand is becoming weaker and weaker.

No deviation in laboratory findings. Cranium and cervical spine display no MR deviation. ENG test confirmed motor neuron disease. We started treatment using the BEMER Professional device with the patient as out-patient 3-4 times per week (mat PI and 1). After 2 weeks of therapy, his mother reported that he was no longer urinating overnight. After 2 months of treatment – muscle mass and atrophy visibly remained unchanged – gripping strength was reported in the right hand, the patient's appetite improved and his anxiety levels fell.

Lecture at the BEMER Budapest Congress 2007

More Recent Therapy Modalities for Delayed Speech Development

Dr. med. Szabolcs M. Horváth CSc; Chief Medical Officer, St. Rókus Hospital, Department of Neurology
Dr. med. Csaba Pogány, Assistant Medical Officer

SUMMARY: BEMER treatment resulted in significant clinical improvement in 66.6% of patients studied. The positive change was moderate in 14.8% and no improvement could be measured in 19.2% of cases.

BEMER Therapy Applied in Orthopedics

Support and Movement Apparatus

Kafka W, Schütze N, Walther M; Orthopädische Praxis 41; 1(2005):23-25

SUMMARY: *The focus of this work was to review (in vitro) the influence of molecular regulatory mechanisms of human osteoblasts by special, extremely low frequency (BEMER-type) pulsed low-energy electromagnetic fields based on differential gene expression analyses. Automated micro-titer luminometric ATP tests show that the rate of proliferation after only 3 days of incubation (5 stimulations at time intervals of 12 hours, each lasting for 8 minutes) was significantly enhanced up to five fold for those probes. The product osteoblast cell material obtained from this incubation was used for RNA isolation for subsequent differential analysis of the up-and down-regulated protein production using gene chip analysis. Interestingly no differences were found referring to Cancer related oncogen expressions. Currently performed Polymerase Chain Reactions (PCR) analyses fully support these findings.*

The studies can thus help to better understand the therapeutic success already achieved elsewhere using the BEMER 3000 system based on its form, which is used here and to optimize its use particularly in orthopedics (e.g. osteoporosis or bone healing) as well.

Offizielles Organ der Vereinigung Süddeutschland Orthopäden e.V. [Official Organ of the Association of Southern German Orthopaedists]

Editorship
Prof. Dr Siebert, Kassel
Priv.-Doz. Dr. Stein, Magdeburg Prof. Dr. Rossak, Karlsruhe Publisher
Dr. Clemens, Karlsruhe Prof. Dr. Rompe, Heidelberg
Einsatz extrem niederfrequent (BEMER-typisch) gepulster schwacher elektro-- magnetischer Felder im Bereich der Orthopädie [Application of Extreme Low Frequent (BEMER-type) Pulsed Electromagnetic Fields in Orthopaedics]
Issue 1. January 2005 41st year, ISSN 0030 S88X Orthopädische Praxis 41. 1 (200S) Medizinisch Literarische Verlagsgesellschaft MHB Uelzen

Introduction
Different individual observations and reports from the literature (1-10) suggest that the biological effect of electromagnetic field effects result from the influence of molecular regulatory mechanisms (7, 8). These effects be objectified by the use of extremely low frequency (BEMER-type) pulsed, low- energy electromagnetic fields (Fig. 1) in (in vitro) genesis of human osteoblasts through proliferation and DNA GeneChip analyses. The study should also provide clues in detail as to in which clinical areas further studies on therapeutic application of this special form of electromagnetic stimulation appear useful (e.g. osteoporosis, fracture healing). Under the influence of these electromagnetic fields, osteoblast cell material should be initially obtained for RNA isolation for the study of differential gene expression for reviewing up-and down-regulations. A further review of the results of the test chip based on the polymerase chain reaction is currently underway. So far, this has not led to any different results.

Material and method
The studies on proliferation were performed (by control) in breeder reactors suitably equipped for electromagnetic stimulation. Electromagnetic stimulation was carried out immediately after incubation in the three consecutive days, with breaks of 12 hours each, five times for a duration of 8 hours each via a

specially controlled oval (approx. 48/42 cm) flat coil (INNOMED International AG. FL-Triesen, pulse rate 30 Hz) with an average maximum flux density of up to 100 micro tesla that is dependent on the given sample positioning, Fig. 1, 2). The proliferation rates were determined by means of an automatic, microtiter-supported, luminometric ATP test.

RNA extraction was carried out for chip analysis immediately after the last stimulation. In the case of GeneChip analysis, it allows simultaneous acquisition of about 15,000 genes (Altymetrix system; hybridization by color- labeled RNA) – only samples positioned in the region of maximum flux density were taken. – The selection of the primers for the subsequent PCR was based on results from the GeneChip analysis. Orthopädische Praxis 41.1 (2005)

Results
Proliferation: With respect to control, significant increases in proliferation rates with increasing flux density (but with high clamping width) resulted after a relatively short time by up to five times in the region of maximum average flux density (Tab. I), GenChip

Analysis: The GeneChip analysis revealed significant changes for the up-and down-regulations of gene products for the samples positioned in the region of maximum flux density. They are summarized in Table II along with their biochemical functions.

Conclusion
It can be assumed that the DNA GeneChip analyses provide important insights into the underlying mechanisms of action. The studies can help to better understand the widely achieved success of therapeutic application – especially with the BEMER 3000 system used here – (2) based on its form and to optimize its therapeutic aims in orthopedics as well (e.g. osteoporosis, fracture healing). Regarding the unaffected oncogene activities, these studies contribute significantly to refuting the concern about the carcinogenicity of electromagnetic fields used in this therapy linked fourfold to increased rates of proliferation.

Tab. I: Osteoblasts - GeneChip analysis, electromagnetically indexed up-and down-regulation of gene expression.

Up Regulation	Function
Intersection 2	Protein Transport
Core promoter element binding protein	Transcription factor
Solute carrier family 16. Member 7	Monocarboxylic acid transporter
Myosin VI	Vesicle and organelle transport
Chemokine (C-X-C mottif) lignad 12	Stomal stop signal factor
Chloride channel 4	Ion channel
Osteoprotegerin	Signal factor
ring finger protein (C3H2C3 type) 6	Transcription factor
hypothetical protein FLI21106	unknown
Down Regulation	
karyopherin beta 2b transportin	RNA transport
ras homolog gene family, member 1	G-Protein, Signal transduction
amine oxidase, copper containing 2	Metabolism
hypothetical gene CG018	unknown

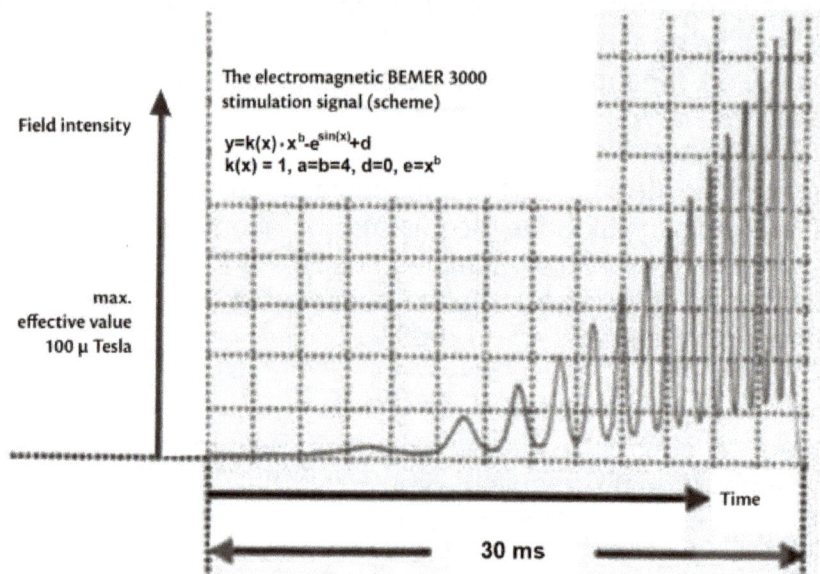

Fig. 1: The BEMER signal masks its peculiarities (After bioelectromagnetic field effects are ultimately always attributed to the influence of molecular interactions and these interactions are essentially dependent on the mass and the charge distribution of the interaction partner (7), a broad-as-possible spectrum of molecular interactions should be addressed by the particularly broadband BEMER signal with respect to the conventional (so-called narrow- band direct field or sinusoidal, trapezoidal and sawtooth) stimuli (BEMER = Bio-Electro-Magnetic Energy Regulation).

0 cm vertkaler Abstand zur Spulenmade											
0	2	6	56	67	15	24	36	24		3	0
2	9	25	105	80	80	60	0	28	29	13	4	0
0	2	5	80		79	80	68	39	25	23	8	0
4	8	24	5	39	88	88	84	94	59	18	5	0
0	4	14	26	19	40	79	99	106	71		3	0
0	3	7	12	20	26	7	29	41	9	18	4	0
0	1	8	7	10	15	21		15	18	11	2	0
0	0	0	0		0	0	0	0	0	0	0

Fig. 2: Sample positioning on the field coil (scheme). Figures: average max. flux density in micro tesla.

836	836	836	836	836
836	2922	4814	2489	836
836	1088	1098	2548	836
36	2512	984	1031	836
836	836	836	836	836

Tab. I: Increase in osteoblast proliferation rates by up to a factor of 5 in the areas of maximum flux densities (see Fig. 2).

SUMMARY: The focus of the present work was the (in vitro) verification of the influence of the molecular regulatory mechanisms on human osteoblasts by special, extremely low frequency (BEMER-type) pulsed low-energy electromagnetic fields, which was performed based on differential gene expression analyses. Automated micro-titer plate supported luminometric ATP tests show that the proliferation rate increased significantly by up to 5 times after only 3 days of incubation (a total of 5 days, with an interval of approximately 12 hours each for a period of 8 minutes) for the conducted applications compared to the control. The osteoblast cell material obtained from this incubation was used for RNA isolation for the subsequent differential analysis of the 'up-and down- regulated' protein production by means of gene chip analysis. Interestingly, no differences in the production of cancer-related oncogenes were observed. Ongoing studies based on the polymerase chain reaction (PCR) support the current findings. Thereby, the studies can help to better understand the therapeutic success already achieved elsewhere with the BEMER 3000 System by reason of its form and to optimally use it in orthopedics (e.g., osteoporosis, fracture healing)

Summary

Aimed at gaining information on the bio molecular processes and the Potential applications in orthopedics, the study examines the electromagnetically induced differences in gene expressions. It was performed by methods of (in vitro, thermo controlled incubator) proliferation studies by micro titer luminometric ATP teste and differential (Affymetrics) GenChip analysis.

Referring to bio molecular regulation processes of human osteoblasts the tests were performed by applying specially designed pulsed inhomogeneous electromagnetic fields with a weak and extremely low frequency (BEMER- ELF-PEMS. generated by an electronic device via a 43/42 cm oval flat coil, at pulsrates of 30 Hz and an amplitude-time (y-x) course of one pulse according to: y=x e, with b=sin(x) with a mean magnetic flux intensity up to 100 microTesla). Despite very short stimulation periods of in total merely 40min (5 stimulations at time intervals of 12 hours, each lasting for 8 mm) proliferation rates were enhanced up to five fold tor those probes which were positioned at higher magnetic flux intensities within the coil. Compared to non treated control osteoblasts the latter probes revealed significant differences of gene expressions due to the application of the BEMER-ELF-PEMS as revealed by clear-cut up and down regulations of protein synthesis Interestingly no differences were found referring to Cancer related oncogen expressions. Currently performed Polymerase Cham reactions (PCR) analyses fully support these findings. Aside from enlightening the underlying molecular principles of the BEMER induced widespread therapeutic results, elsewhere reported, these studies might thus initiate promising developmental footsteps of future bio molecular applications e. g. in orthopedics (osteoporosis or bone healing) as well.

Literature

Brighton, W., R Sektes. G Zhang S. R. Pollack: Signal transduction in electrically stimulated bone cells. J. Bone Joint Surg. Am. 83-A (2001) 1514- 1523.
Bohn. W.WA Kafka Energie und Gesundheit BEMER 3000 Bio- Elektro- Magnetische- Energie- Regulation nach Prof. Dr. Wolf A. Kafka. Haug Vertag. Stuttgart (Thieme Verlagsgruppe). ISBN 3-8304-7199 8 (2004) 1-130.
Coyly A., G.E. Ndebele. K. Jenkins, J. J. Thompson. J. Angel Effects of static electromagnetic fields on characteristics of MG-63 osteoblasts grown in culture. Biomed. Sci Instrum. 39 (2003) 454-159.
Diniz N., K. Sbomura, K. Soejima, G. Ito: Effects of pulsed electromagnetic field (PEMF) stimulation on bone tissue like formation are dependent on the maturation stages of the osteoblasts. Bioelectromagnetics 23 (2002) 398-405.
Lohmann, N. , Z. Schwartz, Y. Liu, H. Guerkov, D. D. Dean, B. Simon, B. D. Boyan:

Pulsed electromagnetic field stimulation of MG83 osteoblast-like cells affects differentiation and local factor production J. Orthop. Res. 18 (2000) 637-646.Lohmann, N., Z. Schwartz, Y. Liu, Z. Li, B. J. Simon, V. L. Sylvia, D.

D. Dean, L. F. Bonawald, H. J. Donahue, B. D. Boyan: Pulsed electromagnetic field effect phenotype and connexin 43 protein expression in MLO-Y4 osteocyte-like cells and ROS 17/2.8 osteoblast-like cells. J. Orthop. Res. 21 (2003) 326-334.

Kafka, W. A.: Extremely low, wide frequency range pulsed electromagnetic fields tor therapeutical use Emphyspace. 2 (2000) 1-20.

Kafka, W. A., K. Spodaryk: The influence of extremely weak, BEMER 3000 type pulsed, electromagnetic fields on ratings of perceived exertion (RPE) at ventilatory threshold. 8th Congress of EFRR. Ljubljaria, i press, 2004.

Klopp, R.: Forschungsbericht zum vitalmikroskopischen und reflexions- spektrometrischen Nachweis der Verbesserung der humanen Mikrozirkulation unter dem Einfluss BEMER 3000-typisch gepulster elektromagnetischer Felder. Institut für Mikrozirkulation, Berlin, 2004.

Torricelli, F., M. Fini, G. Giavaresi, R. Botter, D. Beruto, R. Giardino: Biomimetic.

PMMA-based bone substitutes: A comparative in vitro evaluation of the effects of pulsed electromagnetic field exposure. J. Biomed. Mater. Res. 64 (2003) 182-188.

Treatment of Various Orthopaedic Diseases with the BEMER 3000 System

Dr. Hans Härtling; Specialist in Orthopaedics

SUMMARY: In summary, we can say that with a treatment time of about 2 to 3 weeks – the length I treated patients on average – the best results, in addition to trauma, were found in radicular and pseudo-radicular diseases. In the "various diseases" group, tendinopathy or bursitis came in first followed by arthritis.

As the BEMER device came on the market in late 1998, I developed a questionnaire with which I particularly wanted to document the impact on the occurrence of pain. In the process, three types of pain were recorded, specifically pain at rest, pressure pain and the stress or movement pain.

Improvement in function was also associated with pain reduction. Local changes to joints such as swelling and effusion were considered as well as concomitant therapy. If possible, the previous therapy was not changed. The patients thus retained their medication. At the beginning and at the end, all patients graded how they originally felt their pain and what success electro- magnetic field treatment brought. In practice, the patients were questioned about their health three to four days if possible and rated this on a scale of 0 - 100 percent was recorded.

Various diagnostic groups were evaluated.

I labelled the first major group as "various diseases", perhaps not a happy name, but it includes a lot of diseases that I did not want to divide into separate categories because of their small number, such as arthrosis, with the exception of knee osteoarthritis, arthritis, diseases of the small joints, arthritis such as polyarthrosis, Heberden arthrosis, Bouchard arthrosis, the abundance of tendomyoses, bursitis, heel spurs, etc.

The second major group was osteoarthritis of the knee. Here I examined 80 patients. The largest group, and also the most successful, were patients with pseudoradicular or radicular pain syndromes, i.e.: Cervical syndromes, cervicobrachial neuralgia, cephalgia, lumbago or lumbo sciatica.

The best results we found in traumas. Here we have a recovery rate or remission of 80 percent. BEMER therapy is therefore indispensable in a traumatology ward or emergency hospital. The other groups still demonstrated shoulder diseases as well as epicondylitis as the smallest group. Here the results were satisfactory. I saw the least success in the case of epicondylitis.

The following must be said about pain assessment: All patients displaying an improvement of more than 70 percent were categorized as symptomless.

Those groups displaying between 30 and 70 percent improvement were categorized as satisfactory and all patients with an improvement of up to 30 percent were categorized as unchanged as this width lies in the placebo- control area.

In summary, we can say that with a treatment time of about 2 to 3 weeks – the length I treated patients on average – the best results, in addition to trauma, were found in radicular and pseudo-radicular diseases. In the "various diseases" group, tendinopathy or bursitis came in first followed by arthritis.

Follow-up examination: The shortest follow-up was 4 months, the longest 18 months after the last treatment. The results were very encouraging even after a treatment-free interval of 1 1/2 years. In general, we can conclude that patients who did not respond well during the treatment to electromagnetic field therapy subsequently showed no improvement.

Application of pulsed electromagnetic fields at very low frequency (BEMER- type) in orthopedic proteomics Markus Walther, Prof. Dr., Centre for Sports Medicine and Foot Surgery, Schön Clinics in Munich.

SUMMARY: The results confirm the results of other analyses carried out using polymerase chain reaction (PCR) that are currently taking place. These studies could therefore lead to other promising steps in future biomolecular applications, for example in orthopaedics (osteoporosis and bone healing), in addition to the clarification of molecular principles that describe the wide range of treatment results accomplished with BEMER therapy (described elsewhere).

It was the aim of this study to obtain information about biomolecular processes and possibilities of their use in therapeutic applications, particularly for orthopaedics; the study explored electromagnetically induced differences in the expression of genes. Methods from proliferation studies (in vitro, incubator with controlled temperature) were used in the study with the use of microtitration luminometric examination of ATP and differential technology (Affymetrix) of the GeneChip analysis. Special pulsed inhomogeneous, weak electromagnetic fields at very low frequency were used to influence biomolecular regulation processes of human osteoblasts.

This concerned BEMER ELF PEMS, which was generated with an electronic device by an oval flat coil with dimensions of 48/42 cm, with a pulse frequency of 30 Hz and an amplitude-time curve (y-x) of a pulse according to: $y = x3c(sinb)$, where $b = sin(x3)$, with an average intensity of magnetic flux density, which amounted to 100 micro tesla).

Even with very short stimulation times that were a total of 40 minutes, (i.e. 5 stimulations at intervals of 12 hours, each lasting 8 minutes), the rate of proliferation of osteoblasts could be accelerated up to five times namely in the probes, which were higher in intensity of the magnetic flux in the coil. In comparison with non-affected control osteoblasts, significant differences in the expression of genes were detected in the above probes, which materialized through the effect of BEMER-ELF-PEMS and manifested themselves in the form of a clear acceleration and deceleration of protein synthesis.

It was interesting that no differences were found in relation to the expression of oncogenes, which are associated with malignant tumors.

These results confirm the results of other analyses carried out using polymerase chain reaction (PCR), which are currently taking place. These studies could therefore lead to other promising steps in future biomolecular applications, for example in orthopaedics (osteoporosis and bone healing), in addition to the clarification of molecular principles that describe the wide range of treatment results accomplished with BEMER therapy (described elsewhere).

Fibromyalgia – Reduction of Pain and Increase in Quality of Life as a Result of Standard Therapy Supported by BEMER 3000-Type Pulsed Electric-Magnetic Treatment: A Quantitative Comparative Multi-Centric Pilot Clinical Study on 150 Patients

Freitag-Perez K; Ambesa N; 2002; Universidad Complutense de Madrid

SUMMARY: As a summary of this study, the application of BEMER 3000 electromagnetic field therapy can be seen as an effective and important tool in the therapeutic treatment of this syndrome, which is confronted by doctors with great uncertainty.

FIBROMYALGIA - Reduction of pain and increase quality of life as a result of a standard therapy supported by BEMER 3000-type pulsed electromagnetic field treatment: A quantitative comparative, multicenter pilot clinical study in 150 patients

Abstract: As part of an ongoing quantitative comparative clinical study conducted at various centers, the success of a therapy supported by the success of a special (BEMER 3000-type) pulsed electromagnetic field (by 1. Cyclobenzapin and Tryptizol, 2. Recupteration. (sodium citrate, potassium chloride, sodium chloride, magnesium carbonate and calcium phosphate). 3. Samet 200 (S-adenomsilmetionina). 4. Ozone therapy, 5. Rehabilitation treatment with ultrasound at all points of pain) and the resulting improved quality of life is examined to reduce chronic painful suffering associated with fibromyalgia. The results currently obtained from 150 patients based on the evaluation of laboratory values (CPK, LDH, aldolase, calcium, phosphorus, alkaline phosphatase, plasma serotonin and plasma cortisol), thermographic analyses (after the 3rd, 6th and 12th month of the examinations), and standardized health questionnaires (SF36, before and after the examination) already show significantly increased improvement of the usual therapeutic successes.

As a summary of this study, the application of BEMER 3000 electromagnetic field therapy can be seen as an effective and important tool in the therapeutic treatment of this syndrome, which is confronted by doctors with great uncertainty.

Introduction
Fibromyalgia is a clinical syndrome of rheumatic diseases of the soft tissues and is characterized by general pain, asthenia (weakness) and accompanying insomnia, often produced by tension, paresthesia (prickling, numbness, tingling) anxiety, depression, and irritable bowel syndrome.

It occurs in a ratio of 3:1 in women and its prevalence increases with age. Several hypotheses have been created about the etiology of this disease and it is associated with a deficit of serotonin, the neurotransmitter that regulates pain and NREM sleep (non-REM-phase without rapid eye movement).

With regard to the muscles, the only finding was dysfunction of the muscles and a deficit of somatomedin C, growth hormone mediator, which intervenes in the repair process of the muscles and increase of substance P, which contributes to the spread of pain.

The latest studies are aimed at pathological changes in vascularization. Clinical diagnosis takes place by evaluating 18 trigger points, 11 of which are necessary for diagnosis according to the criteria of the American College of Rheumatology.

Description of the Problem
Because of the described characteristics of this difficult-to-define syndrome, diagnosis is difficult and treatment is often unsuccessful. Patients visit a myriad of specialists, ranging from clinical traumatologists, internal specialists and psychiatrists, up to any kinds of alternative medicine, such as a

vegetarian diet, homeopathy, phytotherapy, acupuncture, aromatherapy, Chi Kung, Feng Sui, yoga, etc. Add to that the inability to work, which affects nearly 10-25% of these patients.

Objective
The aim of this study is to find an effective medical treatment, which possibly in addition to other therapies will provide these patients with an acceptable quality of life.

Study design
Within the framework of a comparative, multicenter clinical trial of the Rheumatology Department and the Department of Pain Management at the Universidad Complutense de Madrid, the therapeutic success of a combined treatment conducted according to the following regimen should be examined in a 2-year practical research study:
- Cyclobenzapin and Tryptizol depending on weight. Stature and age 10 - 75mg/day,
- Recuperation, 2 doses per day (sodium citrate, potassium chloride, sodium chloride, magnesium carbonate and calcium phosphate),
- Samet 200 (S-adenomsilmetionina), once a month,
- Ozone therapy. 15-20 sessions (5 cervical, lumbar 5),
- Rehabilitation treatment with ultrasound at all points of pain,
- BEMER 3000, Electromagnetic field therapy

The study began in October 2001 and includes patients up to March 2002 where the subjects are aleatory, divided into three groups:
- Group for infiltration
- Group with rehabilitation treatment
- Group with BEMER 3000 and recuperation

All patients receive treatment with Cyclobenzapin and Tryptizol. Dr. Albesa (Unidad de Dolor from the Ruber Clinic) applies the protocol with ozone infiltrations. Dr. Freitag performs "rehabilitation" treatment.

Materials and methods
Laboratory: CPK, LDH, aldolase, calcium, phosphorus, alkaline phosphatase, plasma serotonin and plasma cortisol

Thermography: before and after 3 and 6 months during the study Health questionnaire: SF-36 before and after the study

Evaluation and evaluation criteria:
Subjectively using the SF 36 health questionnaire
Objectively by means of thermography and muscle biopsy after the 3rd, 6th and 12th month of the study.

Purpose:
To create a statistically significant correlation by means of a statistical analysis between subjective and objective improvement in the health of three study groups among themselves and to therefore make a conclusion as to which of the three therapies (ozone therapy, electromagnetic field therapy or the restoration of ionic balance therapy) can be recommended as an effective treatment for fibromyalgia.

Preliminary Discussion:
We currently have 150 patients in this study who were divided into 3 equal groups. The study is still ongoing. So far, statistically significant improvement has been shown in all patients who were treated with BEMER electromagnetic field therapy with the P 4 program and recuperation (Fig 1). Because of the current status of this study, these results should nevertheless be interpreted as preliminary.

As a summary of this study, the application of BEMER 3000 electromagnetic field therapy can be seen as an effective and important tool in the therapeutic treatment of this syndrome, which is confronted by doctors with great uncertainty.

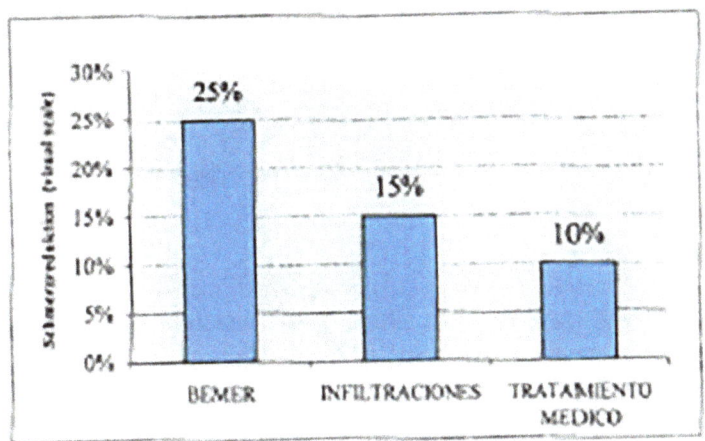

Fig 1: Fibromyalgia: Therapeutic improvement in pain reduction by the additional use of BEMER 3000 electromagnetic field therapy. Results after 6 months: April 1, 2002 n= 150 patients; (Copyrights: Dra. Freitag & Dra. Albesa Madrid (Spain)

Activity of Electromagnetic Fields in Treatment of Knee Osteoarthritis

Sabsabi Y; Hamadi W; Faculty of Medicine, Aleppo University; 2005

ZUSAMMENFASSUNG: Das positive Ergebnis einer Behandlung ist direkt proportional der Anzahl der täglichen Anwendung des BEMER 3000 Intensivapplikators. Demzufolge ist der Einsatz der BEMER-Systeme sehr vielversprechend und eine effektive therapeutische Möglichkeit in der Behandlung der Kniegelenksarthrose.

Sabsabi. Y and Hamidi. W. Department of Orthopedic and Physiotherapy Faculty of medicine, Aleppo University, Syria Arab Republic

Objectives:
This study was undertaken to examine the effects of electromagnetic fields (low intensity, broad spectrum and multiple frequency) in the treatment of knee Osteoarthritis (KO) by using BEMER 3000.

Patient inclusion criteria:
One hundred patients (40 male and 60 female) ranging in age from 40-60 years of old had a history of knee osteoarthritis taken their medical consultant at the department of orthopedic and physiotherapy at the hospital of Aleppo University, enrolled in the study. These patients were divided on their clinical and X-ray examination onto four groups:

61 patients were suffering of narrowing in the joint space between the femur and the tibia / Stage (1).
28 patients were suffering of sub-chondral Sclerosis / Stage (2).
Patients have Osteophytes and calcification in the soft tissues / stage (3).
Patients have absence of joint space and have deformity of joint / Stage (4).

Patient data including age, sex, history with knee Osteoarthritis and other complications like diabetic and obesity has been taken for every patient. However, patients with trauma were excluded. All these patients were treated by using BEMER 3000 intensive applicator for 6 months. The placebo treatment was applied on 25 patients with knee Osteoarthritis.

Table 1: Number of KO Patients in respect of their age

Age. Years	>40	40-50	51-60	61-70	>70
No. of patients (%)	18 (18)	36 (36)	14 (14)	30 (30)	2 (2)

Figure 1: Number of KO Patients in respect of their age

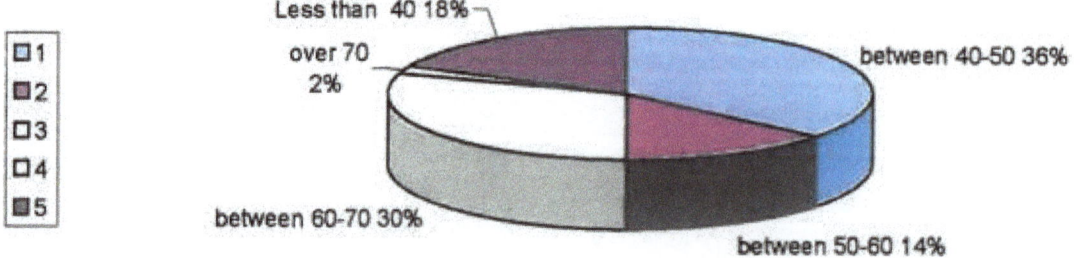

Table 2: Number of KO Patients in respect of there complaints date.

Years of complaint	<1	1-5	5-10	>10
No. of Patients (%)	14 (14%)	54 (54%)	28 (28%)	4 (4 %)

Figure 2: Number of KO Patients in respect of their complaints date.

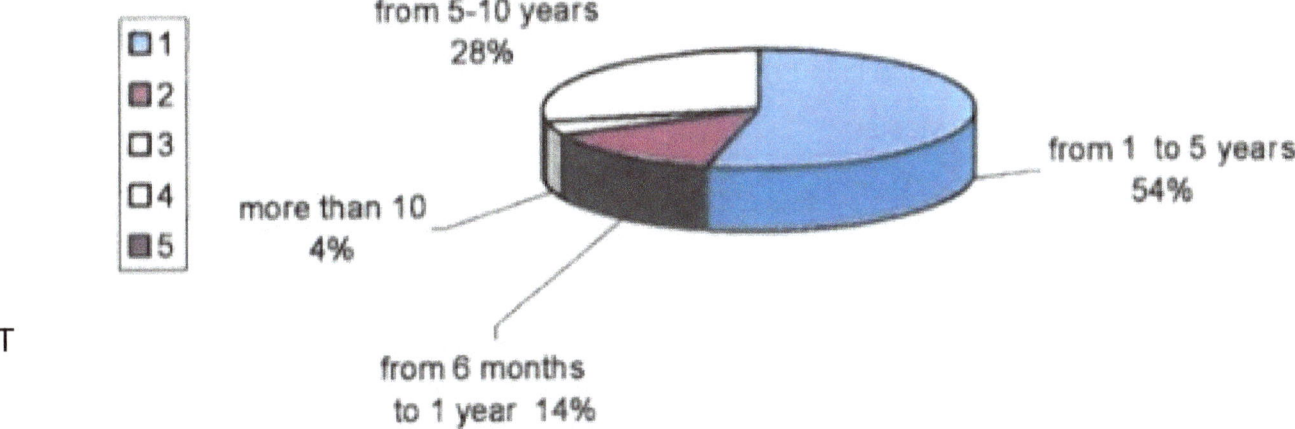

T

Table 3: Number of KO Patients with other complications:

Complication	Diabetes	Obesity	Free of complications
No. of Patients (%)	53 (53%)	33 (33%)	14 (14%)

Figure3: Number of KO Patients with other complications:

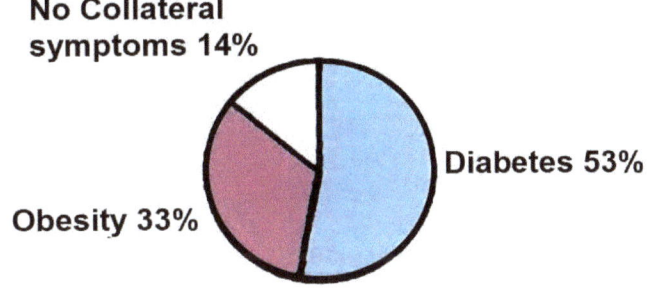

Diagnosis	No. of Patients (%)
Injury degree according to the radiological diagnosis	61 (61%)
Narrowing of the joint space between the femur and the tibia/ stage 1	28 (28%)
sub-chondral Sclerosis / Stage 2	7 (7%)
Osteophytes and calcification in the soft tissues / stage (3).	4 (4%)

Table 4: Number of KO Patient» in respect of their diagnosis by using X ray.
Patients Classification in respect of the injury degree and radiological diagnosis of osteoarthritis

Injury degree according to the radiological	No.	
Narrowing of the joint space between the femur and the tibia / stage 1	61	61 %
Osteophytes and calcification in the soft tissues / stage (3).	7	7%
Complete absence of joint space and deformity of joint / Stage (4).	4	4%

Table 5: Number of KO Patients in respect of their site and degree of complains.

Degree	Femur joint and the tibia / Stage(1)	Femur tibiotarsal / stage (2)		
	Medial	Lateral	Both	
I	11	2	48	0
II	7	2	19	1
III	7	0	0	5
IV	4	0	0	4

Table 6: Personal evaluation of KO recovery.

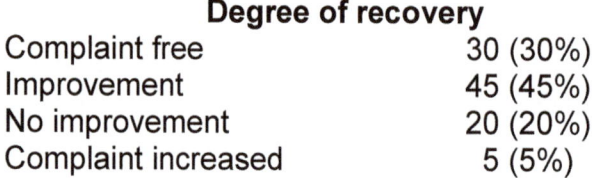

Degree of recovery
Complaint free — 30 (30%)
Improvement — 45 (45%)
No improvement — 20 (20%)
Complaint increased — 5 (5%)

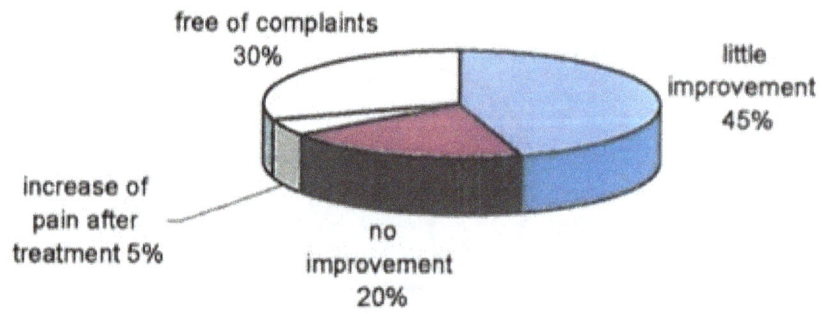

Table 8: Relationship between degree of treatment and patients age.

Age (years)	Complaint free	Good improvement	Improvement	No improvement	Total
<40	12 (67%)	3 (16.5%)	3 (16.5%)		18 (100%)
40-50	21 (21%)	10 (28%)	3 (8%)	2 (6%)	36 (100%)
51-60	9 (9%)	3 (22%)		2 (14%)	14 (100%)
61-70	6 (6%)	18 (60%)	3 (10%)	3 (10%)	30 (100%)
>70			1 (50%)	1 (50%)	2 (100%)
Totals	48 (48%)	34 (34%)	10 (10%)	12 (67%)	100 (100%)

Table 9: Relationship between degree of treatment and patients sex.

Sex	Complaint free	Good improvement	Improvement	No Improvement	Total
Male	19 (48%)	13 (33%)	5 (12%)	3 (7%)	40 (100%)
Female	29 (48%)	21 (35%)		5 (8.5%)	60 (100%)

Figure 9: Relationship between degree of treatment and patients sex.

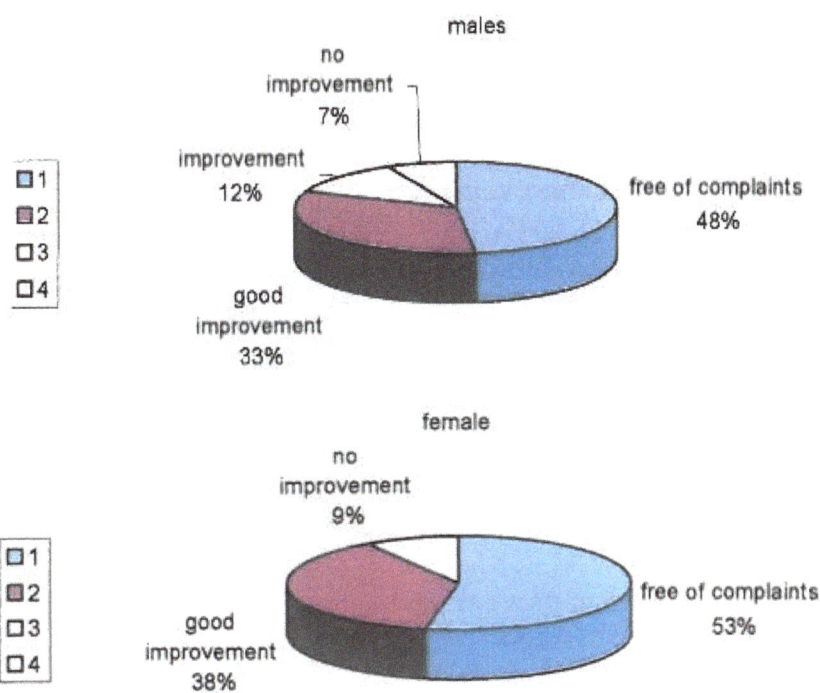

Table 10: Relationship between degree of treatment and complain period

Years	Complaint free	Good improvement	Improvement	No improvement	Total
<1	9 (64%)	4 (29%)	1 (7%)	0	14 (100%)
1 bis 5	28 (52%)	19 (35%)	3 (6%)	4 (7%)	54 (100%)
6 bis 10	11 (39%)	9 (32%)	5 (18%)	3 (11%)	28 (100%)
>10		2 (50%)	1 (25%)	1 (25%)	4

Figure 10: Relationship between degree of treatment and complain period

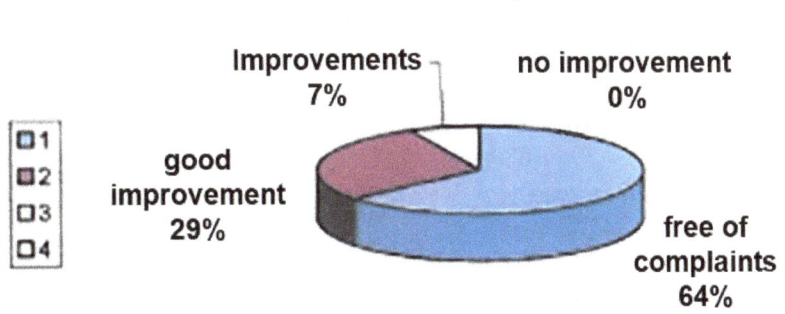

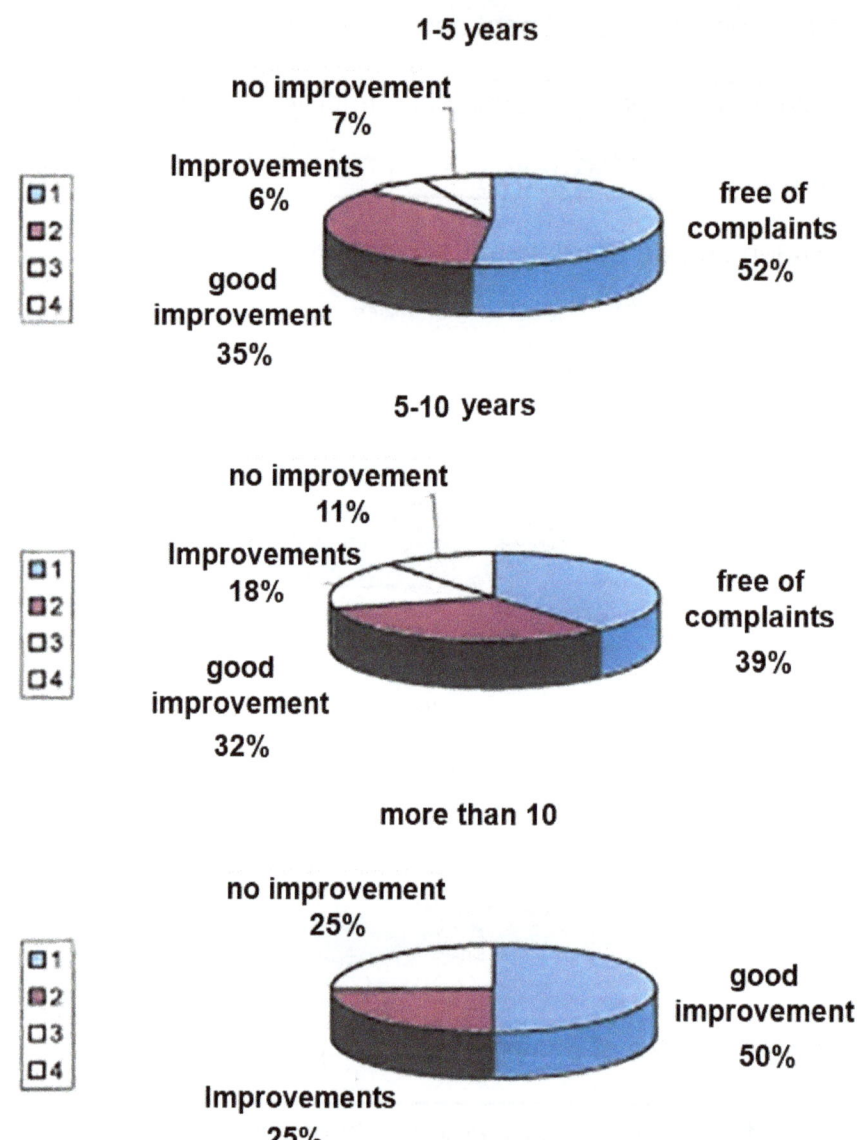

Table 11: Relationship between degree of treatment and concomitant diseases.

Disease	Complaint free	Good Improvement	Improvement	No Improvement	Total
Diabetes	19	25 (47%)	6 (11%)	3 (6%)	53
Obesity	6 (18%)	12 (37%)	10 (31%)	4 (14%)	33 (100%)
None	7 (50%)	4 (29%)	2 (14%)	1 (7%)	14 (100%)

Figure 11: Relationship between degree of treatment and concomitant diseases.

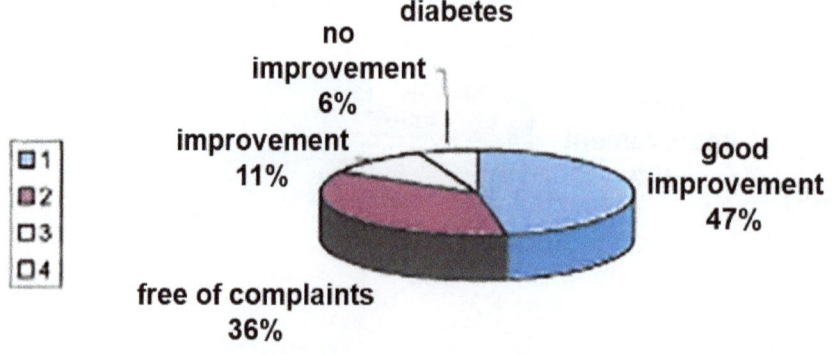

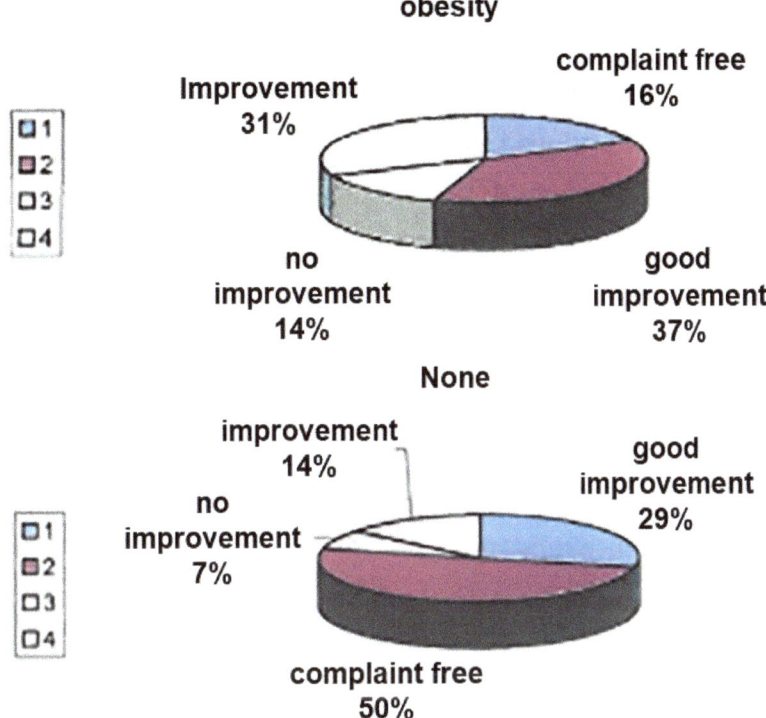

Table 12: Outcome of treatment with BEMER 3000 intensive applicator depending on X-ray use.

Degree	Complaint free	Good Improvement	Improvement	No Improvement
I	36(59%)	25(41%)	0	0
II	12(43%)	8(29%)	7(25%)	1(3%)
III	0	1(14%)	3 (43%)	3 (43%)
IV	4(100%)	0	0	0

Table 14: Outcome of treatment with placebo.

	Complaint free	Good Improvement	Improvement	No Improvement
No. Of Patients	0	9	5 (20%)	20 (80%)

Figure 14: Outcome of treatment with placebo.

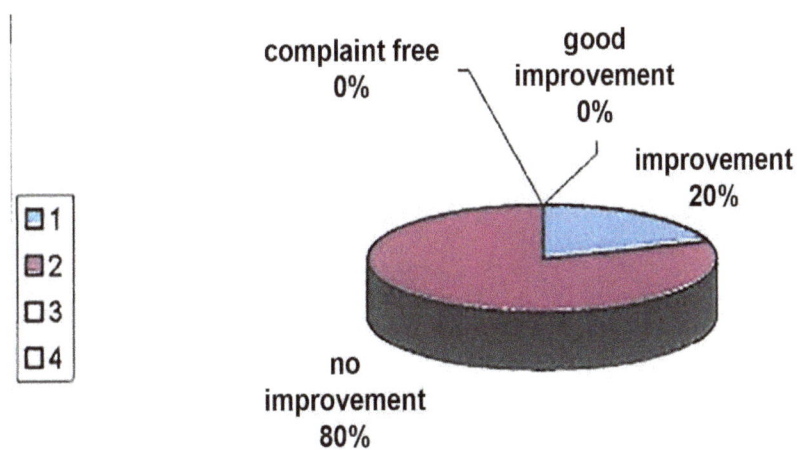

Table 14: Outcome of treatment of knee osteoarthritis with BEMER 3000 intensive applicator.

Complaint free	Good Improvement	Improvement	No Improvement
48 (48%)	34 (34%)	10 (10%)	8 (8%)

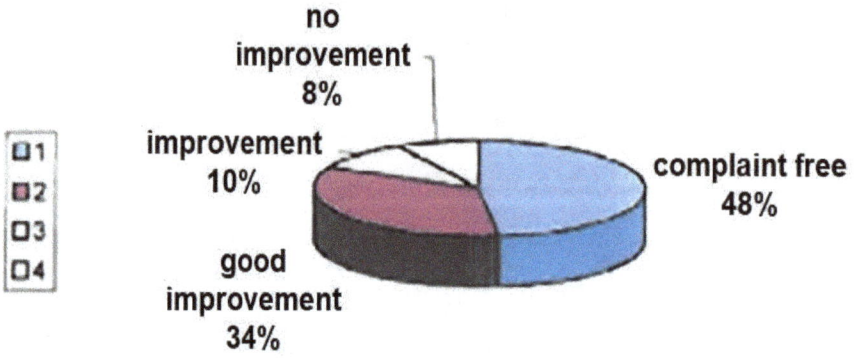

Conclusions:

As stated earlier, the applied impulses and intensities electromagnetic fields by using BEMER 3000 intensive applicator reveal that the effects of age, sex and diabetes on treatment outcome were insignificant. Whereas, the degree of complain significantly affects treatment outcome. In addition, obesity decreased the patient response to the treatment. However, the positive outcome of treatment directly proportional with the number of daily application of BEMER 3000 intensive applicator. Therefore, BEMER System is a very promising and effective therapeutical application to promote recovering from knee osteoarthritis.

BEMER Therapy Applied in Physiology

Immediate Effect of a Suitable Electromagnetic AC Field (BEMER) on the Surface Microvessel Networks of the Subcutis and the Intestine

Klopp R; Microcirculation in the Focus of Research [Mikrozirkulation im Fokus der Forschung]; ISBN 978-3-033-01464-0; 421-424; 2008

SUMMARY: Following application of a specific pulsed electromagnetic field (BEMER), the investigated sample demonstrated the following characteristic behavior in the microcirculation of the subcutaneous and intestinal target tissue:

1. Complex changes in the functional status of the microcirculation to a biologically relevant extent (increased venular flow out of the microvascular networks, extended distribution of the plasma/blood cell mix in the capillary networks, and increased spontaneous arteriolar vasomotion). This equates to a greater local range of control of the microcirculation resulting in increased venule-side oxygen saturation.

2. Owing to the increased venular outward flow and the perfusion of a greater number of microvessels, the micro-hemodynamic general conditions improve for unhindered performance of the first steps in the immunological reactions in the subjects exposed to infection.

3. Parallel characteristic changes occur in the subcutis and intestine. I.e., the identified characteristic changes affect two organs that are representative of the circulation and are immunologically active. They are therefore relevant with regard to the entire organism.

4. The identified characteristic changes are temporary (supplementary investigation showed that the initial values were re-established after approx. 15 mins).

To assess the effects of a suitable changing electromagnetic field on the microcirculation we look at the main characteristics that determine its functional state. First we will focus on the immediate effects of a suitable changing electromagnetic field on the microcirculatory network close to the surface in the subcutis and in the intestine for a biometrically defined sample test group of subjects exposed to stress and infection of middle age. For the selection of the therapy system the test results from figure 282 above were the deciding factor.

Research Design

Test Sample	Test sample size N_{total} =36 Male test subjects, age ~30 years of age, no pathological abnormalities Exposure to stress and infection
Partial Test Samples	2 equal partial test samples of n=18: ▶ Control group: no treatment (placebo) ▶ Test Group: treatment with a changing pulsed electromagnetic field
Test System, Application	Blind study, GCP criteria Pulsed changing electromagnetic field BEMER 3000 One-time treatment of 2 minutes (intensity level 3)

Measurement Intervals and Timing	Observation time of 8 minutes, equidistant measurement intervals: Zero minutes (determination of base values immediately prior to the application), subsequent 2-minute treatment, with data measurements following in the 2nd, 4th, 6th, and 8th minute.
Target Tissue	Synchronized measurements in two target tissues: Sub-cutis (abdomen, regio epigastr.) Intestine (rectum, lamina muscolaris)
Measurement Methods	▶ Intravitalmicroscopy with computer assisted image processing. (documentation of findings: high-speed camera, 35 mm film, high resolution, up to 120 pictures per second). ▶ Vitalmicroscopic reflection spectrometry. ▶ Laser-DOPPLER-microflow-measurement and white light spectroscopy. Capture of complete interconnected micro-vascular networks with defined tissue volume V=1200µm3 (diameter of vessels d≤200µm).
Parameters	▶ Number of blood cell perfused nodal points nNP. ▶ Changes in the venular flow rate ΔQ_{ven}. ▶ Area below the envelope of the amplitude-frequency-spectrum of the (spontaneous) arteriolar vasomotion Avm. ▶ Oxygen utilization in the venules ΔpO_2. ▶ Number of white blood cells adhering to a defined venular wall nWBC/A. ▶ Localized change in concentration of ICAM-1.
Statistical Analysis	WILCOXON rank-sum test (MWW), a = 5%

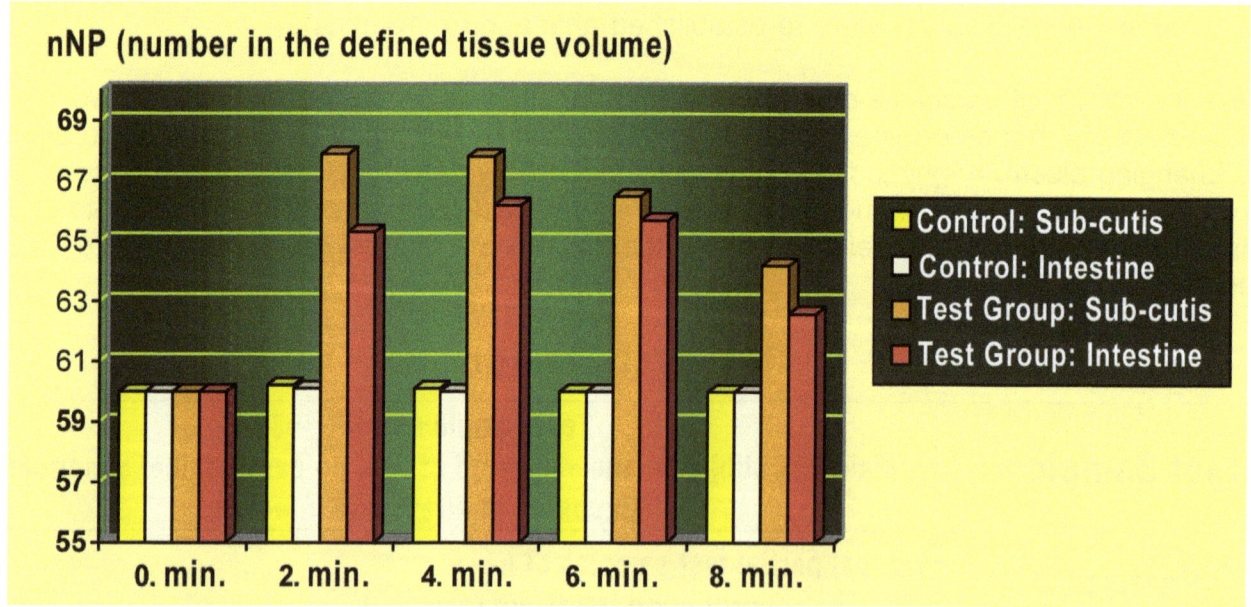

Figure 283
Measurements for the parameter "number of blood cell perfused nodal points nNP" (mean values) in the target tissues sub-cutis and intestine after 2 minutes of treatment with a certain pulsed electromagnetic field (BEMER) for test subjects exposed to stress and infection compared to a non-treated control group.

No significant parameter changes in the control group. The measurement data of the test group show a significant change from the base values and from those of the control group after 2 minutes.

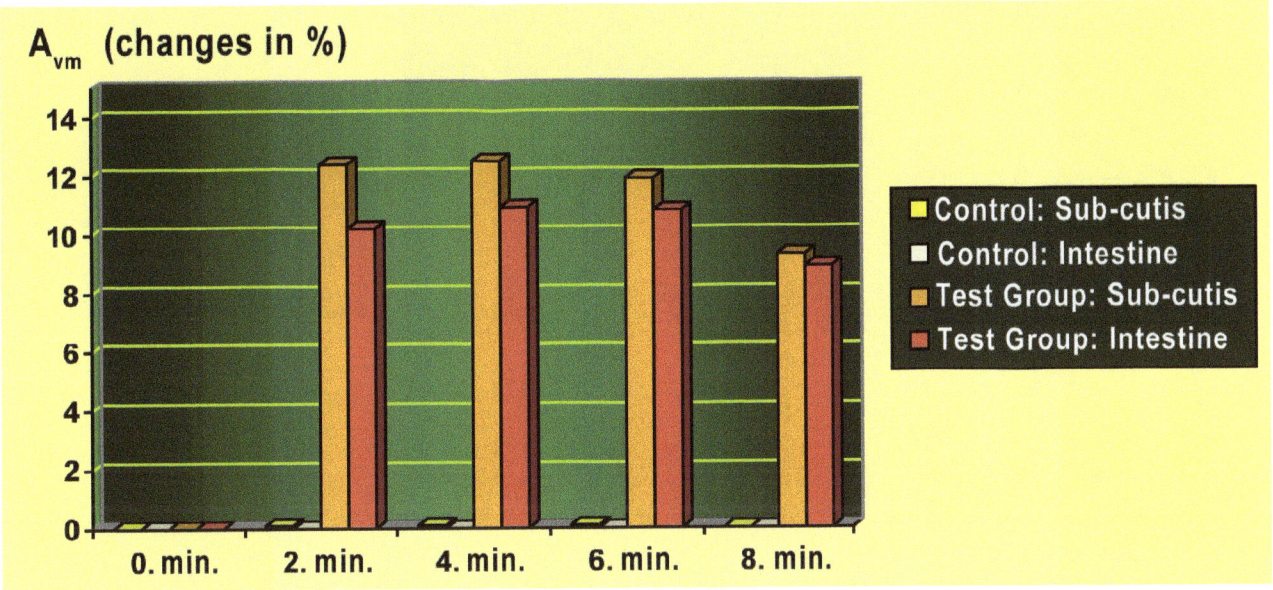

Figure 285
Measurements for the parameter "area below the envelope of the amplitude-frequency spectrum of the (spontaneous) arteriolar vasomotion Avm" (mean values) in the target tissues sub-cutis and intestine after 2 minutes of treatment with a certain pulsed electromagnetic field (BEMER) for test subjects exposed to stress and infection compared to a non-treated control group. No significant parameter changes in the control group. The measurement data of the test group show a significant change from the base values and from those of the control group after 2 minutes.

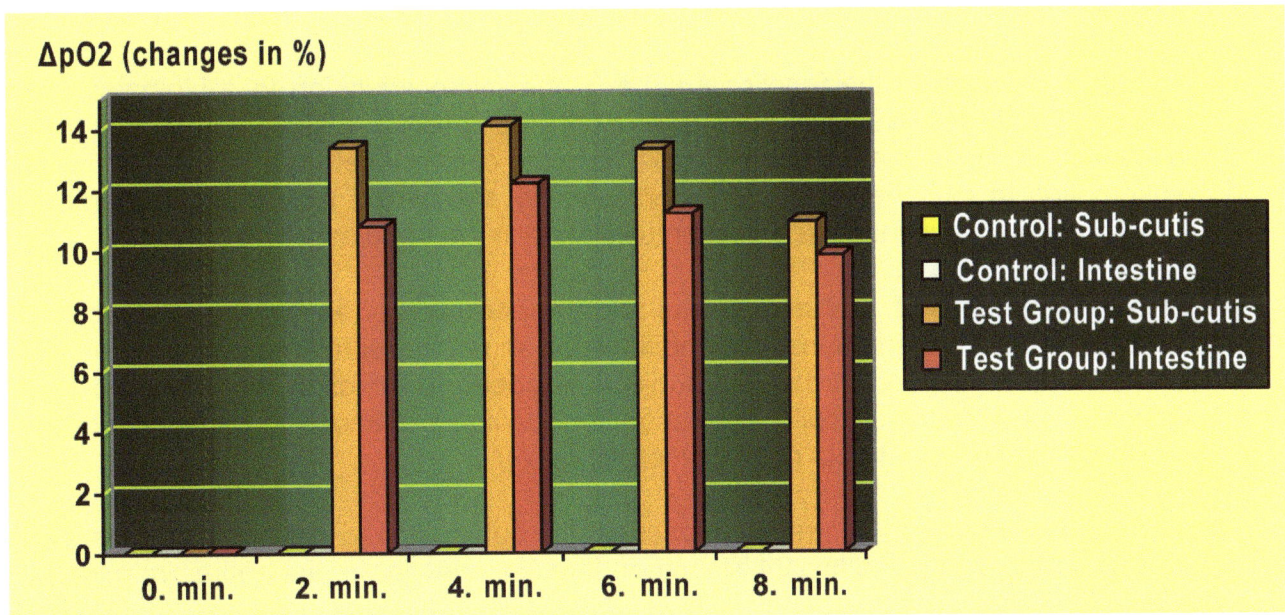

Figure 286
Measurements for the parameter "oxygen utilization in the venules $\Delta pO2$" (mean values) in the target tissues sub-cutis and intestine after 2 minutes of treatment with a certain pulsed electromagnetic field (BEMER) for test subjects exposed to stress and infection compared to a non-treated control group. No significant parameter changes in the control group. The measurement data of the test group show a significant change from the base values and from those of the control group after 2 minutes.

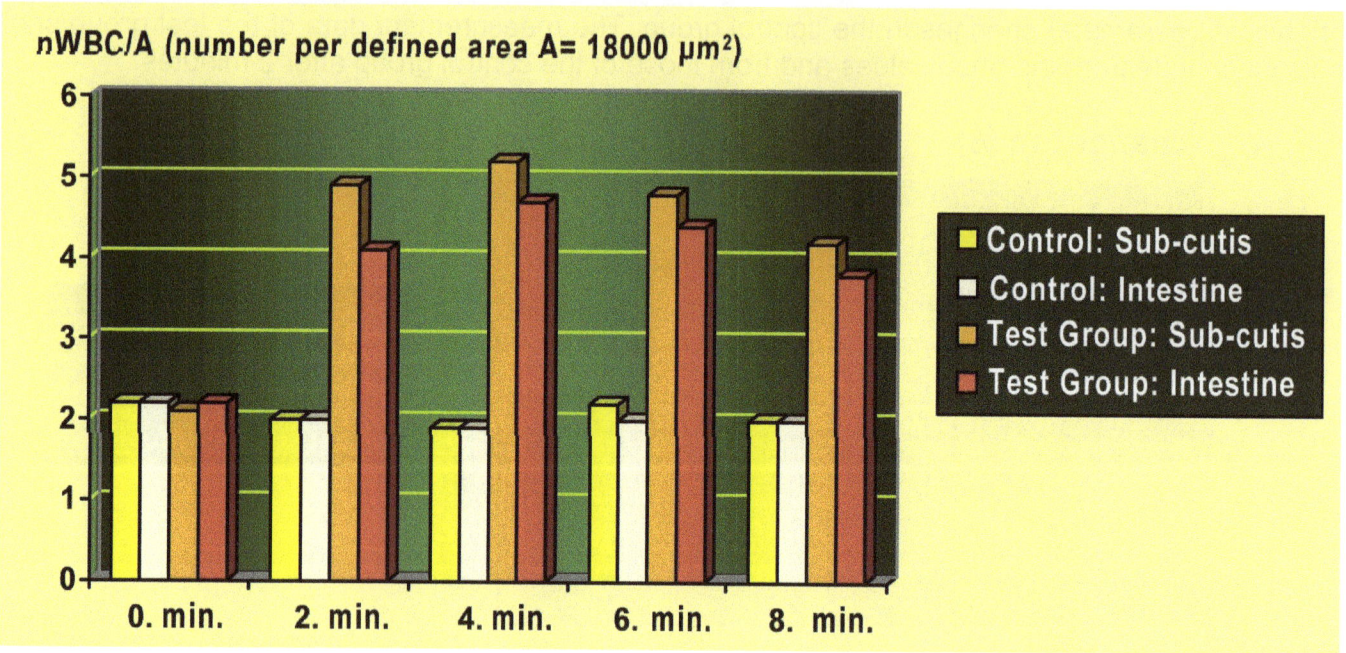

Figure 287
Measurements for the parameter "number of white blood cells adhering to a defined venule wall nWBC/A" (mean values) in the target tissues sub-cutis and intestine after 2 minutes of treatment with a certain pulsed electromagnetic field (BEMER) for test subjects exposed to stress and infection compared to a non- treated control group. No significant parameter changes in the control group. The measurement data of the test group show a significant change from the base values and from those of the control group after 2 minutes.

The test sample showed the following behaviors of microcirculatory characteristics in the subcutaneous and intestinal target tissues after the application of a certain pulsed electromagnetic field (BEMER):

- Complex changes in the functional state of the microcirculation to a biologically relevant degree (increased venular flow rate from the micro- vascular networks, expanded distribution of the plasma-blood cell mixture in the capillary network, increased spontaneous vasomotion in the arterioles). This translates to a localized extension of microcirculatory function, resulting in increased oxygen utilization in the venules.

- Due to the increased venular flow rate and the perfusion of an increased number of micro vessels, the micro-hemodynamic conditions for an uninterrupted sequence of the first steps of an immune reaction in the test subjects exposed to infection are improved (increased adhesion of white blood cells, corresponding localized changes in concentration levels of ICAM-1 [measurement data not represented here]).

- Two parallel changes in parameters occur in the sub-cutis and the intestine. This means the criteria changes apply to two 24 They therefore are relevant for the entire organism.

- The criteria changes are temporary (additional tests show a return to the base values after about 15 minutes). One considers: The data refer to the investigation (Design) of a certain selected sample (Responder/Non Responder) and to the research methods here used. The effects of varying therapy durations and varying intensity levels within the flux density levels of the therapy system used (see figure 281) on the degree of change in parameters and the time it takes for the changes to subside can be gathered from the following research series.

Test Sample	Test sample size Ntotal =30 Male test subjects, ~35 years of age, no pathological abnormalties, Exposure to stress and infection Participation in two test series at least 3 days apart
Test Series, Partial Test Samples	**Variation of the length of therapy (one time) with identical intensity level(level 3):** 3 equal partial test samples of n=10 ▶ Therapy time 2 minutes ▶ Therapy time 10 minutes ▶ Therapy time 20 minutes **Variation of the intensity level with identical length of therapy (one time 10 minutes):** 2 equal partial test samples of n=15 ▶ Therapy with intensity level 3 ▶ Therapy with intensity level 10
Test System, Application	Blind study, GCP-criteria Pulsed, changing electromagnetic field BEMER 3000 Single therapy session each
Measurement Intervals and Timing	Observation time of 30 minutes. Equidistant measurement intervals: Zero minutes (determination of base values immediately prior to the application), subsequent treatment, with data measurements following in the 2nd, 4th, 6th, 8th, 10th, 12th, 14th, 16th, 18th, 20th, 22nd, 24th, 26th, 28th, and 30th minute.
Target Tissue	Sub-cutis (abdomen, region epigastr.)
Measurement Methods	▶ Laser-DOPPLER-microflow measurement and white light spectroscopy
Parameter	▶ Oxygen utilization in the venules ΔpO_2
Statistical Analysis	WILCOXON rank-sum test (MWW), a = 5%

Figures 288 and 289 provide information on the measurement data collected. Longer therapy times do not result in added contributions to the parameter changes, however, they prolong the time it takes for the changes to subside.

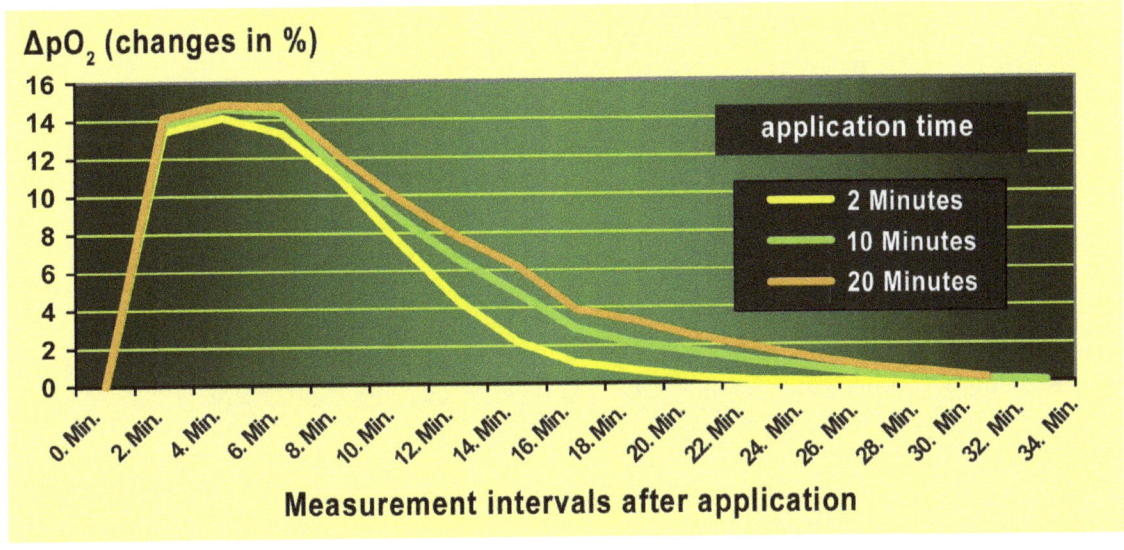

Figure 288
Measurements for the parameter "oxygen utilization in the venules $\Delta pO2$" (mean values) in the subcutaneous target tissue after treatment with a certain changing pulsed electromagnetic field (BEMER) of varying application times (2 min., 10 min., 20 min.; intensity level 3) for test subjects exposed to stress and infection.

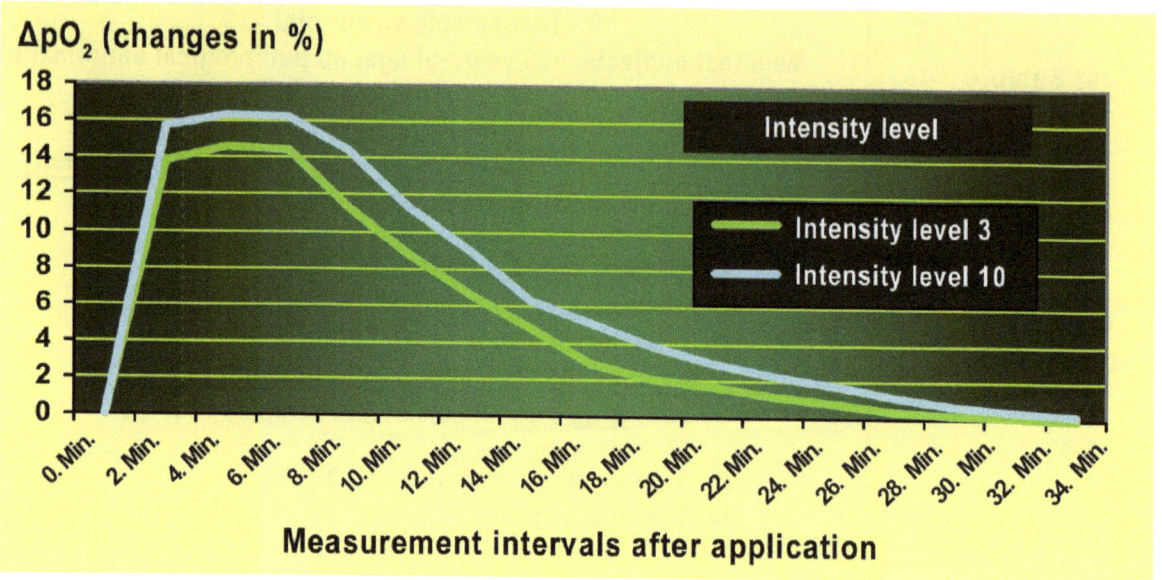

Figure 289

Measurements for the parameter "oxygen utilization in the venules ΔpO2" (mean values) in the subcutaneous target tissue after treatment with a certain changing pulsed electromagnetic field (BEMER) of varying intensities (10 minute application, intensity levels 3 and 10) for test subjects exposed to stress and infection.

Please note: The data refer to the research (design) for a specific selected test sample and to the applied research method.

The following figures 290 to 293 display selected vitalmicroscopic findings from the subcutaneous and intestinal target tissues regarding the effects of a certain changing electromagnetic field (BEMER) on the microcirculation.

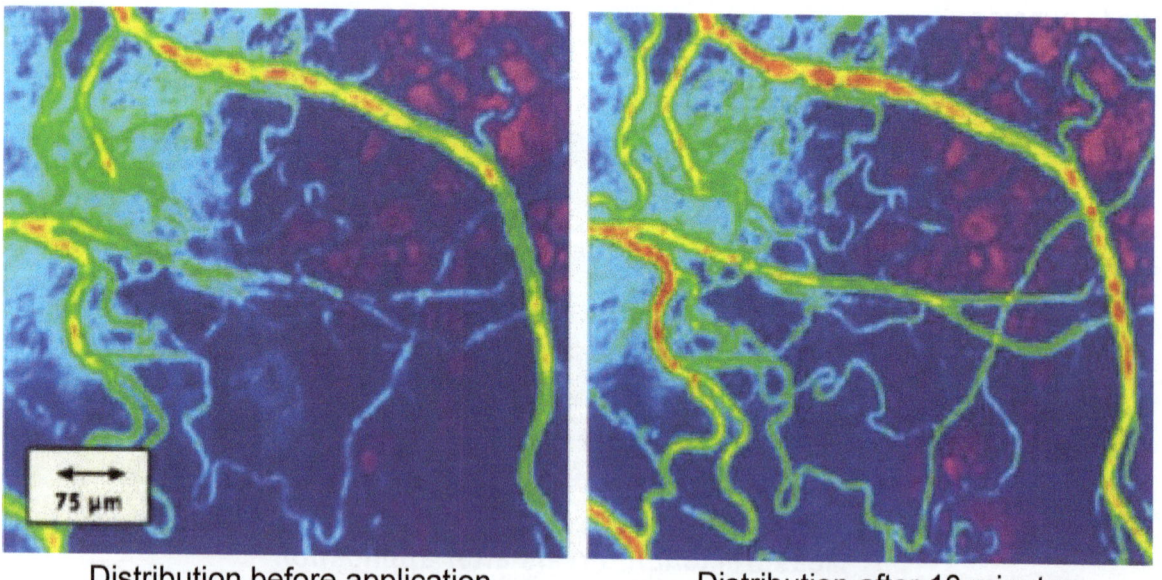

Distribution before application · Distribution after 10 minutes of application

Figure 290

Change in the distribution of the plasma-blood cell mixture in the micro- vascular networks of the subcutis after a 10 minute application of a certain changing electromagnetic field (BEMER, intensity level 3). (Example of vitalmicroscopic findings, 1/1000 second; capillaries, arterioles and venules). Pseudo-transformation of color of the primary images (the blood cell perfused micro vessels are marked in red).

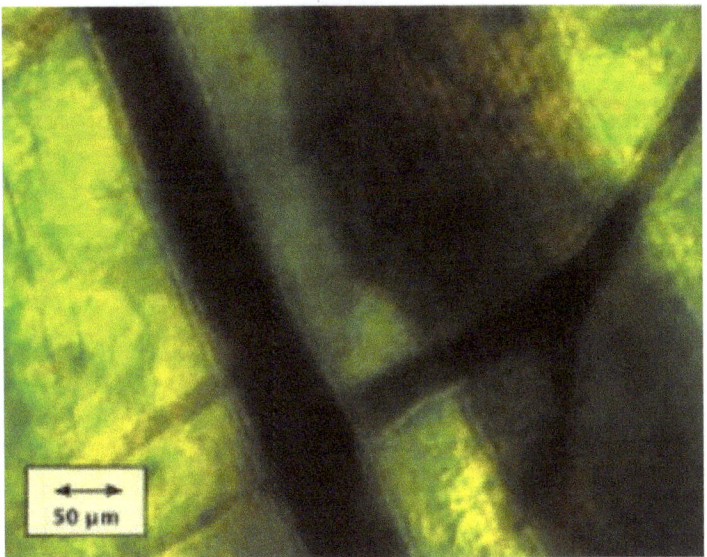 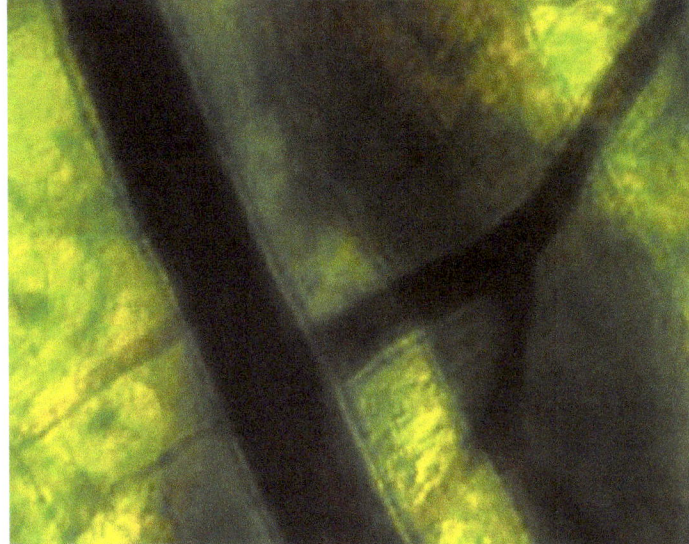

Perfusion level before application | Perfusion level after 10 minutes of application

Figure 292
Change in the perfusion level at micro-vascular nodal points in the sub- cutaneous network after a 10 minute application of a certain changing electromagnetic field (BEMER, intensity level 3). (Example of vitalmicroscopic findings, 1/1000 second; capillaries, arterioles and venules).
  a: Perfusion level before application.
  b: Perfusion level after 10 minutes of application One considers the changes of diameter.

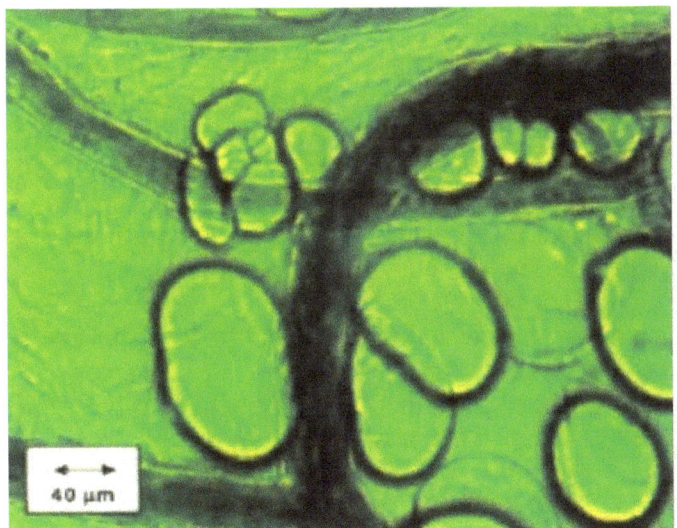 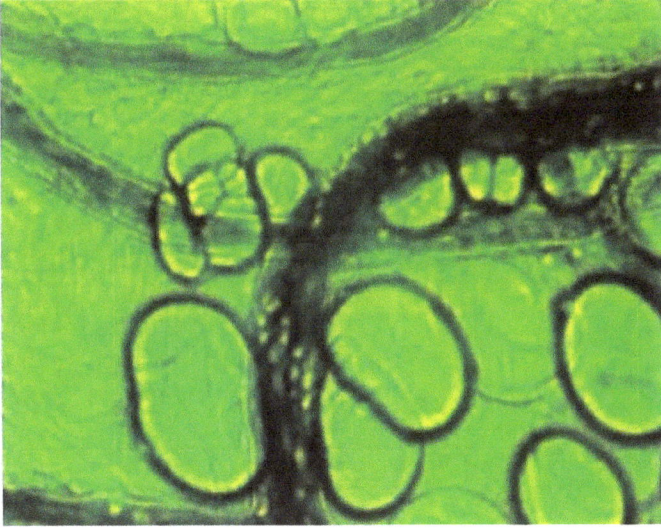

Figure 293
Change in the level of vasomotion and the tonus of intestinal micro vessels after a 10 minute application of a certain changing electromagnetic field (BEMER, intensity level 3). (Example of vitalmicroscopic findings, 1/1000 second; capillaries, arterioles and venules). a: Accumulation of few white blood cells before application. b: Increased accumulation of white blood cells after 10 minutes of application.

The effects of the repeated application of a suitable electromagnetic AC field (BEMER) on the superficial microvessel networks of the subcutis of the intestineKlopp R; Microcirculation in the Focus of Research (Mikrozirkulation im Fokus der Forschung); ISBN 978-3-033-01464-0; 432-436; 2008

A "potency effect" and reduced speed of decay of the characteristic changes occur when 2 applications at an interval of 2 hours are apply even 2 days on three treatment days within a week.

SUMMARY: *Frequent applications at short time intervals on one day have no increased influence on the behavior of the microcirculatory functional characteristics.*

We now turn to the question if, and in which way repeated applications can result in increased parameter changes.

Research Design

Test Sample	Total test sample N_{total} =36 Male test subjects, ~40 years of age, no pathological abnormalities Exposure to stress and infection
Test Series, Partial Test Samples	➡ Test series A 　　One-time application on one day ➡ Test series B 　　Three applications 2 hours apart on one day ➡ Test series C 　　Two applications per day 2 hours apart, within one week on Two equal partial test sample groups of n=18 for each partial test group ▶ Control group: No treatment (placebo) ▶ Test group: treatment with a changing electromagnetic field
Test System, Application	Changing pulsed electromagnetic field BEMER 3000 Applications of 2 minutes each (intensity level 3) Blind study, GPC criteria
Measurement Intervals and Timing	Observation time of 30 minutes each. Equidistant measurement intervals: Test series A: Zero minutes (determination of base values immediately prior to the application), subsequent 2-minute treatment with data measurements following in the 2nd, 4th, 6th, and 8th minute. Test series B: Zero minutes (determination of base values immediately prior to each application), subsequent 2-minute treatment with data measurements after each application following in the 2nd, 4th, 6th, and 8th minute. Test series C: Zero minutes (determination of base values immediately prior to each application on each treatment day), subsequent 2-minute treatment with data measurements following after each application on each treatment day in the 2nd, 4th, 6th, and 8th minute.
Target Tissue	Sub-cutis (abdomen, regio epigastr.)
Measurement Methods	▶ Intravitalmicroscopy with computer-enhanced image processing ▶ Vitalmicroscopic reflectionspectrometry ▶ Laser-DOPPLER-microflow measurement and white light spectroscopy Capture of complete interconnected micro-vascular networks with defined tissue volume V=1200µm³ (diameter of vessels d≤200µm). Defined conditions of macro-circulation and
Parameters	▶ Number of blood cell perfused nodal points nNP ▶ Changes in the venular flow rate ΔQ_{ven} ▶ Area below the envelope of the amplitude-frequency-spectrum of the (spontaneous) arteriolar vasomotion Avm ▶ Oxygen utilization in the venules ΔpO_2 ▶ Number of white blood cells adhering to a defined venule wall nWBC/A ▶ Localized change in concentration of ICAM-1
Statistical Analysis	WILCOXON rank-sum test, a = 5%

Research results:

The data from test series A are used for comparison, they are literally identical to the data of another research series named above (see fig. 283-287).

Test series B (3 applications two hours apart on the same day) displays parallel parameter changes for all applications, however with differing values. After the 2nd application the measurement values were somewhat increased compared to the 1st application; the changes in measurement values after the 3rd application however were slightly lower than after the 1st application. This means the documented (slight) "potentiating effect" occurring after a 2nd application on the same day does not continue with subsequent applications.

Conclusion:

Multiple applications within a short time frame on the same day do not have a positive effect on the behavior of functional parameters of the microcirculation. A "potentiating effect" and a slower subsiding of the parameter changes occur when applications are conducted 2 day apart, twice a day, 2 hours apart, within one week on three different days (test series C). The measurement data depicted in figure 294 for the parameter "oxygen utilization in the venules $\Delta pO2$" give a visual illustration of how application frequency affects the change in microcirculatory parameters.

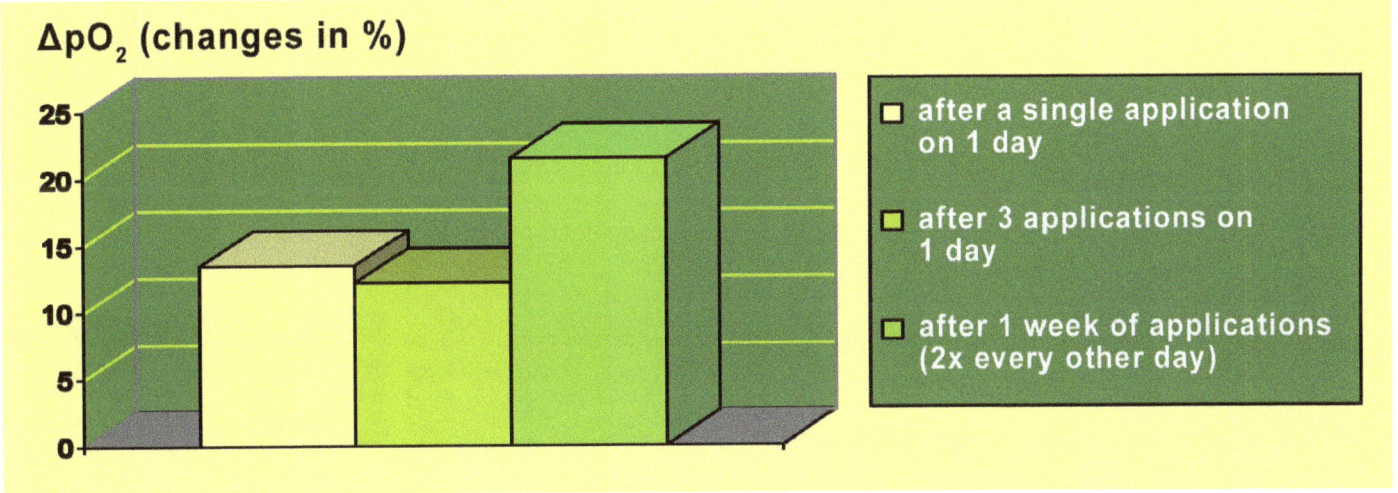

Figure 294
Measurements for the parameter "oxygen utilization in the venules $\Delta pO2$" (mean values) in the target tissue sub-cutis for test subjects exposed to stress and infection after applications with varied frequencies.

Test Series A: Collection of measurements immediately after the 2 minute application.

Test Series B: Collection of measurements immediately after the 3rd application (2 minutes) on the day of treatment.

Test Series C: Collection of measurements immediately after the 2nd application on the last treatment day after 1 week of treatments (2x2 minutes every other day).

The influence of a beneficial therapy frequency on increased and prolonged microcirculatory effects (test series C) can be seen in the data displayed in figures 295 through 298.

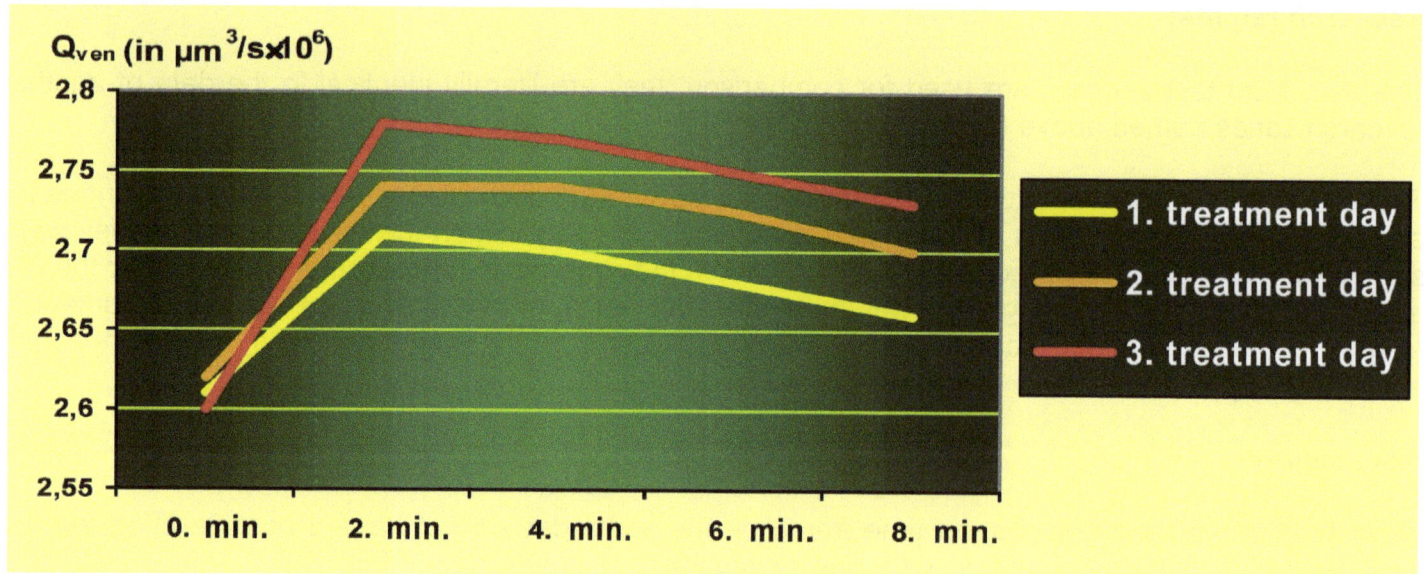

Figure 296
Measurements for the parameter "venular flow rate Qven" (mean values) in the target tissue sub-cutis after 1 week of treatment with a certain pulsed electromagnetic field (BEMER) for test subjects exposed to stress and infection. 3 treatment days at intervals of 2 days with 2 applications each (2 min., intensity level 3), 2 hours apart. Measurements taken after the 2nd treatment each day. Results of the statistical evaluation: Significant differences in parameters after the 2nd minute for all 3 days of therapy.

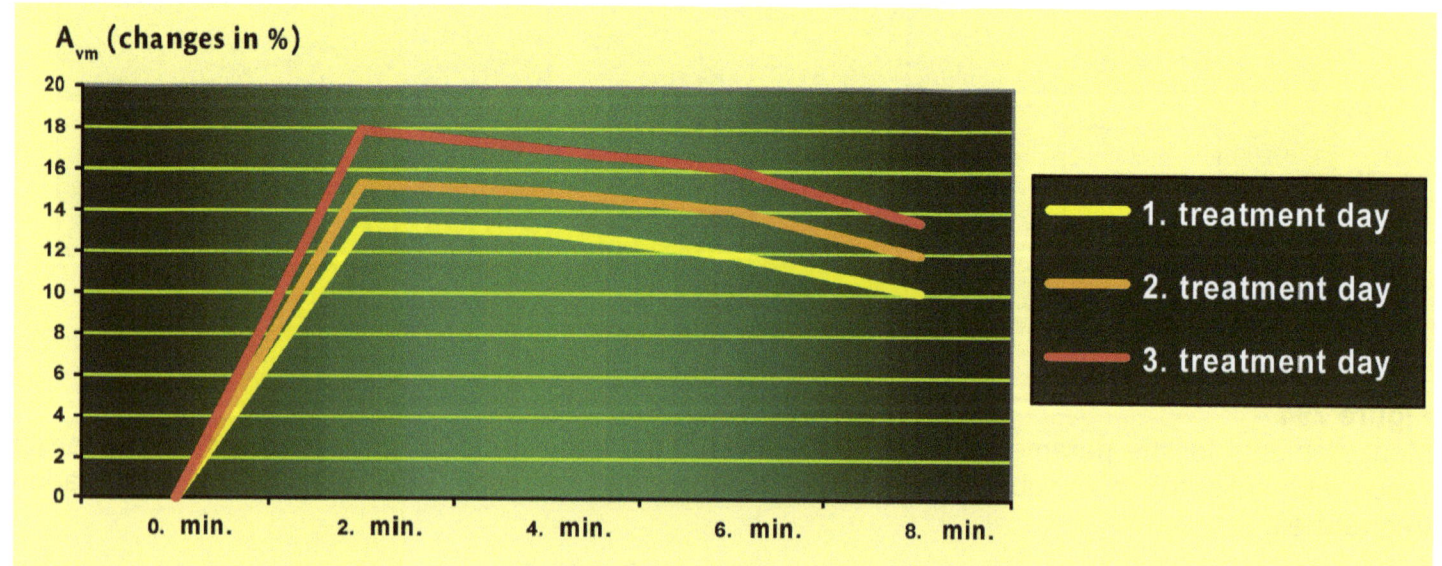

Figure 297
Measurements for the parameter "area under the envelope of the amplitude- frequency spectrum of spontaneous vasomotion in the arterioles Avm" (mean values) in the target tissue sub-cutis after 1 week of treatment with a certain pulsed electromagnetic field (BEMER) for test subjects exposed to stress and infection. 3 treatment days at intervals of 2 days with 2 applications each (2 min., intensity level 3), 2 hours apart.

Measurements taken after the 2nd treatment each day. Results of the statistical evaluation: Significant differences in parameters after the 2nd minute for all 3 days of therapy.

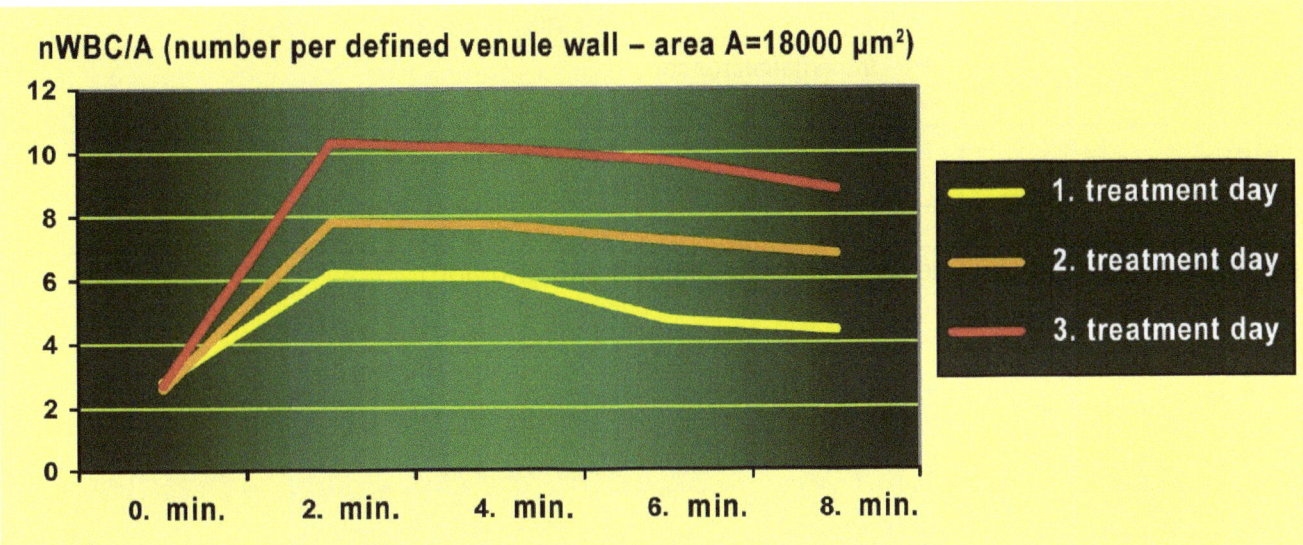

Figure 298
Measurements for the parameter "number of white blood cells adhering to a defined venule wall nWBC/A" (mean values) in the target tissue sub-cutis after 1 week of treatment with a certain pulsed electromagnetic field (BEMER) for test subjects exposed to stress and infection. 3 treatment days at intervals of 2 days with 2 applications each (2 min., intensity level 3), 2 hours apart. Measurements taken after the 2nd treatment each day. For additional explanation refer to the legend for figure 295. Results of the statistical evaluation: Significant differences parameters after the 2nd minute for all 3 days of therapy.

The effects of a suitable electromagnetic AC field (BEMER) on the characteristic changes in the microvessel network of the subcutis and intestine at varying tissue depth (penetration depth), Klopp R; Microcirculation in the Focus of Research [Mikrozirkulation im Fokus der Forschung]; ISBN 978-3-033-01464-0; p1; 20

SUMMARY: The results of the investigation support the following conclusion: In the microvessel networks of deep tissue regions, higher values and longer-lasting microcirculatory characteristic changes occur after application of a specific electromagnetic AC field (BEMER) than in the superficial regions. The fact that the layers of tissue and therefore the position of the microvessel networks each vary must be taken into account.

So far, we have observed microcirculatory characteristic changes at tissue depths close to the surface. The characteristic behavior at varying tissue depths (penetration depths) is investigated below.

Research Design

Test Sample	Total sample Ntotal =14 Male test subjects, ~30 years of age, no pathological abnormalities
Test Series	Simultaneous measurement in two depths of penetration: ▶ Depth of penetration 3mm ▶ Depth of penetration 8mm
Test System, Application	Changing pulsed electromagnetic field BEMER 3000 One-time application (2 minutes, intensity level 3)
Measurement Intervals and Timing	Observation time 14 minutes. Equidistant measuring intervals: Zero minutes (determination of base values immediately prior to the application), subsequent 2-minute treatment, with data collection following in the 2nd, 4th, 6th, 8th, 10th, 12th, 14th minute

Target Tissue	Sub-cutis / infra-cutis (left forearm)
Measurement Methods	▶ Intravitalmicroscopy ▶ Laser-DOPPLER-microflow measurement and white light spectroscopy
Parameters	▶ Number of blood cell perfused nodal points nNP ▶ Venular flow rate $Q_{ven.}$
Statistical Analysis	WILCOXON rank-sum test, a = 5%

The measurements show an unexpected result (figures 299 and 300).

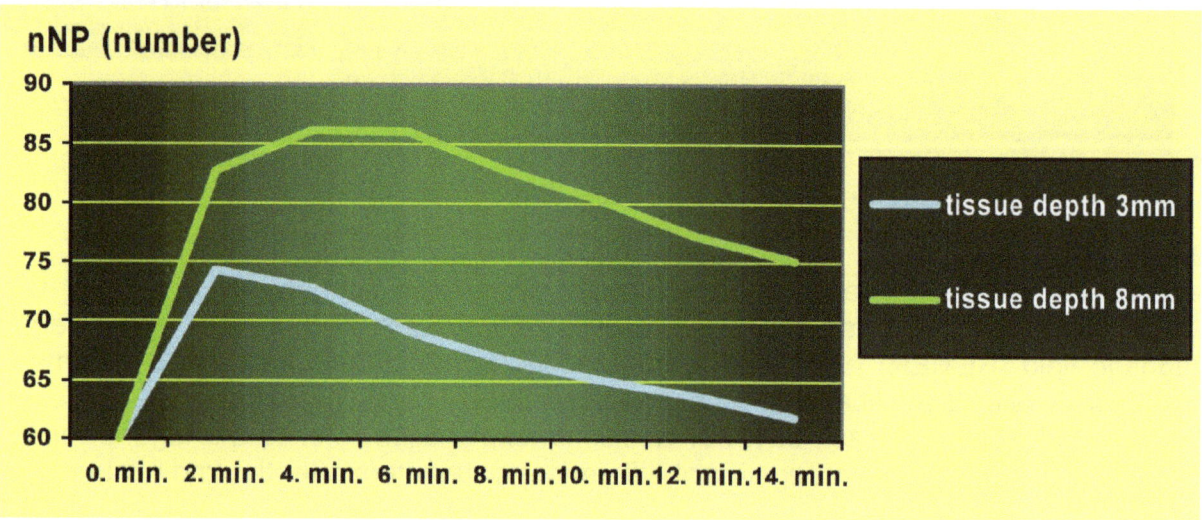

Figure 299
Measurement data for the parameter "number of blood cell perfused nodal points nNP" (mean values) in sub-cutaneous and infra-cutaneous target tissues at varying tissue depth after a one-time treatment with a certain pulsed electromagnetic field (BEMER, intensity 3, 2 minute application). Results of the statistical evaluation: Significant differences in the parameters after the 2nd minute between the two tissue depths.

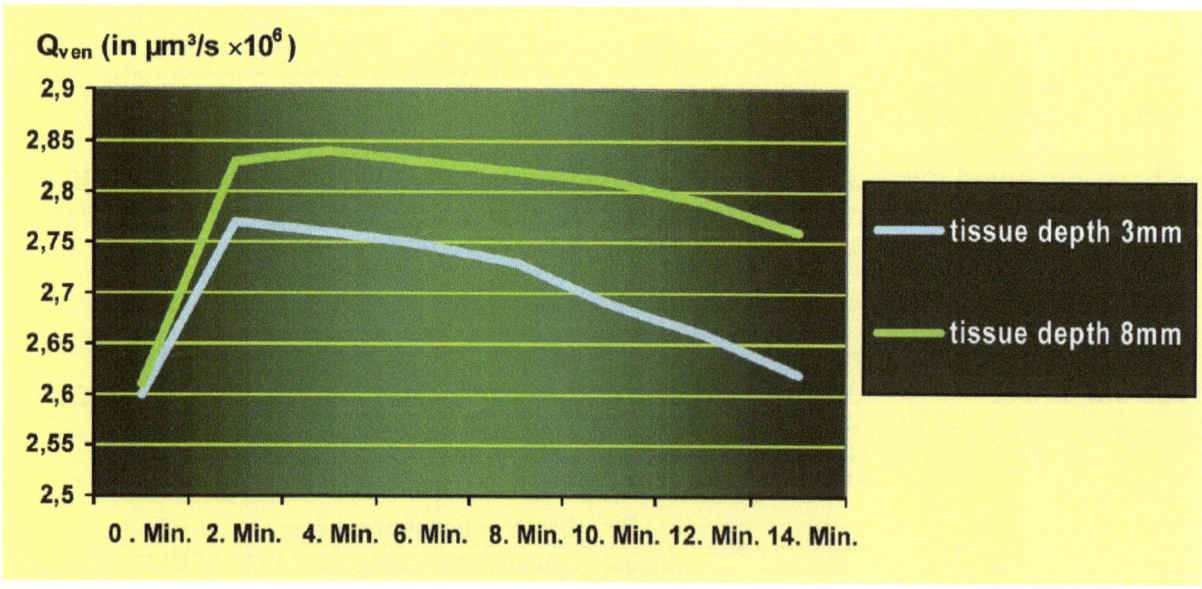

Figure 300
Measurement data for the parameter "venular flow rate" (mean values) in sub- cutaneous and infra-cutaneous target tissues at varying tissue depth after a one- time treatment with a certain pulsed electromagnetic field (BEMER, intensity 3, 2 minute application). Results of the statistical evaluation: Significant differences in the parameters after the 2nd minute between the two tissue depths.

The findings lead to the following conclusion: The micro vessel networks of deeper lying tissues show higher and longer lasting changes in microcirculatory parameters after the application of a certain changing electromagnetic field (BEMER) than areas closer to the surface. Please bear in mind that the tissue layers and with them the location of the micro-vessel networkswill vary for each individual.

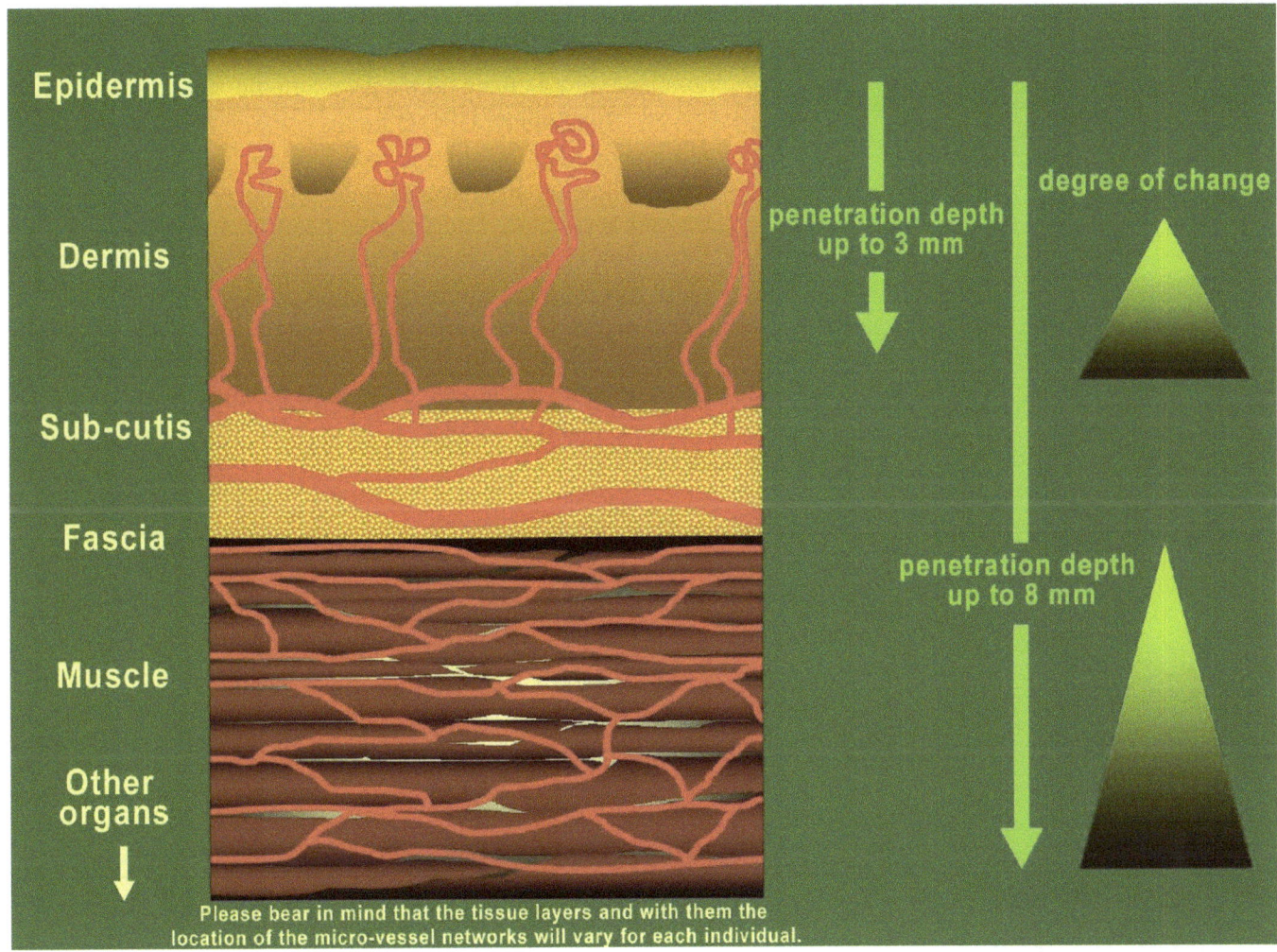

Please bear in mind that the tissue layers and with them the location of the micro-vessel networks will vary for each individual.

At the close of this chapter we would like to pay attention to the effects of a certain changing electromagnetic field on an area of tissue that is distinguished by its extraordinary immunological activity: the gingiva or gums. In the outspread flow pattern of the venules of the gumtissue that borders the teeth, stimulations of immunological behavior of the white blood cells can be observed impressively.

SUMMARY: The increased adhesion behavior of white blood cells after application of the pulsed electromagnetic field is considered to be one consequence of the extended distribution of the plasma/blood cell mix in the gingival microvessel networks at increased venular outward flow and is viewed as indirect stimulation of the body's own defense mechanisms. At the close of this chapter, we would like to consider the effects of a specific electromagnetic AC field in a tissue region that demonstrates particular immunological activity: the gingiva. Stimulation of the immunological behavior of white blood cells can be observed in an exceptional way in the richly branched venular flow pathways of the gingiva, which adheres directly to the tooth.

To illustrate this, we introduce the following results and selected vitalmicroscopic findings from two test series conducted.

Research Design

Test Sample	Total test sample Ntotal =28 Male test subjects, ~35 years of age, no pathological abnormalities
Partial Test Samples	2 equal partial test samples of n=14 ▶ Control group: no treatment (placebo) ▶ Test group: treatment with a changing electromagnetic field
Test System, Application	Blind study, GPC criteria Changing pulsed electromagnetic field BEMER 3000 One-time application of 2 minutes (intensity level 3)
Measurement Intervals and Timing	Observation time 6 minutes. Equidistant measurement intervals Zero minutes (determination of base values immediately prior to the application), subsequent 2-minute treatment, with data collection following in the 2nd, 4th and 6th minute.
Target Tissue	Gingiva (upper jaw, labial side, incisor)
Measurement Methods	▶ Intravitalmicroscopy with computer assisted image processing Documentation of findings: high-speed camera, 35 mm film, high resolution, up to 120 pictures per second. ▶ Vitalmiroscopic reflectionspectrometry ▶ Laser-DOPPLER-microflow measurement and white light spectroscopy Capture of complete interconnected micro-vascular networks with defined tissue volume V=1200µm3 (diameter of vessels d≤200µm). Penetration depth 3 mm maximum
Parameters	▶ Number of blood cell perfused nodal points nNP ▶ Changes in the venular flow rate ΔQ_{ven} ▶ Number of white blood cells adhering to a defined venule wall nWBC/A ▶ Localized changes in concentration of ICAM-1
Statistical Analysis	WILCOXON rank-sum test, a = 5%

The results are represented in figure 301.

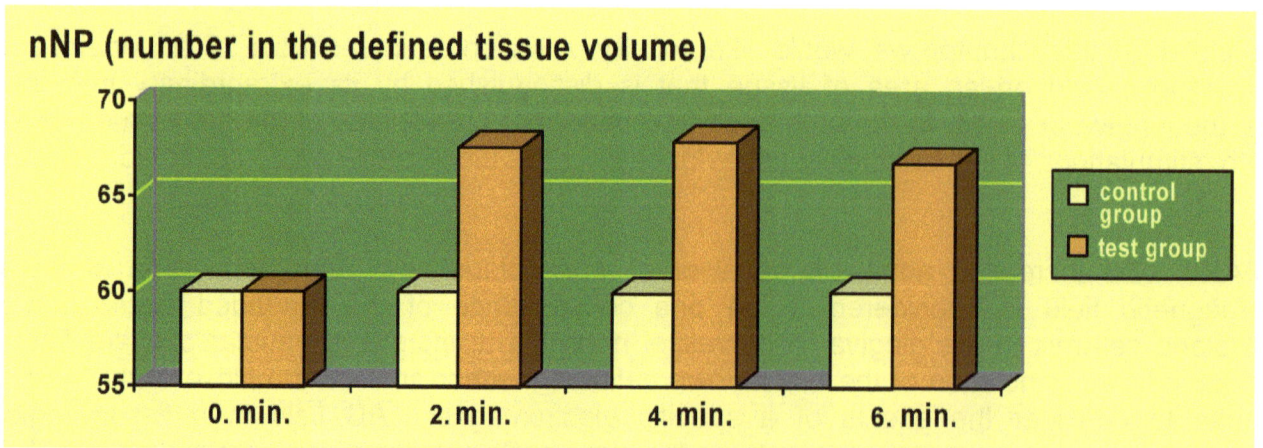

Figure 301
Measurements for the parameter "venular flow rate Qven" (mean values) in the target tissue gingiva after a one-time application of a certain pulsed electromagnetic field (BEMER, intensity level 3, 2-minute application). Results of the statistical evaluation: Significant differences in the parameters after the 2nd minute between the control group and the test group.

The heightened adhesion factor of the white blood cells after application of the pulsed electromagnetic field is assumed to be the result of the increased distribution of the blood-plasma mixture in the microvessel network of the gingiva when flow in the venules is increased and regarded as indirect stimulation of the body's own defense mechanisms. In the larger area of the intestines a parallel change in characteristics is to be expected (rectum, tunica muscularis, see figures 283 through 287). The significance of such an impact on the immunologic properties of white blood cells (e.g. adhesion to the endothelium) becomes apparent when a certain changing electromagnetic field is used for the treatment of experimental gingivitis. Experimental gingivitis constitutes a reversible, moderately developed acute-inflammatory process in younger, healthy subjects with otherwise healthy teeth. The experimental gingivitisis induced by forgoing all dental hygiene for 3 days.

Research Design

Test Sample	Total test sample $N_{total} = 24$ Male test subjects, ~20-25 years of age, no pathological abnormalities, healthy teeth
Partial Test Samples	2 equal partial test samples of n=14 ▶ **Control group:** no dental hygiene for 3 days, with standard oral hygiene afterwards (placebo). ▶ **Test group:** no dental hygiene for 3 days, with standard oral hygiene afterwards plus treatment with a changing electromagnetic field. day-3 day-2 day-1 day-0 day-1 day-2 day-3 day-4 day-5 day-6 no dental hygiene dental hygiene (control group) dental hygiene plus changing electromagnetic field (test group)
Test System, Application	Blind study, GPC criteriria Changing pulsed electromagnetic field BEMER 3000 **Test group: additional application of a changing electromagnetic field on day 1 and day 3** (2 treatments of 2 minutes each, 2 hours apart, intensity level 3 per treatment day)
Measurement Intervals and Timing	**Observation time 10 days.** Equidistant **measurement intervals:** Day -3, day -2, day -1 (experimental gingivitis) Day 0 (restart dental hygiene) Subsequent days 1,2,3,4,5,6 Starting day 0, data collection 1 hour after treatment (dental hygiene and dental hygiene plus changing electromagnetic field respectively).
Target Tissue	**Gingiva** (upper jaw, labial side, incisor)
Measurement Methods	▶ Intravitalmicroscopy with computer assisted image processing Documentation of findings: high-speed camera, 35 mm film, high resolution, up to 120 pictures per second. ▶ Laser-DOPPLER-microflow measurement and white light spectroscopy Capture of complete interconnected micro-vascular networks with defined tissue volume V=1200µm3 (diameter of vessels d≤200µm). Penetration depth 3 mm maximum Defined conditions of macro-circulation and temperature regulation.
Parameters	▶ Changes in the venular flow rate ΔQ_{ven} ▶ Number of white blood cells adhering to a defined venular wall area nWBC/A
Statistical Analysis	WILCOXON rank-sum test, a = 5%

The collected data are displayed in figures 304 and 305.

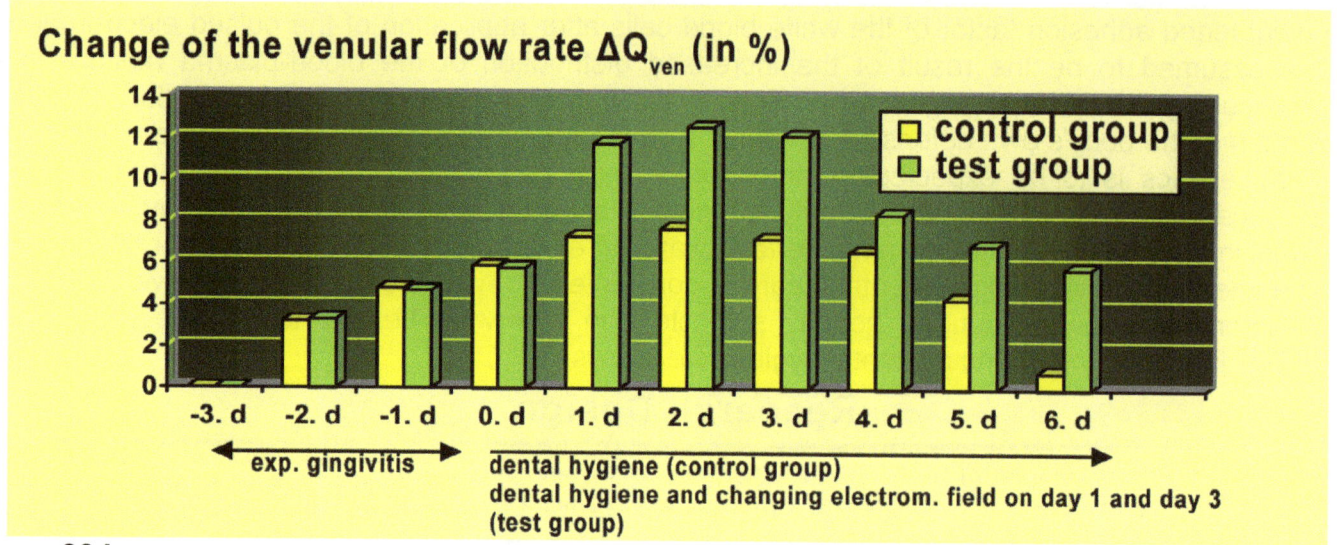

Figure 304
Measurements for the parameter "change in venular flow rate ΔQ_{ven}" (mean values) in the target tissue gingiva for subjects with experimental gingivitis before and after application of a certain pulsed electromagnetic field (test group) in comparison to a control group not treated with the changing electromagnetic field. Results of the statistical evaluation: Significant differences in the parameters after the 1st day between the control group and the test group.

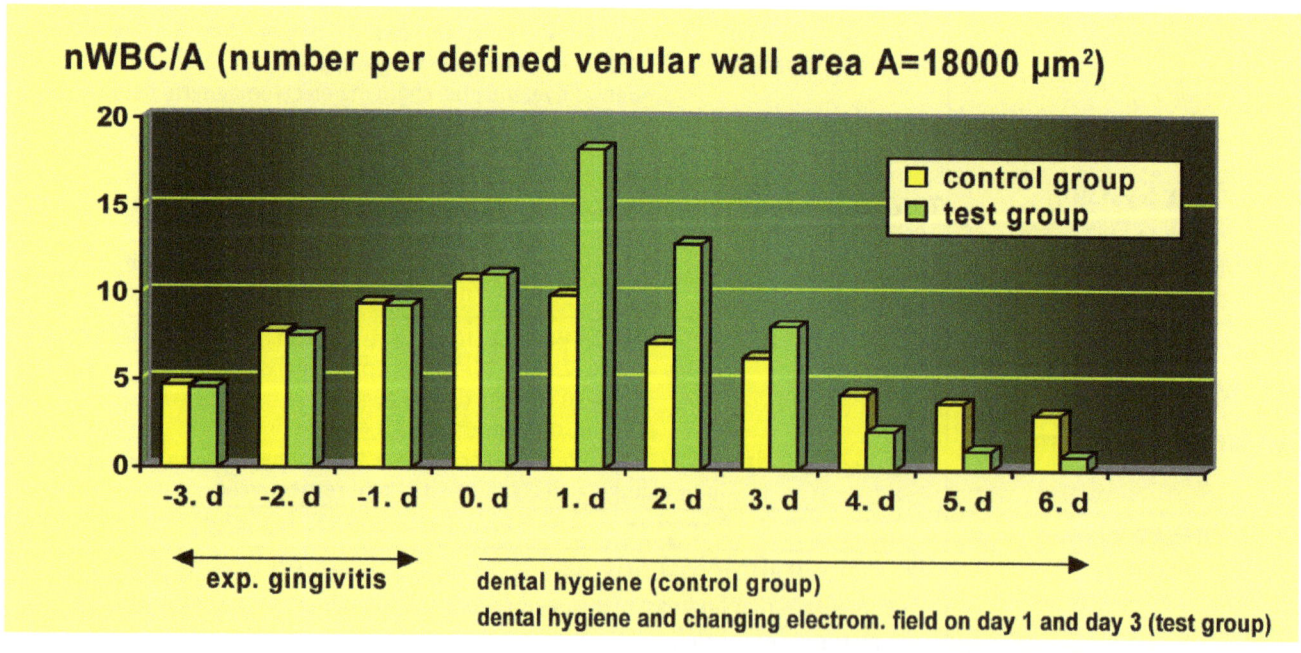

Figure 305
Measurements for the parameter "number of white blood cells adhering to a defined area of a venular wall nWBC/A" (mean values) in the target tissue gingiva for subjects with experimental gingivitis before and after application of a certain pulsed electromagnetic field (test group) in comparison to a control group not treated with the changing electromagnetic field. Results of the statistical evaluation: Significant differences in the parameters after the 1st day between the control group and the test group.

Figures 306 through 308 show selected findings from the gingival tissue for (indirect) stimulation of immunological criteria in white blood cells under the influence of a certain changing electromagnetic field.

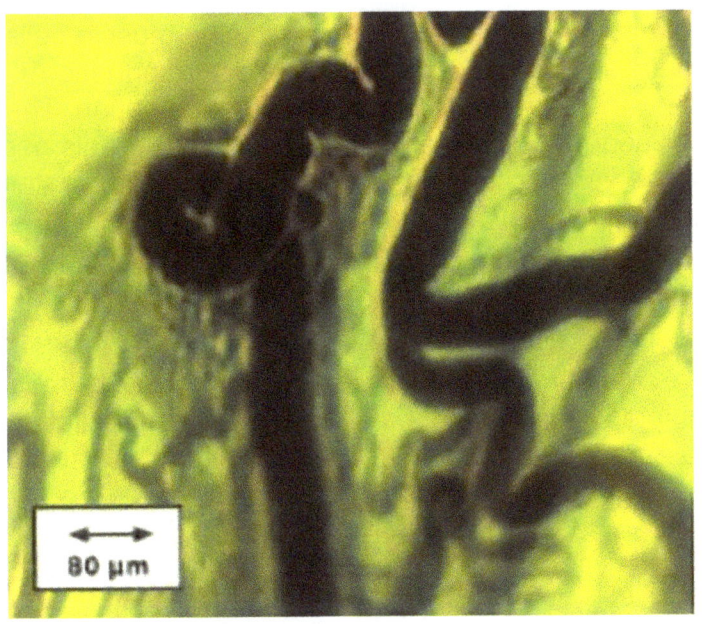 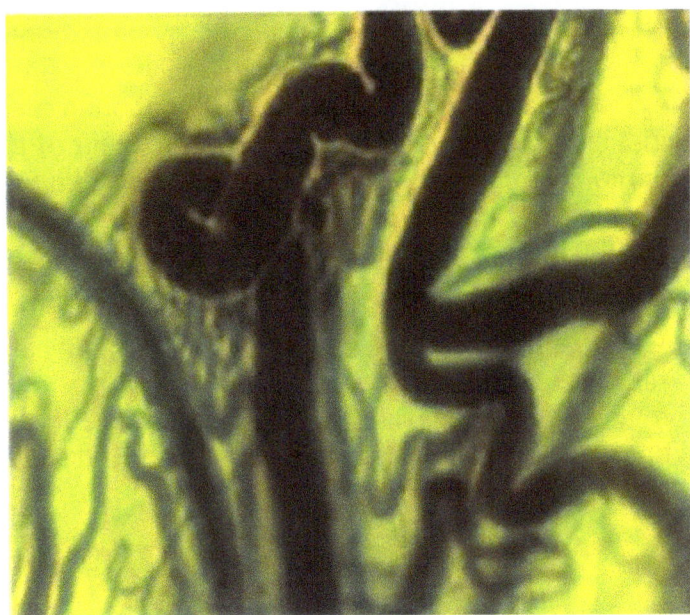

Figure 306
Changes in the venular flow rate and the blood distribution in the gingival microvessels for a test subject with experimental gingivitis before and after application of a certain changing electromagnetic field (BEMER). Vitalmicroscopic findings, 1/1000 second

    a: functional state of the gingival micro-circulation on the 3rd day of experimental gingivitis (day -1 in figures 304 and 305).

    b: functional state of the gingival micro-circulation on the 2nd day of treatment with a certain changing electromagnetic field (day 3 in figures 304 and 305).

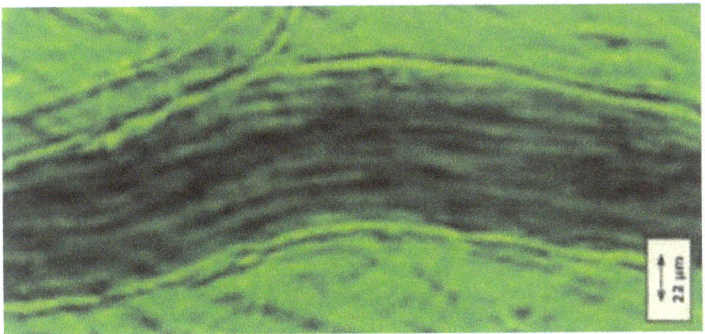 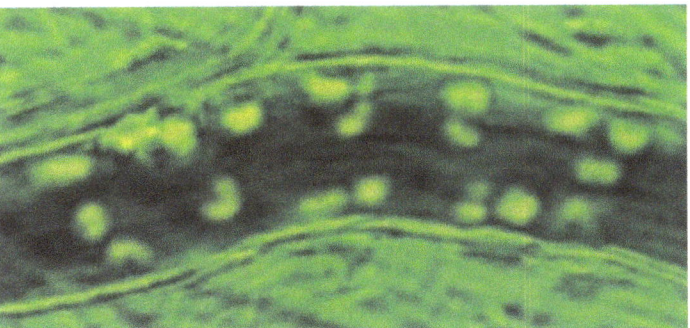

Comparison of the direct effect of a suitable electromagnetic AC field (BEMER) and of a suitable electromagnetic AC field with a special vasomotion-stimulating signal (BEMER Plus) on the characteristic changes in the superficial microvessel networks of the subcutis

Figure 307
Changes in the adhesion properties of white blood cells in the gingival micro- vessels for a test subject with experimental gingivitis before and after application of a certain changing electromagnetic field (BEMER). Vitalmicroscopic findings, 1/1000 second, venular flow.

    a: segment of a venule in the gingival micro-circulation on the 1st day of experimental gingivitis (day - 3 in figures 304 and 305).

    b: identical segment of a venule on the 1st day of treatment with a certain changing electromagnetic field (day 1 in figures 304 and 305). Numerous white blood cells are aggregated, some of them adhering to the endothelium of the venule.

SUMMARY: Stimulation of the autorhythmic contraction movements of the smooth vessel muscle cells in the smaller arterioles occurs directly after an 8-minute application of a specific electromagnetic AC field with additional vasomotoric stimulation in a sample with extensive loss of arteriole vasomotion. The most significant characteristic changes occur at a signal sequence frequency of 3 additional signals per minute. On the basis of the characteristic behavior of the venular flow, Figure 313 shows that greater vasomotoric stimulation effects have a greater influence on the functional status of the microcirculation.

The development of a therapy device that utilizes a certain changing electromagnetic field with added vasomotion stimulation (BEMER PLUS) is an innovative achievement of INNOMED INTERNATIONAL AG in Liechtenstein.

This therapy option makes use of the proven impulse configuration (see chapter 25, figure 281) and provides the possibility of adding a signal that stimulates vasomotion (frequency of the stimulation impulse 3/min.). The configuration of the added signal for vasomotion stimulation follows the principle illustrated in figure 281.

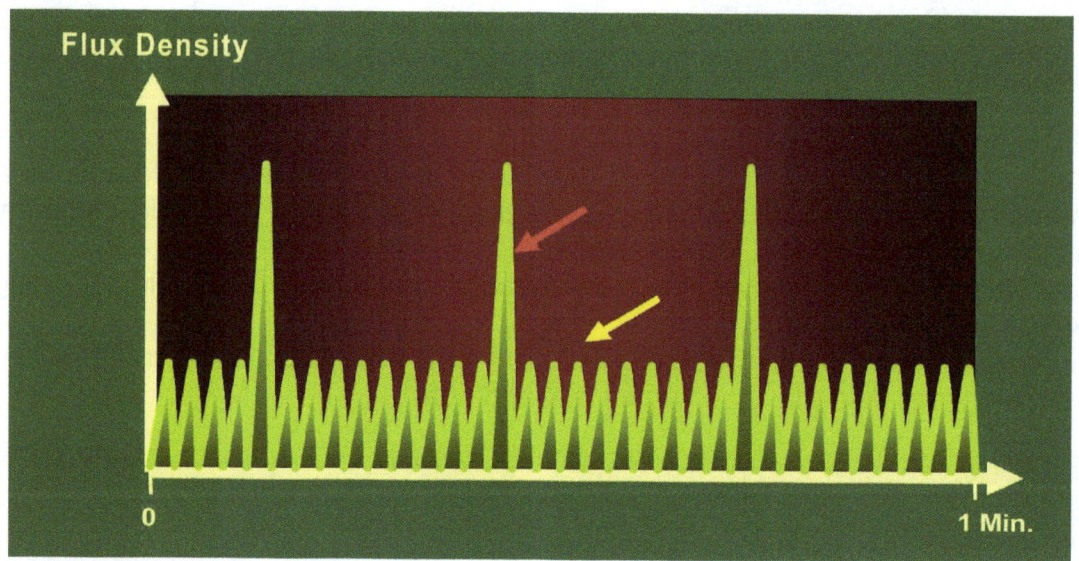

Figure 311 (following) Schematic illustration of the electromagnetic stimulation signals of the BEMER PLUS therapy device:

Basic stimulation identical to BEMER 3000 (yellow arrow), pulse width 33ms. Added signals for vasomotion stimulation (red arrow), pulse width 165 ms, consisting of 5 single impulses each. Added signals are 20 seconds apart.

When using the mat: Flux densities correspond to an intensity level range of ~5 µT to ~35 µT

The following test results show confirmation of this concept. We can see that this kind of stimulation is "recognized" by the biological system and elicits increased therapy-relevant results.

Research Design

Test Sample	Total test sample N_{TOTAL} =54 Multi-morbid male test subject, -70 years of age, no aculte ailments, vasomotion frequency ≤ 0.1/min
Partial Test Sample	3 equal partial test samples of n=18; treated with a certain changing electromagnetic field (BEMER). ▶ Additional vasomotion stimulation signal frequency 1/min ▶ Additional vasomotion stimulation signal frequency 2/min ▶ Additional vasomotion stimulation signal frequency 3/min

Test System, Application	Blind study, GPC criteria Changing pulsed electromagnetic field BEMER 3000 One-time treatment of 8 minutes (intensity level 3, on the mat) plus added stimulation signal
Measurement Intervals and timing	Observation time 8 minutes. Equidistant measurement intervals Zero minutes (determination of base values immediately prior to the application), subsequent 8-minute treatment, with data collection following immedi-
Target Tissue	Sub-cutis (left forearm)
Measurement Methods	▶ Intravitalmicroscopy with computer assisted image processing ▶ Laser-DOPPLER-microflow measurement in combination with white light spectroscopy Depth of penetration 3 mm maximum. Capture of arteriolar diameters in defined tissue volume
Parameters	▶ Number of vasomotion oscillations per minute ▶ Venular flow rate
Statistical Analysis	WILCOXON rank-sum test, a = 5%

The measurement data gathered are displayed in figures 312 and 313.

The data displayed in figure 312 indicate that a stimulation of the auto-rhythmic contractions of the smooth muscle cells in the smaller arterioles happens immediately after an 8-minute application of a certain changing electromagnetic field with added vasomotion stimulation in a test sample of persons with almost nonexistent vasomotion.

The most significant changes in characteristics occur with a frequency of 3 additional signals per minute. We can gather from figure 313, based on the parameter changes in the venular flow rate, that the effects of stronger stimulation of the vasomotion result in a more pronounced influence on the functional state of the microcirculation. We can interpret this as a confirmation of the signal configuration with added vasomotion stimulation that is used in the BEMER PLUS therapy system.

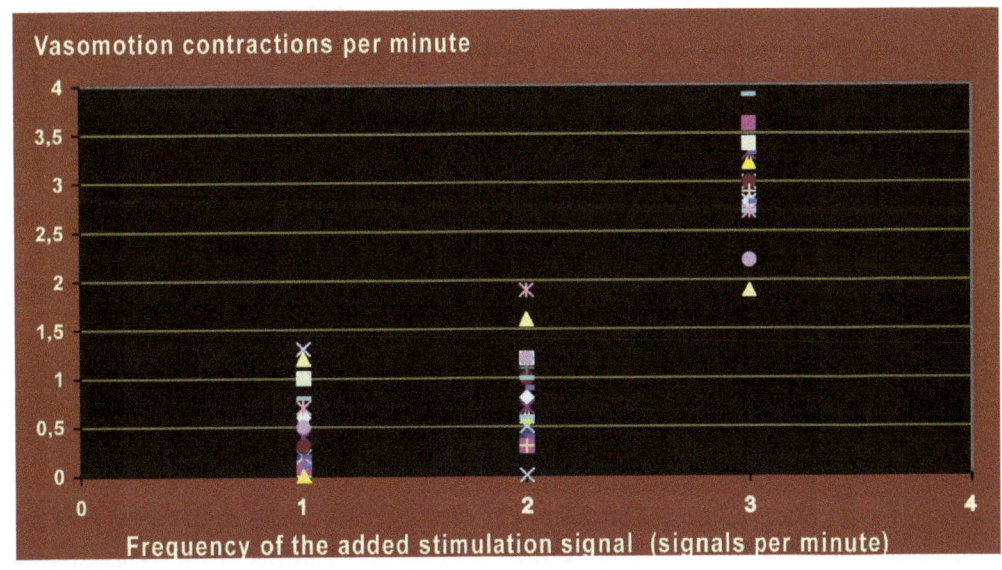

Figure 312
Stimulated vasomotion contractions after an 8-minute application of a certain changing electromagnetic field with added vasomotion stimulation of varying signal sequence frequency in 3 partial test samples (n=18) of multi-morbid older patients. Abscissa: Varying signal sequence frequencies of the added signal used in the 3 partial test samples. Ordinate: Related, in part overlying data points of the individual vasomotion contractions

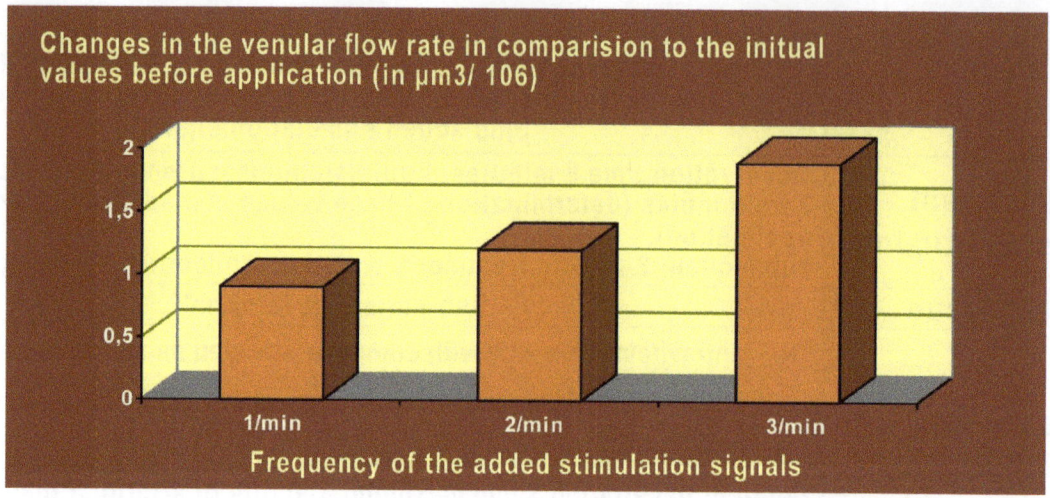

Figure 313

Changes in the venular flow rate in the sub-cutaneous target tissue subject to the impulse sequence frequency of the added signal immediately after an 8-minute application. (Difference of the venular flow rate between the times t=0 before treatment and t= t immediately after an 8-minute application; mean values, significant differences in parameters).

Comparison of the direct effect of a suitable electromagnetic AC field (BEMER) and of a suitable electromagnetic AC field with a special vasomotion-stimulating signal (BEMER Plus) on the characteristic changes in the superficial microvessel networks of the subcutis (infracutaneous, regio epigastrica)

SUMMARY: *The results clearly show increased characteristic changes in the group of patients in which a specific electromagnetic AC field with additional vasomotoric stimulation (BEMER Plus) was applied. The temporal behavior of the characteristic changes is of significantly greater duration compared to a specific electromagnetic AC field without additional vasomotoric stimulation (BEMER 3000). The measurement results show clearer changes at greater tissue depth.*

Below we will address the behavior of functional microcirculatory parameters after the application of a certain changing electromagnetic field with added vasomotion stimulation (BEMER PLUS) for two patient samples whose local microcirculation is restricted in differing degrees: a test sample of middle aged individuals exposed to stress and infection, and a test sample of high-risk geriatric with cardio-vascular patients (therapy controls).

Test	Test sample size N_{TOTAL} =48 Male test subjects, 35-45 years of age, no pathological abnormalties Exposure to stress and infection

Partial Test Samples	3 equal partial test samples of n=18; treated with a certain changing electromagnetic
	➡ Partial test sample A
	    Application of a certain changing electromagnetic field <u>without</u> added vasomotion stimulation (BEMER 3000).
	➡ Partial test sample B
	    Application of a certain changing electromagnetic field <u>with</u> added vasomotion stimulation (BEMER Plus).

Test System,	Pulsed changing electromagnetic field BEMER 3000 and BEMER Plus Application: 2 application each, 2 hours apart (8 minutes, intensity level 3, on the mat).

Measurement Intervals and	Observation time of 60 minutes, equidistant measurement intervals: ▶ Zero minutes (determination of base values immediately prior to the 1st application), subsequent 8-minute treatment. ▶ Data collection immediately following the 2nd treatment in the 4th, 8th, 12th, 16th, 20th, 24th, 28th, 32nd, 36th, 40th, 44th, 48th, 52nd, 56th, and 60th
Target Tissue	Sub-cutis/ infra-cutaneous tissue (abdomen, region epigastr.).
Measurement Methods	Simultaneous measurements at 2 different tissue depth: Penetration depth 3 mm Penetration depth 8 mm ▶ Intravitalmicroscopy with computer assisted image processing ▶ Vitalmicroscopy with computer assisted image processing. ▶ Laser-DOPPLER-microflow-measurement and white light spectroscopy. Capture of complete interconnected micro-vascular networks with defined tissue volume V=1200µm³ (diameter of vessels d≤200µm). Defined conditions of macro-circulation and temperature regulation.
Parameters	▶ Number of blood cell perfused nodal points nNP. ▶ Changes in the venular flow rate ΔQ_{ven}. ▶ Area below the envelop of the amplitude-frequency-spectrum of the (spontaneous) arteriolar vasomotion A_{vm}.
Statistical Analysis	WILCOXON rank-sum test (MWW), a = 5%

Figures 314 through 316 show a summary of the data collected.

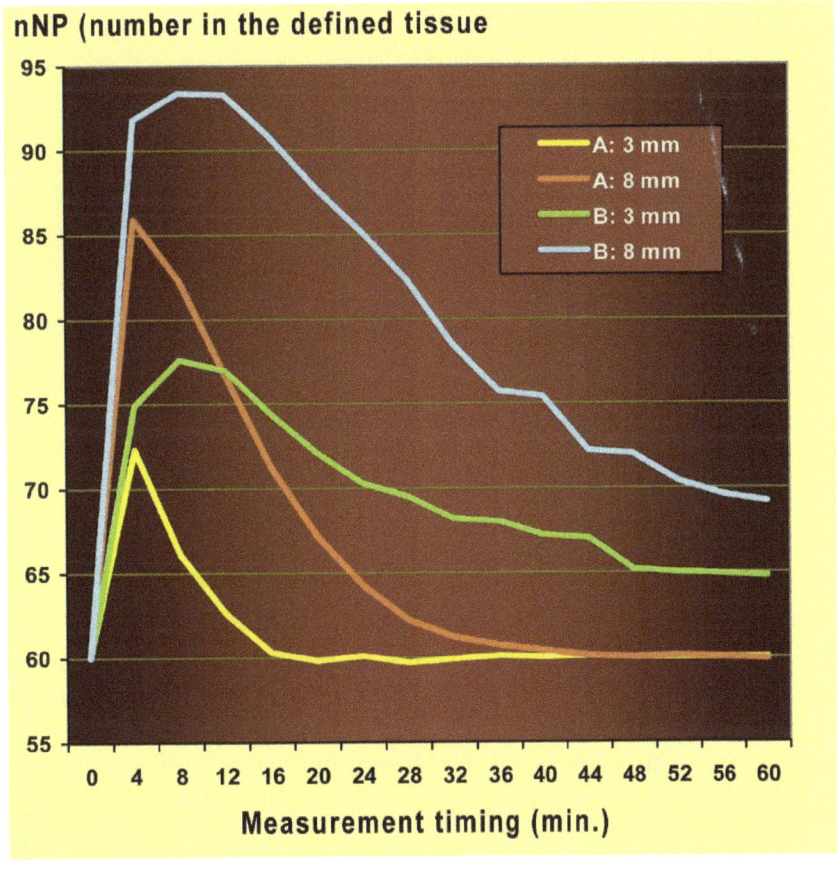

Figure 314
Measurements for the parameter "number of blood cell perfused nodal points nNP" (mean values) in the target tissue sub-cutis after application of a certain pulsed electromagnetic field with and without added

vasomotion stimulation for test subjects exposed to stress and infection. Partial test sample A: no added vasomotion stimulation (BEMER)

Partial test sample B: with added vasomotion stimulation (BEMER PLUS) Measurement values taken at 2 different penetration depths: 3 mm and 8 mm.

Two applications of 8 minutes each, 2 hours apart (intensity level 3). Measurement timing: 0 minutes: initial values prior to the first application. Every four minutes up to 60 minutes after the 2nd application. Significant differences in measured parameters after the 4th minute between the wo partial sample groups.

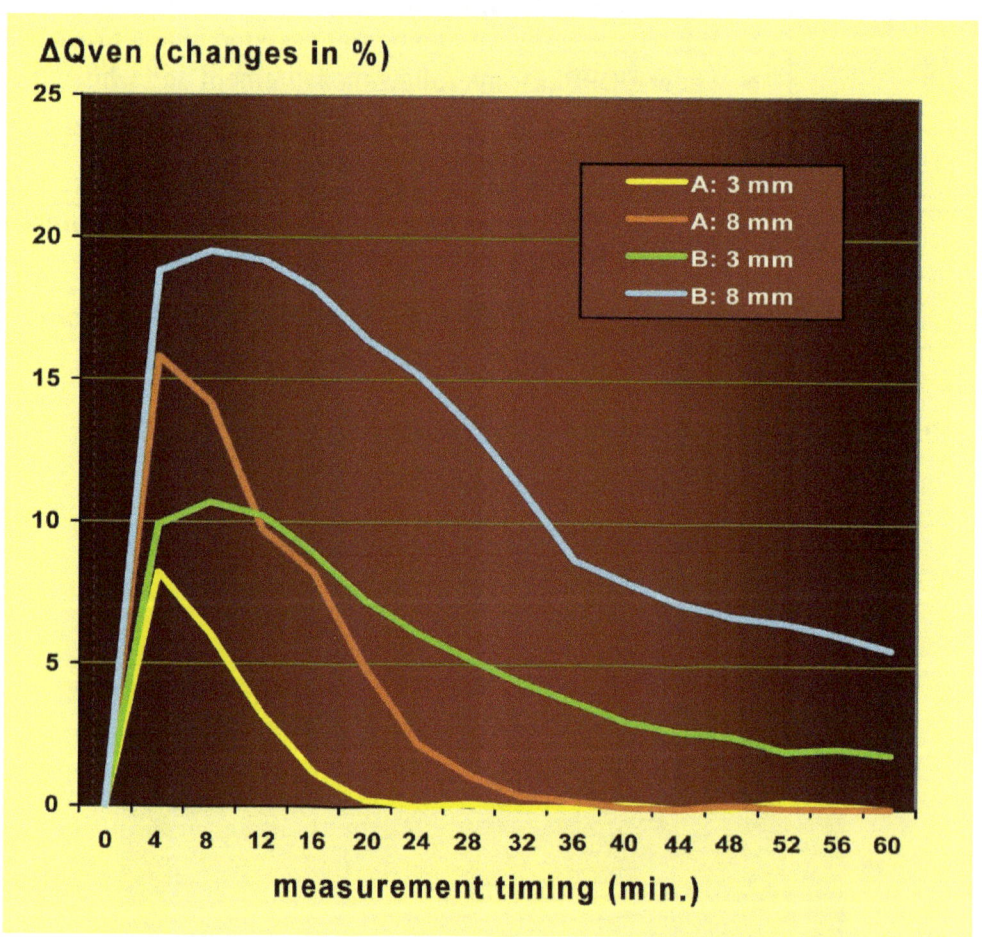

Figure 315
Measurements for the parameter "changes in the venular flow rate ΔQven" (mean values) in the target tissue sub-cutis after application of a certain pulsed electromagnetic field with and without added vasomotion stimulation for test subjects exposed to stress and infection. Partial test sample A: no added vasomotion stimulation (BEMER) Partial test sample B: with added vasomotion stimulation (BEMER PLUS) Measurement values taken at 2 different penetration depths: 3 mm and 8 mm. Two applications of 8 minutes each, 2 hours apart (intensity level 3). Measurement timing: 0 minutes: initial values prior to the first application. Every four minutes up to 60 minutes after the 2nd application.

Significant differences in measured parameters after the 4th minute between the two partial sample groups.

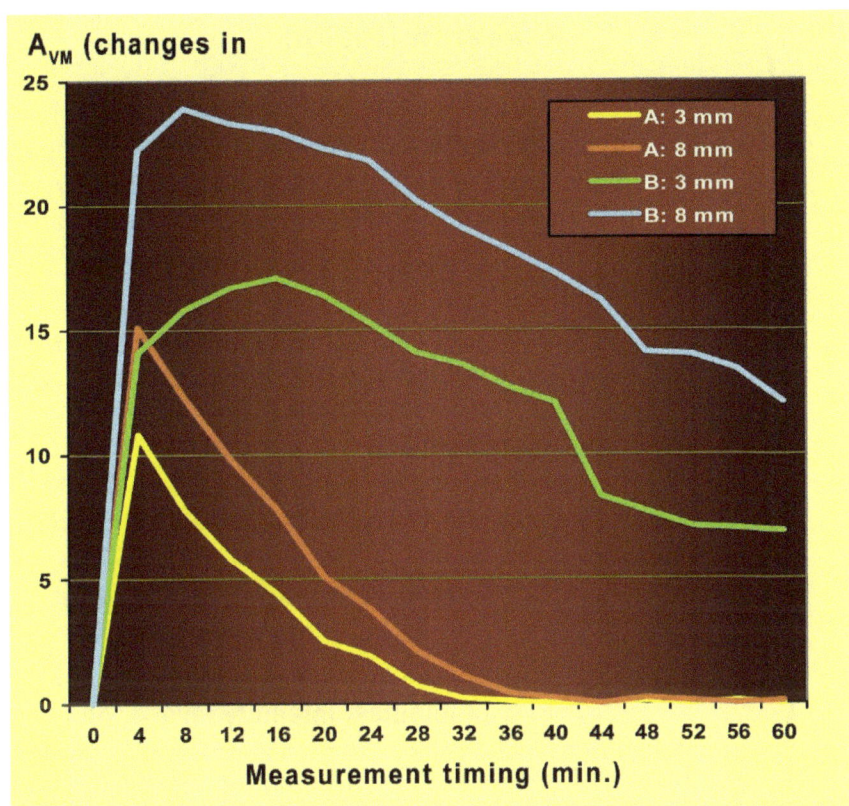

Comparison of the effect of long-term application of a suitable electromagnetic AC field (BEMER) and of a suitable electromagnetic AC field with a special vasomotion-stimulating signal (BEMER Plus) on the characteristic changes in the superficial microvessel networks of the subcutis (infracutaneous, regio epigastrica) at varying tissue depth (penetration depths of 3 mm and 8 mm)

Figure 316
Measurements for the parameter "area under the envelope of the amplitude frequency spectrum of spontaneous arteriolar vasomotion Avm" (mean values) in the target tissue sub-cutis after application of a certain pulsed electromagnetic field with and without added vasomotion stimulation for test subjects exposed to stress and infection. Partial test sample A: no added vasomotion stimulation (BEMER) Partial test sample B: with added vasomotion stimulation (BEMER PLUS) Measurement values taken at 2 different penetration depths: 3 mm and 8 mm. Two applications of 8 minutes each, 2 hours apart (intensity level 3). Measurement timing: 0 minutes: initial values prior to the first application. Every four minutes up to 60 minutes after the 2nd application. Significant differences in measured parameters after the 4th minute between the two partial sample groups.

SUMMARY: The following is a summary of the presented results of investigation into the effects of specific electromagnetic fields with additional vasomotoric stimulation in the field of microcirculation:

The functional status of the microcirculation can be influenced to a physiologically relevant extent by applying specific electromagnetic AC fields. In stressed and diseased conditions associated with disrupted spontaneous vasomotion, additional vasomotoric stimulation signals increase therapy-relevant effects in the microcirculation. Comparison with other treatment options shows that the application of specific electromagnetic AC fields should be given a place in the spectrum of effective prophylactic and complementary therapeutic measures.

The increased effects of a certain changing electromagnetic field with added vasomotion stimulation become impressively evident in the context of long term therapy for ambulant multi-morbid patients suffering from extensive vasomotion disturbances.

Research Design

Test	Total test sample $N_{TOTAL} = 36$ Ambulant male and female patients, 69-78 years of age. Multi-morbid geriatric cardio-vascular at-risk patients. No indication for inpatient treatment (adult onset diabetes)
Partial Test Samples	Two equal partial test samples of n=18 ▶ Partial test sample A Application of a certain changing electromagnetic field <u>without</u> added vasomotion stimulation (BEMER 3000). ▶ Partial test sample B Application of a certain changing electromagnetic field <u>with</u> added vasomotion stimulation (BEMER Plus).
Test System,	Pulsed changing electromagnetic field BEMER 3000 and BEMER Plus Two applications every other day, 2 hours apart (8 minutes, intensity level 3, on the mat).
Measurement Intervals and	Observation time of 60 minutes, equidistant measurement intervals: ▶ Day zero (determination of base values immediately prior to the 1st application), subsequent beginning of treatment. ▶ Data collections 1 day after each application on the 4th, 8th, 12th, 16th, 20th, 24th, 28th, 32nd, 36th, 40th, 44th, 48th, 52nd, 56th, and 60th day.
Target Tissue	Sub-cutis/ infra-cutaneous tissue (abdomen, region epigastr.).
Measurement Methods	Simultaneous measurements at 2 different tissue depth: Penetration depth 3 mm Penetration depth 8 mm ▶ Intravitalmicroscopy with computer assisted image processing Vitalmicroscopy with computer assisted image processing. ▶ Laser-DOPPLER-microflow-measurement and white light spectroscopy. Capture of complete interconnected micro-vascular networks with defined tissue volume $V=1200\mu m^3$ (diameter of vessels $d \leq 200\mu m$). Defined conditions of macro-circulation and temperature regulation.
Parameters	▶ Number of blood cell perfused nodal points nNP. ▶ Area below the envelop of the amplitude-frequency-spectrum of the (spontaneous) arteriolar vasomotion A_{vm}.
Statistical Analysis	WILCOXON rank-sum test (MWW), $a = 5\%$

Figures 317 and 318 provide information on the measurement data collected. Figures 319, 321 and 322 display examples of vitalmicroscopic findings. In figure 320, we use selected individual diagnostic findings to point to the rhythmic character of the changes in microcirculatory parameters after the application of a certain changing electromagnetic field with added vasomotion stimulation.

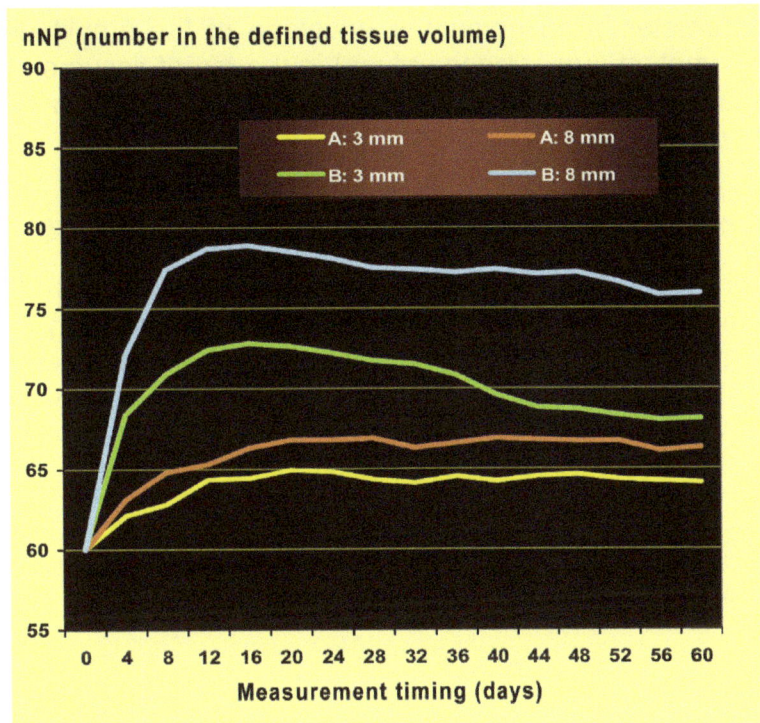

Figure 317
Measurements for the parameter "number of blood cell perfused nodal points nNP" (mean values) in the target tissue sub-cutis after application of a certain pulsed electromagnetic field with and without added vasomotion stimulation for multi-morbid geriatric patients with high cardio-vascular risk factors. Partial test sample A: no added vasomotion stimulation (BEMER) Partial test sample B: with added vasomotion stimulation (BEMER PLUS) Measurement values taken at 2 different penetration depths: 3 mm and 8 mm. Two applications of 8 minutes each, 2 hours apart, every other day (intensity level 3, on the mat). Measurement timing: Day zero: initial values prior to the first application. Day 4 to day 60 of therapy period.

Significant differences in measured parameters after the 8th day between the two partial sample groups.

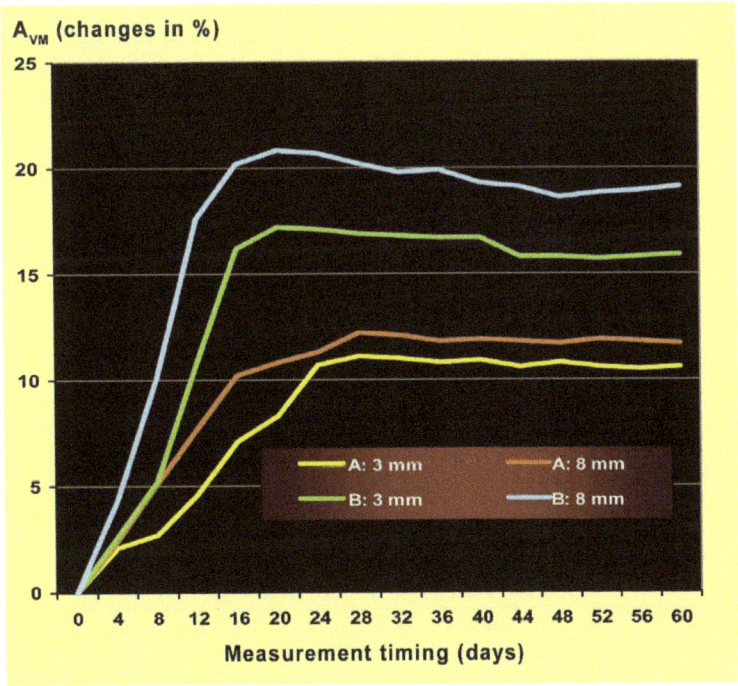

Figure 318

Measurements for the parameter "area under the envelope of the amplitude frequency spectrum of spontaneous arteriolar vasomotion Avm" (mean values) in the target tissue sub-cutis after application of a certain pulsed electromagnetic field with and without added vasomotion stimulation for multimorbid geriatric patients with high cardio-vascular risk factors.

Partial test sample A: no added vasomotion stimulation (BEMER)
Partial test sample B: with added vasomotion stimulation (BEMER PLUS)

Measurement values taken at 2 different penetration depths: 3 mm and 8 mm. Two applications of 8 minutes each, 2 hours apart, every other day (intensity level 3, on the mat). Measurement timing: Day zero: initial values prior to the first application. Day 4 to day 60 of therapy period. Significant differences in measured parameters after the 12th day between the two partial sample groups.

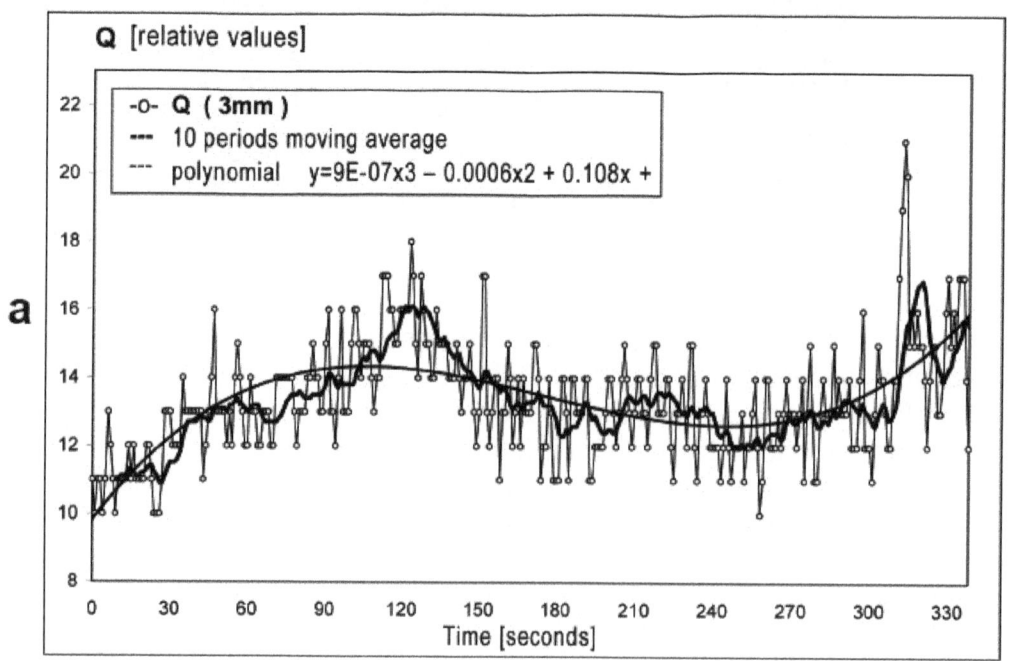

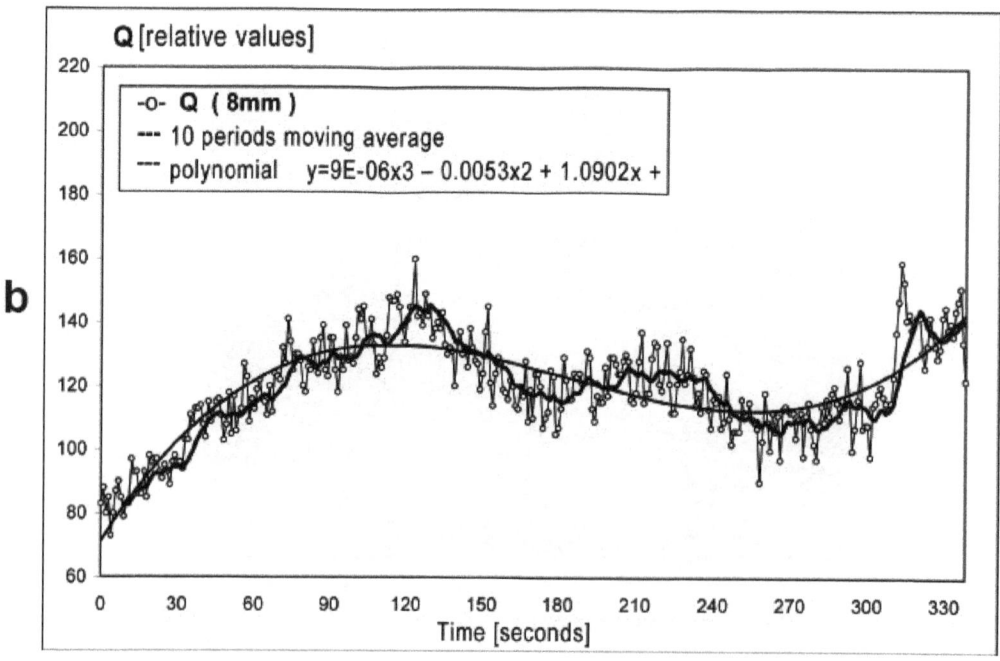

Figure 320

Changes in the venular flow rate in the micro-vessels of the sub-cutaneous target tissue at varying tissue depths (3 mm and 8 mm) under the influence of a certain changing electromagnetic field. Continuous recording within a defined period (beginning with the 2nd minute of the application of a certain changing electromagnetic field). a, b: application of a certain changing electromagnetic field without added vasomotion stimulation (BEMER). c, d: application of a certain changing electromagnetic field with added vasomotion stimulation (BEMER PLUS).

Please pay attention to the differing amounts in parameter changes (ordinate scale!) and the rhythmic course of the graphs. Aside from the daily fluctuations of biological rhythms (circadian rhythms) several other variations of biological characteristics occur. The regulatory processes of microcirculation especially are subject to a changing vibration behavior. One example would be the "swing adjustment" of the microcirculatory flow rate to a different regulatory level under the diction of spontaneous vasomotion.

c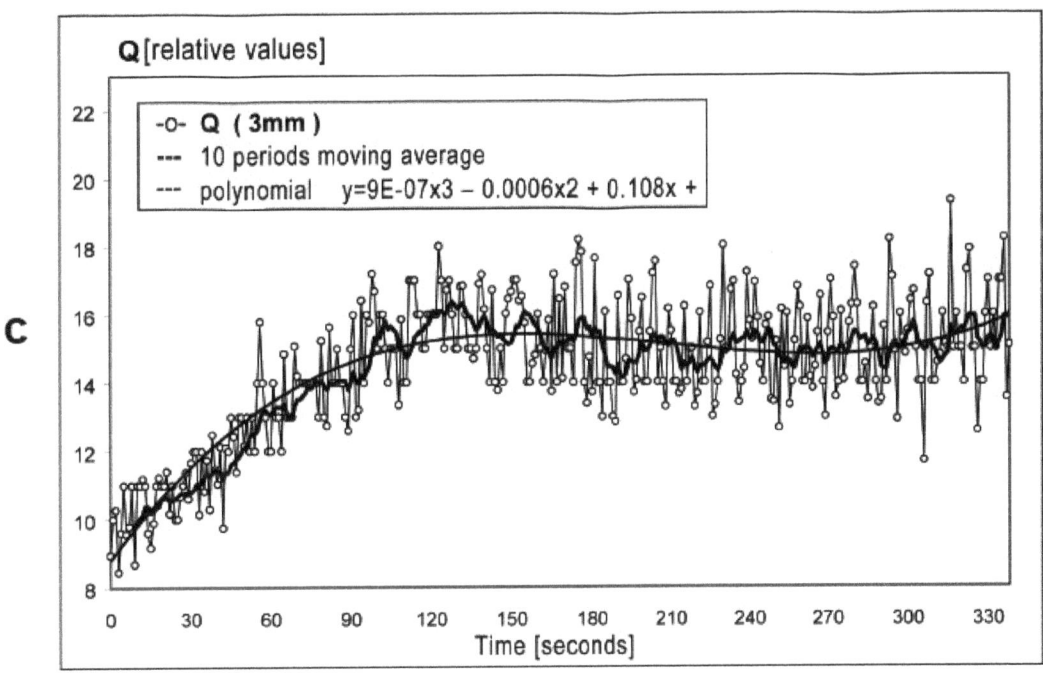

d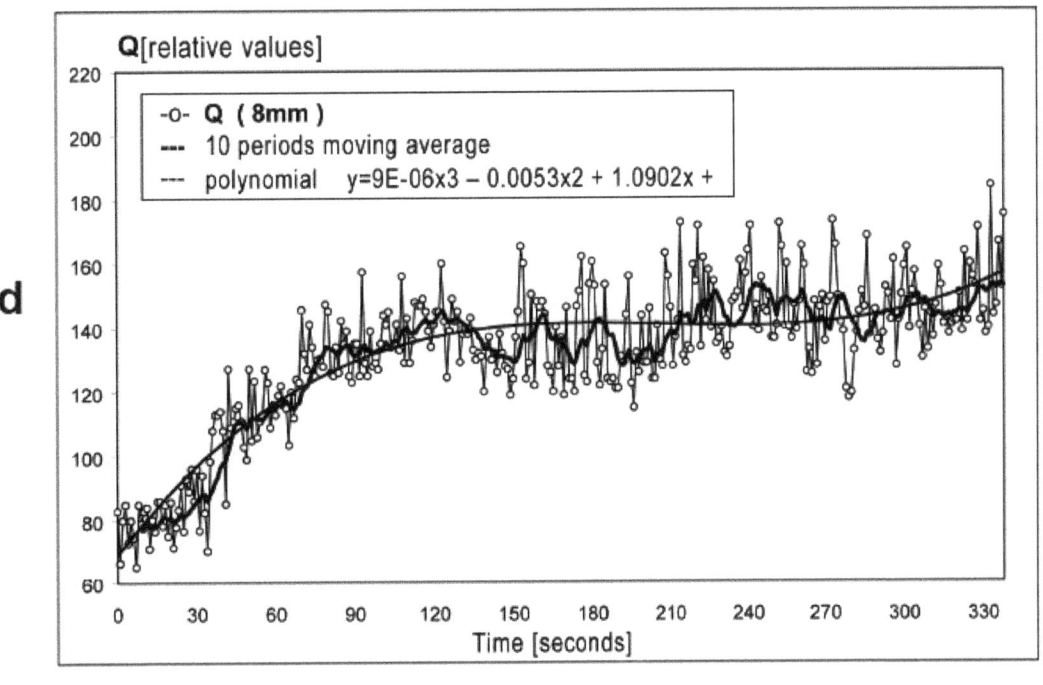

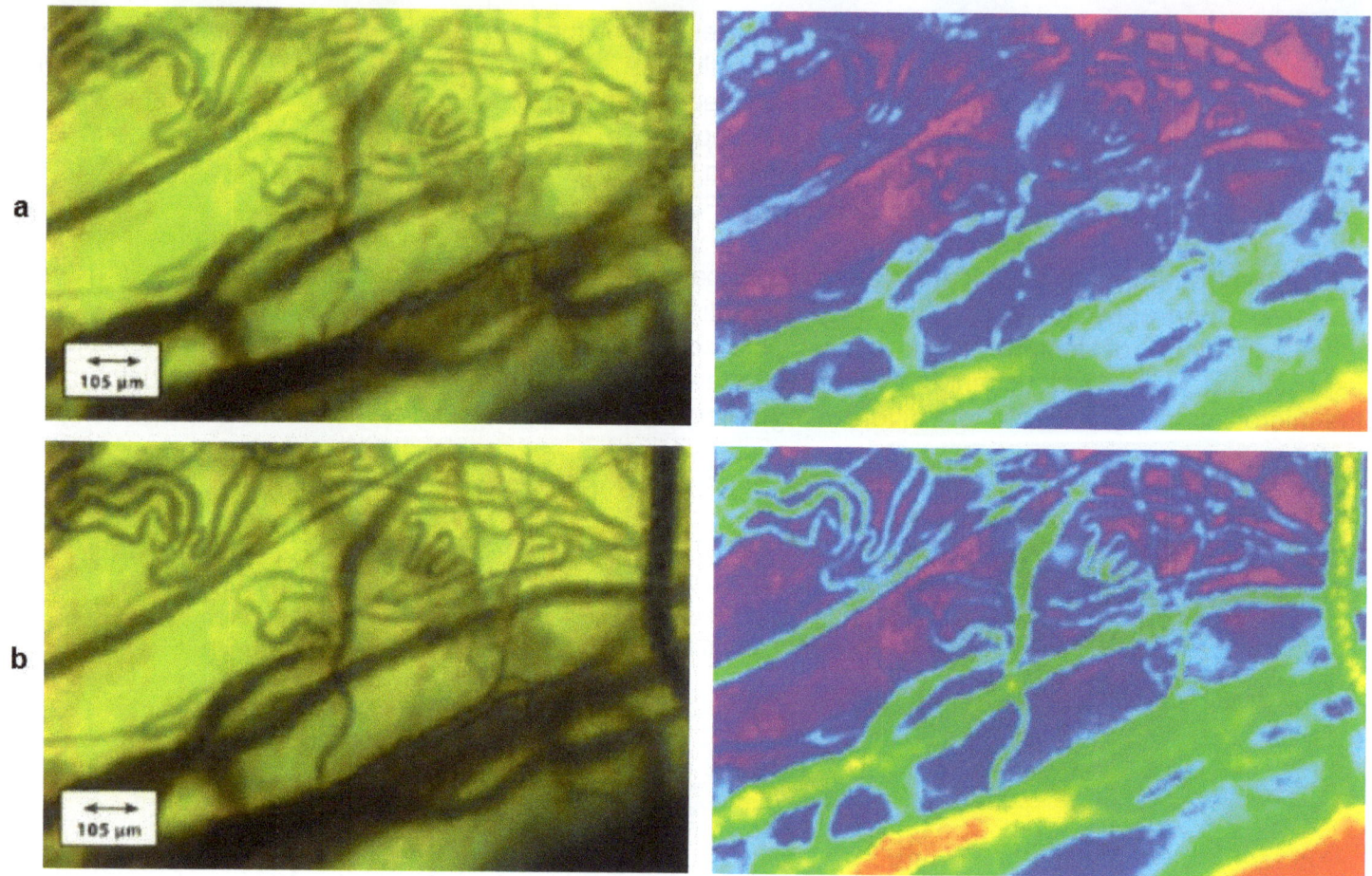

Figure 321
Distribution of the plasma-blood cell mixture in the micro-vessels of the subcutaneous target tissue before and after the application of a certain changing electromagnetic field with vasomotion stimulation. (Example of vitalmicroscopic findings, 1/1000 second; capillaries, venules, arterioles).

    a: distribution before application
    b: distribution after an 8-muinute application

Primary image on left, related pseudo-color-transformation of the primary image on right (the blood cell perfused micro vessels are marked in red). The noticeable increase of blood cell perfused nodal points in the micro-vascular network after the application of a certain changing electromagnetic field with added vasomotorstimulation can be clearly seen.

Figure 322 (following)
Change of the perfusion level in the micro-vessels of the sub-cutaneous target tissue before and after the application of a certain changing electromagnetic field with vasomotion stimulation. (Example of vitalmicroscopic findings, 1/1000 second; capillaries, venules, arterioles). Image sequence a to d: identical region of micro- vessels at different observation times (60 seconds apart)

The functional state of the micro-circulation in this network changes from minute to minute under the influence of the application: Increased speed in the flow of red blood cells, increase of the flow rate in the arterioles and venules, disaggregation of red blood cells, normalized capillary perfusion.

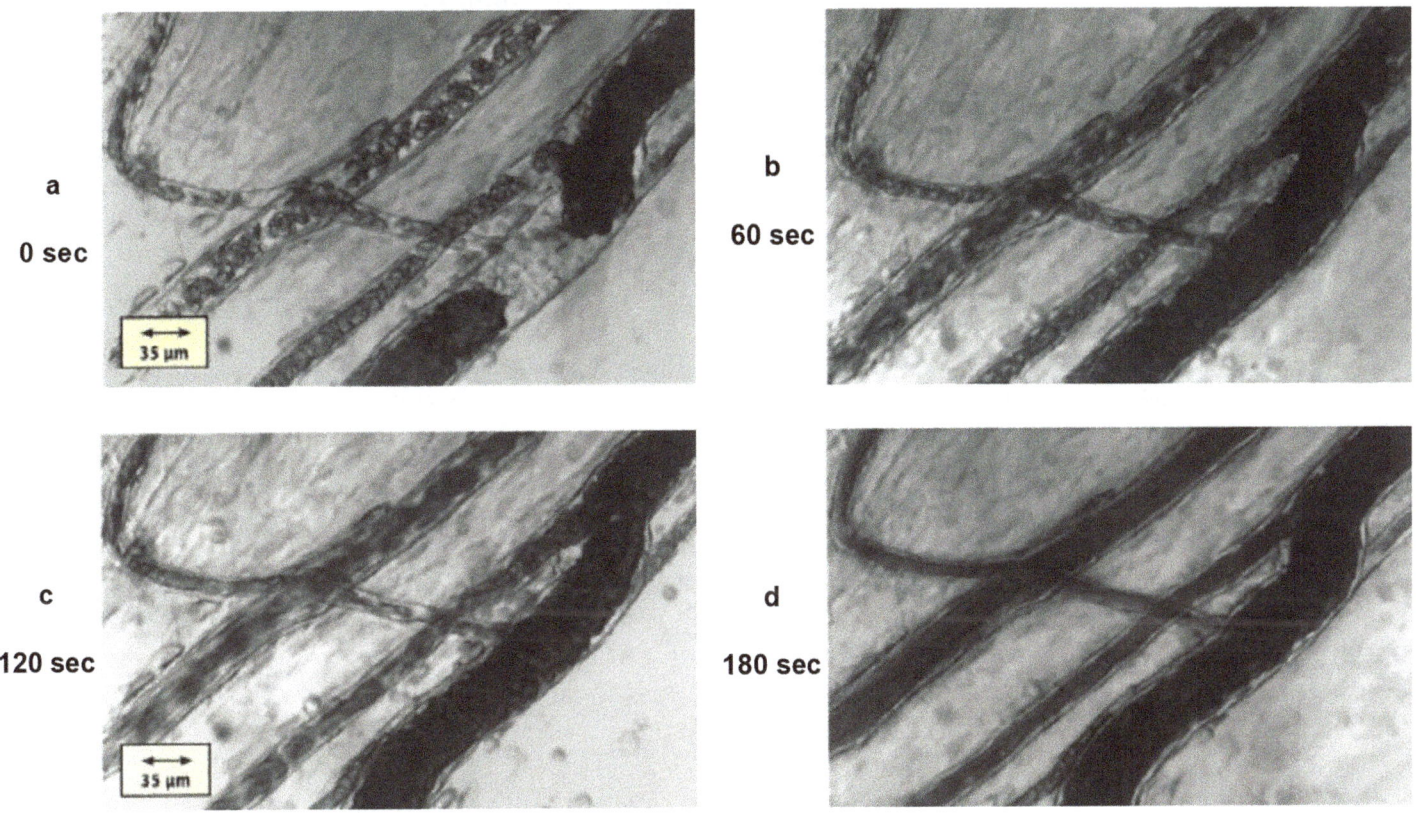

SUMMARY: Micro-circulatory function can be influenced to a physiologically relevant degree by the application of certain changing electromagnetic fields. For conditions of stress and illness that are accompanied by impaired spontaneous vasomotion, added signals for vasomotion stimulation produce increased therapeutic benefits on micro-circulatory function. A comparison to other therapy option shows that the application of certain changing electromagnetic fields has a valid place in the spectrum of effectual prophylactic and complementary therapy options.

The proven possibilities to influence spontaneous vasomotion have revived scientific discussions regarding the hypothesis for possible effects of certain electromagnetic fields in the area of microcirculation. This applies to both endothelial factors of the spontaneous vasmotoric functions and processes during energy provision in the mitochondria.

Complementary Therapeutic Effects of a Defined Electromagnetic AC Field on Local Microcirculation Regulation Mechanisms

Lecture at the 2nd European Congress for Integrative Medicine, Berlin 11.20.2009

Dr.med. Rainer Klopp; Institute for Microcirculation, Berlin, Germany

SUMMARY: The evaluated effect of a defined electromagnetic AC field with a special signal configuration to stimulate spontaneous arteriolar vasomotion (BEMER Plus system) on the microcirculation and the immune system is of a relevant magnitude in terms of prophylactic or complementary therapeutic use.

AIM: Multiple studies in compliance with Good Clinical Practice (GCP) were to demonstrate what effects specific electromagnetic AC fields have when applied preventively or as an additional complementary therapy to improve conventional treatment plans.

MATERIALS AND METHODS: The investigation was performed on 2 samples (each n = 24), divided each into a verum and placebo group. The period of observation and treatment was 30 days in every case. One sample consisted of older patients in rehabilitation; the other sample consisted of middle-aged subjects exposed to stress. The main target parameters were the representative functional characteristics of the microcirculation, as well as the metabolic and immunologic characteristic of white blood cells in the subcutaneous or intestinal target tissue.

The measurement methods included intravital microscopy with subsequent computer-aided imaging and intravital microscopy with reflexion spectrometry, combined with laser microfluidics and white light spectrometry. The Wilcoxon signed-rank test was used for statistical evaluation ($\alpha=5\%$). Comparative investigations were also performed on the different other magnetic or electromagnetic fields of various signal configurations and of varying intensity.

RESULTS: After applying a defined electromagnetic AC field with a special signal configuration to stimulate spontaneous arteriolar vasomotion (BEMER Plus system), the older patients in rehabilitation demonstrated an increase in spontaneous arteriolar vasomotion of 20% compared to the control group. In the group of middle-age subjects exposed to stress, the improvement rates were slightly lower, associated with slower rate of decay.

In addition, similar significant improvements were identified with regard to blood distribution conditions within the microvascular network, the venous outward flow, the venule-side oxygen saturation and the immunological characteristics of the leucocytes.In contrast, extremely lower electromagnetic AC fields with constant periodicity demonstrated a significantly lower effect on the microcirculation characteristics. Weak, static magnetic fields had no effect at all on microcirculation characteristics.

SUMMARY: The evaluated effect of a defined electromagnetic AC field with a special signal configuration to stimulate spontaneous arteriolar vasomotion (BEMER Plus system) on the microcirculation and the immune system is of a relevant magnitude in terms of prophylactic or complementary therapeutic use.

Improvement of Limited or Pathologically Altered Regulation of Organ Blood Flow as a Cause of Impaired Organ Function and Reduced Primary Immunological Processes Effectivity

Lecture at the Budapest Congress 03.26.2011

Dr. med. Wolfgang Bohn; Medical Expert Center, Triesen, Liechtenstein

SUMMARY: BEMER technology systems are able to improve limited or pathologically altered regulation of organ blood flow as a cause of impaired organ function and reduced primary immunological processes effectively and with relevance to therapy.

Systematic basic research into BEMER technology began in 2004 with an initial orientating study on the changes to characteristics in the microcirculation that could be achieved using the weak pulsed electromagnetic fields of the BEMER 3000 system. In subsequent years, the findings on the influence of disrupted microcirculation based on the results of this initial study have been continuously extended.

First, basic knowledge about the actual processes in the microcirculation has been supplemented by recognition of the functional contribution of the vasomotion of Lectures, assessments and observations of small-caliber arterioles and venules and their local autorythmic control. Second, the development of effective signal configurations derived from that knowledge has in turn led to findings with regard to the interaction between these local autorhythmic, controlled vasomotions and the centrally (nerve- and/or humoral-)controlled slower vasomotions in large-caliber arterioles and venules. Only once the exact control and rhythmic differences of the vessels involved in microcirculation were understood was it then possible to design a signal configuration that activated all vasomotions in the vessels participating in microcirculation synergistically. This signal configuration from 2010, now used in the BEMER Classic Set and Pro Set systems, has made it possible to realize long-lasting, therapy-relevant improvement in decisive microcirculation parameters in cases of disrupted microcirculation.

Materials and methods:
The clinical investigations were performed on biometrically defined, largely homogeneous samples of healthy subjects disposed to stress and infection (control and verum) over shorter and longer investigation periods. Non-invasive methods were used to investigate the functional status of the microcirculation in representative target tissues (intravital microscopy, reflexion spectrometry, and combined white light spectroscopy and laser Doppler microflow imaging). The investigated characteristics were: Spontaneous arteriolar vasomotion, venule oxygen saturation, distribution state of the plasma/cell mixture in the microvessel networks, immunological behavior characteristics of white blood cells etc.

Results:
The results of the investigations showed a statistically significant, therapy-relevant effect of BEMER technology on the tissue status in terms of its supply and cleansing and on cellular immune responses, owing to significantly stimulated arteriolar vasomotion first in small-caliber (2006/2007), and later in small- and largecaliber arterioles (2009/2010).

SUMMARY: BEMER technology systems are able to improve limited or pathologically altered regulation of organ blood flow as a cause of impaired organ function and reduced primary immunological processes effectively and with relevance to therapy.

Molecular Biologically and Functional Principles of the BEMER Physical Vascular Therapy (Mitochondrial ATP Production and Arteriolar Blood Flow)

Lecture at the Budapest Congress 03.26.2011

Dr.med. Rainer Klopp; Institute for Microcirculation, Berlin, Germany

SUMMARY: The BEMER system is able to stimulate limited or pathologically altered regulation of blood flow as a cause of impaired organ function and reduced defense against infections effectively and with relevance to therapy. There are now also molecular-biological basic findings in support of this conclusion.

Objective:
New findings regarding the mechanisms of the BEMER system on the functional level (local and higher blood flow regulation of organs) and on the molecularbiological level (results of in vitro tests) will be discussed on the basis of the results of clinical tests, to which reference is made using the example of application of the BEMER system in patients undergoing rehabilitation who are disposed to stress and infection and in patients with diabetic polyangioneuropathy.

Materials and methods:
The clinical investigations were performed on biometrically defined, largely homogeneous samples of older patient in rehabilitation and of patients with diabetic polyangioneuropathy with indication for amputation (control and verum) in a longterm period of investigation, using non-invasive methods to investigate the functional status of the microcirculation in representative target tissues (intravital microscopy, reflexion spectrometry, and combined white light spectroscopy and laser Doppler microflow imaging). The investigated characteristics were: spontaneous arteriolar vasomotion, venule oxygen saturation, distribution state of the plasma/cell mixture in the microvessel networks, immunological behavior characteristics of white blood cells etc. The in vitro tests (pilot test) were performed on defined cell cultures (human tracheal epithelium) using special microscopic and spectrometric procedures (mitochondrial nutrient transport, cellular ATP production, and analysis of ciliary movements).

Results:
The results of the clinical investigations show a statistically significant, therapy-relevant effect of BEMER treatment on tissue nutrition and cellular immune responses as a result of significantly stimulated arteriolar vasomotion, both in largecaliber and small-caliber arterioles.

In accordance with the results of the clinical investigations, the influence, demonstrated in cell cultures, of the BEMER signal configuration on mitochondrial ATP production is a prerequisite (or consequence?) of stimulated vasomotion.

Conclusion:
The BEMER system is able to stimulate limited or pathologically altered regulation of blood flow as a cause of impaired organ function and reduced defense against infections effectively and with relevance to therapy. There are now also molecularbiological basic findings in support of this conclusion.

Wpływ bardzo słabego impulsowego pola elektromagnetycznego typu BEMER 3000 na metabolizm erytrocytów i powinowactwo tlenowe hemoglobiny

Effects of extremely weak pulsed electromagnetic field type BEMER 3000 on red blood cell metabolism and hemoglobin oxygen affinity

Wolf A. Kafka[1], Krzysztof Spodaryk[2]

[1] Międzynarodowe Stowarzyszenie do Badań nad Wpływem Pól Elektromagnetycznych w Normalnych i Ekstremalnych Warunkach (Przestrzennych), Niemcy
International Association on the Research of the Effects of Electromagnetic Fields under Normal and Extreme (Space) Conditions, Germany

[2] Collegium Medicum Uniwersytetu Jagiellońskiego i Akademia Wychowania Fizycznego w Krakowie
Collegium Medicum of Jagiellonian University and Academy of Physical Education, Kraków

Streszczenie

Wiadomo, że niedotlenienie tkanek i narządów zwiększa poziom 2,3-dwufosfoglicerynianu (2,3-DPG) wewnątrz erytrocytów, wpływając na przesunięcie się krzywej dysocjacji oksyhemoglobiny (ODC) w prawo, co postrzegane jest jako mechanizm obronny chroniący tkanki przed niedotlenieniem. Celem pracy było zbadanie, czy krzywa dysocjacji ulega przesunięciu w prawo u 20 badanych mężczyzn, którzy zostali poddani działaniu impulsów elektromagnetycznych (ich przebieg charakteryzowały określona intensywność i czas trwania odzwierciedlające szeroki skład widma — tzw. typ BEMER) oraz czy przesunięcie to łączyło się z jakimikolwiek zmianami poziomu wewnątrzerytrocytowych ligandów tlenowych hemoglobiny, np. adenozynotrójfosforanu (ATP) i 2,3-dwufosfoglicerynianu (2,3-DPG). Krzywe ODC osobników poddanych działaniu promieniowania nie przesunęły się w prawo, jednakże poziom ich ATP i 2,3-DPG wzrósł odpowiednio o 14% i 12%. Nie zaobserwowano znacznego związku między wskaźnikiem P_{50} (ciśnienie O_2 potrzebne do uzyskania 50% saturacji) a poziomem 2,3-DPG. Prawdopodobnie słabe pole elektromagnetyczne ma wystarczającą moc, aby stymulować syntezę ATP i 2,3-DPG, ale jest ona zbyt słaba, aby spowodować przesunięcie się krzywej ODC w prawo. Trzytygodniowy okres ekspozycji całego ciała badanych na strumień indukcji magnetycznej typu BEMER o średniej wartości natężenia 86 µT wywarł korzystny wpływ na produkcję energii przez erytrocyty i wzrost poziomu 2,3-DPG. Zmiany zaobserwowane w metabolizmie erytrocytów uważa się za mechanizm obronny chroniący tkanki przed niedotlenieniem.

Słowa kluczowe: *pole elektromagnetyczne, ATP, 2,3-DPG, krzywa dysocjacji oksyhemoglobiny* (ODC).

Abstract

Hypoxia is known to increase the intraerythocytic 2.3-diphoshoglycerate (2.3-DPG) level and therefore to induce a right shift of the oxyhemoglobin dissociation curve (ODC), which is considered to be a protective mechanism against tissular hypoxia. Our purpose was to assess whether the ODC is shifted to the right in subjects exposed to electromagnetic pulses which are characterized by a special intensity/time course reflecting a wide spectral (so-called BEMER typed) composition and whether this shift correlated with any changes in intraerythrocytic ligands hemoglobin to oxygen, i.e. adenosinetriphosphate (ATP) and 2.3-diphoshoglycerate (2.3-DPG). The ODC of exposed subjects were no shifted to the right but their ATP and 2.3-DPG levels were increased about 14% and 12%, respectively. The was no significant relation in exposed group between their P_{50} (pO_2 necessary to achieve 50% saturation) and their 2.3-DPG. It is likely that weak electromagnetic field is severe enough to stimulate the ATP and 2.3-DPG synthesis but not enough to induce a right shift of the ODC. In summary the three weeks exposition on the mean 86 µT magnetic flux intensity of the BEMER signal at the surface of the mattress (whole body exposition) have a favorable effect on red blood cell energy production and the influence of a high 2.3-DPG level. Observed changes in RBC me-

Key words: *electromagnetic field, ATP, 2.3-DPG, oxygen dissociation curve.*

Leczenie chorób niedokrwiennych i zaburzeń związanych ze starzeniem się jest istotnym problemem klinicznym. Wspólną cechą chorób niedokrwiennych jest zmniejszenie dostaw tlenu powodujące niedotlenienie różnych części ciała i organów, np. nóg, mózgu, serca. Transport tlenu z płuc do tkanek odbywa się za pomocą hemoglobiny zawartej w erytrocytach. Wiązanie się hemoglobiny i tlenu reprezentowane jest przez krzywą dysocjacji tlenu (ODC), a jej przesunięcie w prawo postrzegane jako uruchomienie mechanizmu ochronnego przeciw niedotlenieniu tkanek w warunkach ich niskiego zaopatrzenia w tlen. Często charakteryzuje się ono wzrostem wskaźnika P_{50}, który oznacza ciśnienie tlenu potrzebne do uzyskania 50% saturacji hemoglobiny. Wiele stanów klinicznych wiąże się ze zmianami pozycji krzywej ODC. Jej przesunięcie w prawo, powodujące spadek powinowactwa hemoglobiny do tlenu, postrzega się jako ważny fizjologiczny mechanizm kompensacyjny, gdyż wspomaga on dostarczanie tlenu do tkanek przy wyższych wartościach ciśnienia cząsteczkowego tlenu. Z kolei przesunięcie krzywej ODC w lewo uważane jest za szkodliwe, gdyż ciśnienie cząsteczkowe tlenu musi zostać znacznie zredukowane, aby odpowiednia ilość tlenu mogła zostać uwolniona. Kształt i pozycja krzywej ODC ilustrowane są przez wartości wskaźnika P_{50} i zależą od następujących czynników: równowagi kwasowo-zasadowej (pH, pCO_2), temperatury oraz poziomu metabolitów czerwonych krwinek, takich jak 2,3-DPG i ATP.

Dowiedziono, że wewnątrzkomórkowe stężenie organicznych fosforanów, z których w przybliżeniu 80% to 2,3-DPG i ATP, jest ważnym czynnikiem wspomagającym dostarczanie tlenu. Najważniejszy jest 2,3-DPG, ponieważ jego wewnątrzkomórkowe stężenie jest czterokrotnie większe niż stężenie ATP i niemal równe stężeniu hemoglobiny. Tylko erytrocyty posiadają tak duże stężenie 2,3-DPG. Wzrost stężenia 2,3-DPG w erytrocytach jest widoczny w stanach związanych z niskim tętniczym ciśnieniem tlenu, np. w niedotlenieniu tkanek i narządów, a są nimi między innymi: wrodzone wady serca, choroba obturacyjna płuc, różne formy anemii, adaptacja do dużych wysokości oraz wysiłek fizyczny [1].

Powinowactwo tlenu jest odwrotnie proporcjonalne do wewnątrzkomórkowego stężenia 2,3-DPG. Wysoki poziom stężenia tego metabolitu powoduje przesunięcie krzywej ODC hemoglobiny w prawo, w ten sposób ułatwiając dostawę tlenu do tkanek. Zatem oddziaływanie na metabolizm, czy na powinowactwo tlenu do hemoglobiny można uznać za jeden z mechanizmów sprzyjających natlenieniu tkanek. Wcześniejsze badania wskazują jednak, że impulsowe pole elektromagnetyczne ma wpływ na aktywność niektórych enzymów krwinek czerwonych [2, 3]. Przypuszcza się, że działanie urządzenia BEMER 3000 może prowadzić do zwiększenia stosunku deoksyhemoglobina/oksyhemoglobina.

W pracy opisano badania nad działaniem bardzo słabego impulsowego pola elektromagnetycznego, generowanego przez urządzenie BEMER 3000, na poziom stężenia ATP i 2,3-DPG w erytrocytach oraz nad wpływem działania tego urządzenia na położenie standardowej krzywej ODC u dorosłych, zdrowych mężczyzn.

Treatment of ischemic diseases and disorders associated with ageing remains a major clinical problem. A common factor of these diseases is a decreased oxygen delivery causing a hypoxia of different organ i.e. legs, cerebrum, heart. The oxygen transport from lung to tissues is essentially due to red blood cell (RBC) hemoglobin. The oxygen hemoglobin binding is represented by the oxygen dissociation curve (ODC) and shift to the right of it is considered to be a protective mechanism against tissular hypoxia in conditions of low oxygen delivery. It is often characterized by an increase in P_{50}, which is the pO_2 necessary to achieve a hemoglobin saturation of 50%. A variety of clinical conditions are associated with shifts in the position of the ODC. A shift to the right in the position of the curve, with its decrease in the affinity of hemoglobin for oxygen, is believed to represent an important physiologic compensation because it facilitates oxygen delivery to tissues at higher partial pressures of oxygen. Conversely, a shift to the left in the position of the curve is regarded as deleterious because tissue oxygen tensions must be significantly reduced for adequate oxygen extraction to occur. The shape and position of ODC is described by the oxygen pressure at half hemoglobin saturation (P_{50}) and depends upon several factors: acid-base balance (pH, pCO_2), temperature, and RBC metabolites such as 2,3-diphosphoglycerate (2,3-DPG) and adenosine-triphosphate (ATP).

The intracellular concentration of organic phosphates, approximately 80% of which are composed of 2,3-diphosphpoglycerate and adenosine triphosphate has been shown to be an important factors in facilitating tissue oxygen supply. 2,3-DPG is the most important, as the intra-erythrocyte molar concentration is about four times that of ATP and approximately equal to that of hemoglobin. Erythrocytes are unique in having such a high concentration of 2,3-DPG. In conditions associated with low arterial oxygen pressure, i.e. hypoxemia, an increase in red cell 2,3-DPG levels is seen. Among such conditions are: congenital heart disease, obstructive lung disease, and various types of anemia and high altitude adaptation and also physical exercise [1].

Oxygen affinity is generally inversely proportional to the intracellular levels of 2,3-DPG. The high concentration of this metabolite shifting the oxygen dissociation curve of hemoglobin to the right and thus facilitating oxygen supply to tissues. Then among mechanisms favoring tissue oxygenation, an action on blood red cell metabolism and/or hemoglobin oxygen affinity could be implicated. On the other hand previous study indicated that pulsed electromagnetic field affects the activity of some enzymes of red blood cells [2, 3], so we speculate that this physiotherapeutical modality can lead to increases in the ratio of deoxy- to oxyhemoglobin.

In this investigation we have studied the effect of extremely weak pulsed electromagnetic field typed BEMER 3000 on ATP and 2,3-DPG concentration in red blood cells, and influence of this physiotherapeutic modality on the position of the standard oxygen dissociation curve in healthy adults.

Materials and methods

Subjects

Twenty healthy, non smoking, males (students, age 21.3 ± 2.4 years, $74.3 + 8.4$ kg weight) participated in this study after giving written consent. This study was approved by the Jagiellonian University Research Ethics Committee. Volunteers were informed verbally and in writing of the experimental procedures and, once they had agreed to participate, they signed a consent form. Subjects were screened for current injury or pain, consumption of any form of drugs, diabetes, asthma, weight training, any hematological diseases and participation in similar experiment within the past year. Subject were requested to no attend a hard physical exercise during experiment.

Electromagnetic field generation and exposure conditions

Electromagnetic stimulation was performed by application of the BEMER 3000 (Innomed International AG, FL-Triesen). This physical modality has Polish Ministry of Health permission for therapeutically use no. 28245639. It consists of a signal generator unit (with manual adjusting time of exposition an intensity) and a mattress containing 6 (four circular, $\varnothing 25$ cm and 2 oval 25/40) flat electrical coils as stimulus applicators. The stimulation was mediated via a sequence of extremely low frequent, wide band pulsed weak electromagnetic fields, each pulse being characterized by the formula $y = k(x) * x^a * e^{\sin(x \cdot b)}/c + d$, [e.g. $k(x) = 1$, $x[0, 4)$; $a = b = 3$; $c = 50$; $d = 0$] BEMER 3000® signal. The mean magnetic flux intensity of the signal at the surface of the mattress (0.7×1.7 m^2) was either 18 or 86 µT.

Volunteers were randomly allocated to one of the following two groups under blinded conditions:
- sham treated group (S-T) — subjects in this group received 20 min of pseudotherapy (equipment for generation of electromagnetic field was switched-off);
- treatment group (T) — subjects in this group received total one-day dose 86 µT, 20 min, 6 days per week during 21 days of the experiment.

The local geomagnetic field was measured by an EG & G Geometrics G-866 magnetometer and was 46 µT.

Biochemical determination

Arterial blood has been sampled from volunteers one day before (analysis at D_0) and one after the exposition or sham-exposition on pulsed magnetic field (analysis at D_{21}). Oxygen dissociation curve were determined using a Hemox-Analyzer (TCS-Southampton, USA). This is a continuous method combining a dual wavelength spectrophotometer and a Clark oxygen electrode. The blood samples were suspended in a buffer solution (Tris, pH 7.40) and blood oxygen affinity was analyzed as a P_{50}: partial pressure of oxygen in mm Hg required for 50% saturation of hemoglobin. As inorganic phosphates (P_i) may determine too the positions of the ODC their plasmatic ganiczne (P_i) mogą również mieć wpływ na położenie krzywych ODC, ich stężenia w osoczu zostały określone za pomocą aparatu Technician SMAC II wyprodukowanego w USA.

W celu określenia składu metabolitów czerwonych krwinek krew badanych została przepuszczona przez filtr z α-celulozy i celulozy mikrokrystalicznej (producent: Sigma, St. Louis, USA), który usunął leukocyty i trombocyty z krwi. Określenia stężenia ATP i 2,3-DPG wewnątrz erytrocytów dokonano za pomocą metody spektrofotometrycznej, używając w tym celu odczynników zapewnionych przez firmę Sigma (zestaw odczynników 366 UV dla ATP oraz zestaw odczynników 35 UV dla 2,3-DPG). Wyniki wyrażono w µmol/gHb. Hematokryt (Hct: metoda odwirowywania mikrohematokrytu), wartość stężenia hemoglobiny i nasycenie tlenem (Hb i SO_2: mierzono spektrometrem o podwójnej długości fali z urządzeniem Oxygen Saturation Meter 2 firmy Radiometer), pH całej krwi (pH_{blood}: mierzono urządzeniem Blood Gas Analyser 3 firmy Radiometer), wewnątrzerytrocytowe pH (pH_{RBC}) zmierzono po odwirowaniu beztlenowym w rurkach włoskowatych krzepnącotającyh hemolizatów koncentratu czerwonych krwinek przy użyciu urządzenia BMS2 blood micro-system i urządzenia do pomiaru pH (producent: Radiometer, Dania). Wartości pH krwi z próbek równoważonych zostały określone w opisany sposób. Te wartości pH zostały użyte do skorygowania wartości wskaźnika P_{50} do standardowego poziomu pH osocza, czyli 7,4 (efekt Bohra). Użyty współczynnik Bohra wynosił $-0,48$.

Analiza statystyczna

Do oceny statystycznej otrzymanych wyników użyto analizy wariancji i testu-t. Wartość $p < 0,05$ uznawano za wskazującą na różnicę istotną statystycznie.

Wyniki

Wyniki uzyskane w tym eksperymencie zaprezentowane zostały w tab. 1. Poziomy hemoglobiny (Hb) i karboksyhemoglobiny ($HbCO_2$), ciśnienie tętnicze tlenu (pO_2) i dwutlenku węgla (pCO_2), pH krwi i wewnątrzerytrocytowe (pH_{blood} i pH_{RBC}), stężenie 2,3-DPG i ATP w erytrocytach, stężenie fosforanów nieorganicznych (P_i) oraz średnie korpuskularne stężenie hemoglobiny (MCHC) nie różniły się między grupami na początku badań (D_0). Wskaźnik P_{50}, który wyraża ciśnienie cząstkowe tlenu potrzebne do uzyskania 50% saturacji hemoglobiny, nie różnił się również.

Po 21 dniach ekspozycji na impulsowe pole elektromagnetyczne poziom ATP zmniejszył się o 14,3% ($p < 0,04$, $D_0 = 596,6 \pm 7,1,2$ µmol/L i $D_{21} = 681,1 \pm 64,6$ µmol/L), podczas gdy stężenie 2,3-DPG zwiększyło się o 12,2% ($p < 0,05$, $D_0 = 12,2 \pm 2,0$ µmol/gHb i $D_{21} = 14,8 \pm 1,4$ µmol/gHb). Statystycznie istotne różnice ($p < 0,01$) w poziomie tych związków zaobserwowano między grupą kontrolną i badawczą przy D_{21}.

Średnia wartość P_{50} nie została skorygowana dla pH, ale przy pCO_2 równym 40 mm Hg (5,33 kPa) wy-

levels were determined by a Technician SMAC II apparatus (USA).

For RBC metabolite determination, blood was passed trough α-cellulose and dry microcrystalline cellulose (Sigma, St. Louis, USA), which remove leukocyte and platelets from whole blood. Intraerythrocyte ATP and 2.3-DPG determination were performed by specrophotometric method using reagents supplied by Sigma (366 UV reagent kit and 35UV reagent kit, respectively), and results were expressed as µmol/gHb. Hematocrit value (Hct: microhematocrit centrifugation method), hemoglobin concentration and oxygen saturation (Hb and SO_2: two wavelength spectrophotometer with the Radiometer Oxygen Saturation Meter 2) and whole blood ph (pH_{blood}: Radiometer Blood Gas Analyzer 3). The intraerythrocyte pH (pH_{RBC}) was measured after anaerobic centrifugation in capillaries and freeze-thaw hemolysates of packed red cells by BMS2 blood micro-system and pH-meter (Radiometer, Denmark). Blood pH values of the equilibrated samples were determined as described above. These pH-values were used to correct the P_{50} values to a standard plasma pH of 7.4 (Bohr effect). The Bohr coefficient used was -0.48.

Statistical analysis

For statistical evaluation analysis of variance and t-test analysis were used. A value $p < 0.05$ was considered to indicate significant difference.

Results

Results corresponding to this experiment are represented in Table 1. The hemoglobin (Hb) and carboxyhemoglobin (HbCO) levels, arterial oxygen (pO_2) and carbon dioxide (pCO_2) tension, blood and intraerythrocyte pH (pH_{blood} and pH_{RBC}, respectively), red blood cell concentration of 2.3-diphosphoglycerate (2.3-DPG) and adenosinotriphosphate (ATP), serum inorganic phosphates (P_i) and mean corpuscular hemoglobin concentration (MCHC) did not differ between the two groups at the start of the experiment (D_0). The P_{50}, which is the pO_2 necessary to achieve a hemoglobin saturation of 50%, did not differ also.

After 21 days of exposure on pulsed electromagnetic field the level of ATP increased about 14.3% ($p < 0.04$, $D_0 = 596.6 \pm 71.2$ µmol/L and $D_{21} = 681.1 \pm 64.6$ µmol/L) while 2.3-DPG concentration was 12.2% higher ($p < 0.05$, $D = 12.2 \pm 2.0$ µmol/gHb and $D_{21} = 14.8 \pm 1.4$ µmol/gHb). There were statistical significant differences ($p < 0.01$) in level of these compounds between groups S-T to T at D_{21}.

The mean P_{50} value not corrected for pH, but at a pCO_2 of 40 mm Hg (5.33 kPa) was 27.01 ± 1.27 mm Hg (3.59 ± 0.16 kPa) at D_0, and slightly increased

Table 1. Hematological data, arterial blood gases and intraerythrocyte compounds in sham-treated (placebo) group and in subjects treated with BEMER 3000 86 µT magnetic field (n = 10 for each group)

Wskaźniki Indices	Grupa kontrolna Sham treated group (S-T)		Grupa badawcza Treatment group (T)	
	D_0	D_{21}	D_0	D_{21}
Hb [g/dL]	13,9±1,1	14,1±13	14,3±1,5	14,0±1,0
pCO_2 [kPa]	5,32±0,51	5,28±0,46	5,30±0,44	5,31±0,39
pO_2 [kPa]	12,60±0,75	12,69±0,80	12,58±0,82	12,61±0,74
pH_{blood}	7,411±0,023	7,403±0,032	7,422±0,053	7,416±0,040
pH_{eryth}	7,341±0,019	7,357±0,022	7,329±0,031	7,206±0,024
DPG [µmol/gHb]	12,5±1,7	12,0±2,2	12,2±2,2	14,8±1,4*
ATP [µmol/L]	591,4±72,2	583,1±54,8	596,6±71,2	681,1±64,6*
P_i [mEq/L]	1,8±0,4	1,9±0,3	1,7±0,5	1,8±0,3
P_{50} [kPa]	3,55±0,14	3,52±0,16	3,59±0,16	3,86±0,18
MCHC	33,6±2,4	33,2±2,1	32,9±2,0	33,2±1,8

Dane zaprezentowane są w formie wartości średnich z odchyleniem standardowym:
Data is presented as mean values ±SD:
Hb — hemoglobina, hemoglobin; pCO_2 — ciśnienie cząsteczkowe dwutlenku węgla, partial pressure of carbon dioxide; pO_2 — ciśnienie cząstkowe tlenu, partial pressure of oxygen; pH_{blood} — pH całej krwi, whole blood pH; pH_{eryth} — pH erytrocytów, pH in erythrocytes; DPG — 2,3-dwufosfoglicerynian, 2.3-diphosphoglycerate; ATP — adenozynotrójfosforan, adenosinotriphosphate; P_i — fosforany nieorganiczne, inorganic phosphates; P_{50} — standardowe ciśnienie potrzebne do osiągnięcia 50% saturacji, standard half saturation pressure; MCHC — średnie korpuskularne stężenie hemoglobiny, mean corpuscular hemoglobin concentration; D_0 — dzień przed eksperymentem, one day before the experiment; D_{21} — dzień po 21-dniowej ekspozycji na impulsowe pole elektromagnetyczne lub po pseudozabiegu, one day after the 21 days of exposure or sham-exposure to pulsed electromagnetic field; *p < 0,05 dla D_{21} w zależności od D_0, p < 0.05 for D_{21} vs. D_0

niosła 27,01±1,27 mm Hg (3,59±0,16 kPa) przy D_0, i wzrosła do 29,07±1,38 mm Hg (3,86±0,18 kPa) po ekspozycji na pole elektromagnetyczne. Po korekcji efektu Bohra nie odnotowano różnicy między wartościami początkowymi i końcowymi. Efekt Bohra wyrażono w $\Delta(\log pO_2)/\Delta pH$ wynoszącym −0,06, −0,05 i 0,05 dla poziomów saturacji równych odpowiednio 5%, 50% i 95%. Odpowiadające wartości dla efektu termicznego wyrażonego w $\Delta(\log pO_2)/\Delta T$ wyniosły −0,004, −0,003 i 0,003.

Krzywa ODC przesunęła się w prawo po 21 ekspozycji na pole magnetyczne (grupa T_{86}) z 20% na 95% saturacji, a efekt maksymalny zaobserwowano przy ciśnieniu 4,67 kPa. Jednak przesunięcie to nie było statystycznie istotne (ryc. 1). Nie zaobserwowano żadnych zmian w położeniu krzywej ODC w grupie kontrolnej między D_0 a D_{21}.

to 29.07±1.38 mm Hg (3.86±0.18 kPa) after exposition to electromagnetic field. After correction for the Bohr effect there was no difference between the initial and post-exposition values. The Bohr effect as expressed in $\Delta(\log pO_2)/\Delta pH$ amounted to −0.06, −0.05 and 0.05 for saturation levels equal to 5%, 50% and 95%, respectively. The corresponding values for the temperature effect as expressed in $\Delta(\log pO_2)/\Delta T$ were −0.004, −0.003 and 0.003, respectively.

The oxygen dissociation curve (ODC) was shifted to the right after 21 days of exposition to magnetic field (group T_{86}) from 20 to 95% saturation and the maximal effect was observed at 4.67 kPa. However, this shift was not statistically significant (Figure 1). Any changes in position of ODC were not observed in group S-T between D_0 and D_{21} (not shown).

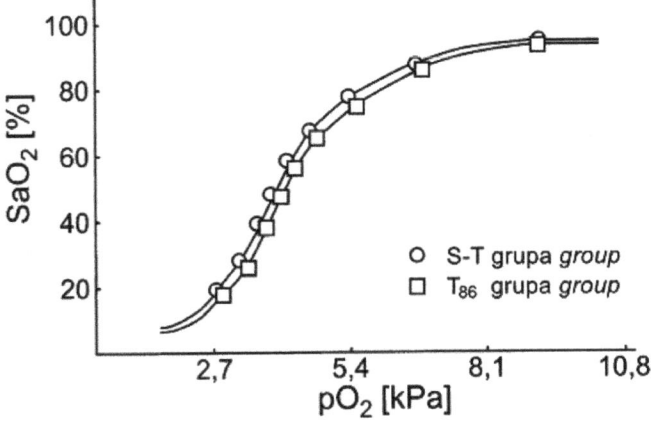

Ryc. 1. Przesunięcia krzywej ODC w obu badanych grupach po 21 dniach badania

Fig. 1. Shifts of the oxygen dissociation curves of the investigated two groups (S-T and T_{86}) after 21 days of experiment

Discussion

The present study focused to the question of whether electromagnetic stimulations might proof aplicable also to support oxygenation of tissues by the changes in red blood metabolism and a oxygen affinity to hemoglobin described by position of oxyhemoglobinn dissociation curve. Especially on the basis of several hypotheses indicating that the primary site of interactions occurs at plasma membranes or, more precisely, adherent molecular or sub-molecular structures [4] the electromagnetic stimulations were performed by application of a novel type of impulse form. Designed to tune the (charge/mass relation dependent) processes of molecular activation these pulses are characterized by a special intensity/time course reflecting a wide spectral (so-called BEMER typed) composition [4]. Referred to the spectral composition these BEMER-pulses exceed the spectral power of sinus-, rectangular- or saw-tooth like pulses of conventional electromagnetic stimulations by more than a factor of 1000, and have already proven effective in accelerated wound healing [5], sedation processes [6], increased ATP synthesis [2], delayed onset of muscle, soreness [7] and stress response activation against teratogens [8]. However extremely weak pulsed electromagnetic field was not previously studied as a effect on RBC metabolism and oxygen affinity of hemoglobin in arterial blood. This results shown that 21 day exposition on electromagnetic field produces statistical significant increase of ATP and 2.3-DPG productions (14% and 12%, respectively) and shifts oxygen curve to the right but not significantly.

The red blood cell can no longer be considered an *effete sac* or *passive carrier* of hemoglobin, since there exists within this cell an intrinsic mechanism for the control of the oxygen affinity of hemoglobin, which enables it to act as on oxygen donor under physiological conditions. This mechanism depends on the interaction of hemoglobin with intraerythrocyte organic phosphates, approximately 80% of which are composed of 2.3-diphosphoglycerate (2.3-DPG) and adenosine troposphere (ATP). In 1967 it was shown that 2.3-DPG alters the oxygen affinity of hemoglobin, such that an increase in the intraerythrocyte 2.3-DPG concentration reduces the affinity of hemoglobin for oxygen and vice-versa [9]. Therefore an increase in 2.3-DPG concentration improves tissue oxygenation whereas a decrease in 2.3-DPG concentration may lead to tissue hypoxia.

Several factors can influence the intracellular concentration of 2.3-DPG. The changes in 2.3-DPG concentration during physical exercise are explained by catecholamine-induced stimulation of red cell glycolysis, increases in the ratio of deoxyto oxyhemoglobin and changes in plasma inorganic phosphate [10]. On the other hand, intensive physical exercise induces changes in blood composition such as hemoconcentration, acid-base status, plasma electrolyte concentration and body temperature. All these factors influence the oxygen binding properties of hemoglobin mainly by decreasing Hb-O_2-affinity via the Bohr and temperature effects. However, the decrease in Hb-O_2 affinity during strenuous exercise depends only on the degree of lactacidosis and temperature elevation because changes in 2.3-DPG and ATP are negligibly low.

W czasie tego eksperymentu wewnątrzerytrocytowe pH zmieniło się podczas ekspozycji na pole elektromagnetyczne, ale obserwowano wzrost stężenia 2,3-DPG spowodowany aktywacją glikolizy. Nasuwa się pytanie, czy zmiany w stężeniach 2,3-DPG i ATP, zaobserwowane w czasie tego eksperymentu, są istotne z fizjologicznego punktu widzenia. Badania wykazały, że niewielki wzrost stężenia fosforanów wewnątrzerytrocytowych nie miał zauważalnego wpływu na poziom powinowactwa tlenowego hemoglobiny.

Synteza i rozpad 2,3-DPG kontrolowane są w cyklu fosfoglicerynianowym Rapporta & Leuberinga (będącego częścią głównej drogi przemian metabolicznych Embdena-Meyerofa). Około 20% strumienia glikotycznego przechodzi przez ten cykl. W normalnych warunkach fizjologicznych czynnikami kontrolującymi poziom stężenia 2,3-DPG są: 2,3-DPG (mechanizm ujemnego sprzężenia zwrotnego hamuje aktywność enzymu 2,3-DPG mutazy), poziom stężenia jonów wodoru (w alkalozie tempo glikolizy jest zwiększone, aktywność 2,3-DPG fosfatazy zahamowana, a stężenie 2,3-DPG zwiększone) oraz poziom stężenia fosforanów nieorganicznych (w hipofosfatemii stężenie 2,3-DPG jest niskie, a w hiperfosfatemii wysokie). Jednak 2,3-DPG jest anionem nieprzenikliwym. Zwiększenie stężenia 2,3-DPG powoduje spadek pH wewnątrzerytrocytowego wskutek zadziałania efektu równowagi membranowej Donnana. Spowalnia on glikolizę, aktywuje 2,3-DPG fosfatazę, redukując stężenie 2,3-DPG. Dlatego też wielkość jakiegokolwiek wzrostu stężenia 2,3-DPG w erytrocytach ograniczana jest przez ten mechanizm i przez inhibicję produktu.

Aby zbadać wpływ pola elektromagnetycznego typu BEMER 3000 na powinowactwo $Hb-O_2$, dokonano pomiaru wskaźnika P_{50}. Otrzymane wyniki wskazują na brak statystycznie istotnej różnicy po 21 dniach ekspozycji na to pole elektromagnetyczne. Autorzy nie odnaleźli w dostępnej literaturze doniesień o wpływie działania pola elektromagnetycznego na zwiększanie się powinowactwa $Hb-O_2$ (Med line library). Wyniki uzyskane wcześniej przez autorów wskazują na występowanie zmian stężenia 2,3-DPG i ATP wewnątrz erytrocytów zależnych od działania pola elektromagnetycznego, można zatem przypuszczać, że taka stymulacja glikolizy w erytrocytach może prowadzić do zwiększenia stosunku deoksyhemoglobina-oksyhemoglobina [3]. Hipotezy autorów nie zostały potwierdzone. Jednak wzrost stężenia tych dwóch, bardzo ważnych, związków komórkowych może sugerować, że pole elektromagnetyczne typu BEMER 3000 działa jako czynnik stymulujący metabolizm erytrocytów.

Uzyskane wyniki pozwalają stwierdzić, że długotrwała ekspozycja na pole elektromagnetyczne prowadzi do lekkiego zwiększenia glikolizy erytrocytów, które jednak nie ma wykrywalnego wpływu na poziom powinowactwa tlenowego hemoglobiny.

In this experiment the intraerythrocyte pH does not changes during exposition on electromagnetic field, than the observed elevation of 2.3-DPG concentration due to activation of glycolysis. The question arises as to whether the changes in 2.3-DPG and ATP concentrations noticed in this experiment are of any physiological significance. The data demonstrated that slightly elevation in intraerythrocyte phosphates had no detectable influence on O_2 binding properties of Hb.

The synthesis and breakdown of 2.3-DPG is controlled in the phosphoglycerate cycle of Rapport & Luebering a side-shuttle off the main Embden-Meyerof pathway). Approximately 20% of the glycolytic flux is via this shuttle. Under normal physiological conditions, factors controlling the concentration of 2.3-DPG are: the concentration of 2.3-DPG itself (a negative feed-back mechanism inhibits the activity of the enzyme 2.3-DPG mutase), hydrogen ion concentration (in alkalosis the rate of glycolysis is increased and the activity of 2.3-DPG phosphatase is inhibited and 2.3-DPG concentration is increased), and inorganic phosphate concentration (in hypophosphataemia 2.3-DPG concentration is low and in hyperphosphataemia it is high). On the other hand, DPG is a non-penetrating anion. Increases in the concentration of 2.3-DPG produce a fall in intraerythrocyte pH via the Donnan membrane equilibrium effect. This slows down glycolysis, activates 2.3-DPG phosphatase and so reduces 2.3-DPG concentration. Therefore the magnitude of any increase in red cell 2.3-DPG concentration is limited by this mechanism as well as by product inhibition.

To examine the impact of electromagnetic field typed BEMER 3000 on affinity $Hb-O_2$ the measurement of P_{50} was done. The obtained data indicate non significant statistical difference after 21 days of exposition on this modality. We found not trace in the literature of electromagnetic fields excess in $Hb-O_2$ affinity (Med line library). Our own previous data showed consistent electromagnetic field-dependent changes in 2.3-DPG and ATP in red blood cells [3], so we speculate that this stimulation of red cell glycolysis can lead to increases in the ratio of deoxy- to oxyhemoglobin. Our hypothesis was not supported in this investigation. However the elevation of concentration of two very important cell compounds suggest that electromagnetic field type BEMER 3000 act as biostimulating agent on red blood cell metabolism.

In summary, the data demonstrate that long term exposition on electromagnetic field let to slightly increased red blood glucolysis, which had no detectable influence on oxygen binding properties of Hb.

Piśmiennictwo

[1] Duhm J., Gehrlach: *On the mechanism of hypoxia induced increase of 2.3-diphosphoglycerate in erythrocytes.* Pflugers Arch., 1971, 326, 254–269.

[2] Spodaryk K.: *Red blood metabolism and hemoglobin oxygen affinity: effect of electromagnetic field in healthy adults.* [In]: Kafka Wolf A. (ed.) 2nd Int. World Congress Bio-Electro-Magnetic-Energy-Regulation. Emphyspace, 2001, 2, 15–19.

[3] Spodaryk K., Kafka W. A.: *Oxidant stress clearance in human erythrocytes by non-invasive stimulation with extremely weak (BEMER Type) pulsed electromagnetic fields: a blinded, randomised, placebo-controlled study.* Arch. Phys. Biochem 2003 (in press).

[4] Kafka W. A.: *Extremely low, wide frequency range pulsed electromagnetic fields for therapeutical use.* Emphyspace, 2000, 2, 1–22.

[5] Kafka W. A., Preißinger M.: *Verbesserte Wundheilung durch gekoppelte, BEMER 3000 typisch gepulste, Elektromagnetfeld- und LED-Licht-Therapie am Beispiel vergleichender Untersuchungen an standardisierten Wunder nach Ovarektomie bei Katzen (felidae)*. [In]: Ganster Edwin (ed.), Österreichische Gesellschaft der Tierärzte (ÖGT), 2002, Kleintiertage-Dermatologie 02.-03. März 2002, Salzburg Congress 72–77.

[6] Michels-Wakili S., Kafka W. A.: *Bemer 3000 type pulsed low-energy electromagnetic fields reduce dental anxiety: a randomised placebo-controlled single-blind Study*. [In:] 10th International Dental Congress on Modern Pain Control IFDAS, 2003, June 2003, Edinburgh, Scotland (in press).

[7] Spodaryk K.: *The effect of extremely weak electromagnetic field treatments upon signs and symptoms of delayed onset of muscle soreness: a placebo controlled clinical double blind study*. Medicina Sportiva, 2002, 6, 19–25.

[8] Jelinek R., Bláha J.: *Preconditioning with repeated exposure to BEMER 3000 signal alleviates the embryotoxic effect of cyclophosphamide*. Bioelectromagnetics 2003, (in press).

[9] Duhm J., Gehrlach: *Metabolism and function of 2.3-diphosphoglycerate in red blood cells*. [In:]: Greenwald T. J., Jamieson G. A. (eds.) *The human red cell in vitro*. Grune & Stratton, New York, 1974, 111–118.

[10] Katz A., Sharp R. L., King D. S.: *Effect of high intensity interval training on 2.3-diphosphoglycerate at rest and after maximal exercise*. Eur. J. Appl. Physiol., 1984, 52, 331–335.

[11] Mairbaurl H., Schobersberger W., Hasibeder W.: *Regulation of red cell 2.3-DPG and $Hb-O_2$ affinity during acute exercise*. Eur. J. Appl. Physiol., 1986, 55, 174–180.

[12] Blank E.: *Electricity and Magnetism in Biology and Medicine*. San Francisco Press, San Francisco, 1993.

[13] Carpenter D. O., Aryapetyan S.: *Biological Effects of Electric and Magnetic Fields: Sources and mechanism (Vol. 1); Beneficial and Harmful Effects (Vol 2)*. Academic Press 1994, San Diego, New York, Boston, London, Sydney, Tokyo, Toronto.

[14] Kafka W. A.: *Device applying electric or magnetic signals for promoting biological processes*. Europaisches Patent Nr 0995463 (16.08.2001).

[15] Polk C., Postow E.: *Handbook of biological effects of electromagnetic fields*. CRC Press Boca Taton, Boston, London, New York, Washington DC.

[16] Quittan M., Schuhfried O., Wiesinger G. F., Fialka-Moser V.: *Klinische Wirksamkeiten der Magnetfeldtherapie — eine Literaturübersicht*. Acta Medica Austriaca 2000, 3, 61–68.

Adres do korespondencji:
Address for correspondence:
Krzysztof Spodaryk
Akademia Wychowania Fizycznego
al. Jana Pawła II 78
31-571 Kraków

In this experiment the intraerythrocyte pH does not changes during exposition on electromagnetic field, than the observed elevation of 2.3-DPG concentration due to activation of glycolysis. The question arises as to whether the changes in 2.3-DPG and ATP concentrations noticed in this experiment are of any physiological significance. The data demonstrated that slightly elevation in intraerythrocyte phosphates had no detectable influence on O_2 binding properties of Hb.

The synthesis and breakdown of 2.3-DPG is controlled in the phosphoglycerate cycle of Rapport & Luebering a side-shuttle off the main Embden-Meyerof pathway). Approximately 20% of the glycolytic flux is via this shuttle. Under normal physiological conditions, factors controlling the concentration of 2.3-DPG are: the concentration of 2.3-DPG itself (a negative feed-back mechanism inhibits the activity of the enzyme 2.3-DPGmutase), hydrogen ion concentration (in alkalosis the rate of glycolysis is increased and the activity of 2.3-DPG phosphatase is inhibited and 2.3-DPG concentration is increased), and inorganic phosphate concentration (in hypophosphataemia 2.3-DPG concentration is low and in hyperphosphataemia it is high). On the other hand, DPG is a non-penetrating anion. Increases in the concentration of 2.3-DPG produce a fall in intraerythrocyte pH via the Donnan membrane equilibrium effect. This slows down glycolysis, activates 2.3-DPG phosphatase and so reduces 2.3-DPG concentration. Therefore the magnitude of any increase in red cell 2.3-DPG concentration is limited by this mechanism as well as by product inhibition.

To examine the impact of electromagnetic field typed BEMER 3000 on affinity Hb-O_2 the measurement of P_{50} was done. The obtained data indicate non significant statistical difference after 21 days of exposition on this modality. We found not trace in the literature of electromagnetic fields excess in Hb-O_2 affinity (Med line library). Our own previous data showed consistent electromagnetic field-dependent changes in 2.3-DPG and ATP in red blood cells [3], so we speculate that this stimulation of red cell glycolysis can lead to increases in the ratio of deoxy- to oxyhemoglobin. Our hypothesis was not supported in this investigation. However the elevation of concentration of two very important cell compounds suggest that electromagnetic field type BEMER 3000 act as biostimulating agent on red blood cell metabolism.

In summary, the data demonstrate that long term exposition on electromagnetic field let to slightly increased red blood glucolysis, which had no detectable influence on oxygen binding properties of Hb.

Piśmiennictwo

[1] Duhm J., Gehrlach: *On the mechanism of hypoxia induced increase of 2.3-diphosphoglycerate in erythrocytes.* Pflugers Arch., 1971, 326, 254–269.
[2] Spodaryk K.: *Red blood metabolism and hemoglobin oxygen affinity: effect of electromagnetic field in healthy adults.* [In]: Kafka Wolf A. (ed.) 2nd Int. World Congress Bio-Electro-Magnetic-Energy-Regulation. Emphyspace, 2001, 2, 15–19.
[3] Spodaryk K., Kafka W. A.: *Oxidant stress clearance in human erythrocytes by non-invasive stimulation with extremely weak (BEMER Type) pulsed electromagnetic fields: a blinded, randomised, placebo-controlled study.* Arch. Phys. Biochem 2003 (in press).
[4] Kafka W. A.: *Extremely low, wide frequency range pulsed electromagnetic fields for therapeutical use.* Emphyspace, 2000, 2, 1–22.

[5] Kafka W. A., Preißinger M.: *Verbesserte Wundheilung durch gekoppelte, BEMER 3000 typisch gepulste, Elektromagnetfeld- und LED-Licht-Therapie am Beispiel vergleichender Untersuchungen an standardisierten Wunder nach Ovarektomie bei Katzen (felidae).* [In]: Ganster Edwin (ed.), Österreichische Gesellschaft der Tierärzte (ÖGT), 2002, Kleintiertage-Dermatologie 02.-03. März 2002, Salzburg Congress 72–77.

[6] Michels-Wakili S., Kafka W. A.: *Bemer 3000 type pulsed low-energy electromagnetic fields reduce dental anxiety: a randomised placebo-controlled single-blind Study.* [In:] 10th International Dental Congress on Modern Pain Control IFDAS, 2003, June 2003, Edinburgh, Scotland (in press).

[7] Spodaryk K.: *The effect of extremely weak electromagnetic field treatments upon signs and symptoms of delayed onset of muscle soreness: a placebo controlled clinical double blind study.* Medicina Sportiva, 2002, 6, 19–25.

[8] Jelinek R., Bláha J.: *Preconditioning with repeated exposure to BEMER 3000 signal alleviates the embryotoxic effect of cyclophosphamide.* Bioelectromagnetics 2003, (in press).

[9] Duhm J., Gehrlach: *Metabolism and function of 2.3-diphosphoglycerate in red blood cells.* [In:]: Grenwald T. J., Jamieson G. A. (eds.) *The human red cell in vitro.* Grune & Stratton, New York, 1974, 111–118.

[10] Katz A., Sharp R. L., King D. S.: *Effect of high intensity interval training on 2.3-diphosphoglycerate at rest and after maximal exercise.* Eur. J. Appl. Physiol., 1984, 52, 331–335.

[11] Mairbaurl H., Schobersberger W., Hasibeder W.: *Regulation of red cell 2.3-DPG and Hb-O_2 affinity during acute exercise.* Eur. J. Appl. Physiol., 1986, 55, 174–180.

[12] Blank E.: *Electricity and Magnetism in Biology and Medicine.* San Francisco Press, San Francisco, 1993.

[13] Carpenter D. O., Aryapetyan S.: *Biological Effects of Electric and Magnetic Fields: Sources and mechanism (Vol. 1); Beneficial and Harmful Effects (Vol 2).* Academic Press 1994, San Diego, New York, Boston, London, Sydney, Tokyo, Toronto.

[14] Kafka W. A.: *Device applying electric or magnetic signals for promoting biological processes.* Europaisches Patent Nr 0995463 (16.08.2001).

[15] Polk C., Postow E.: *Handbook of biological effects of electromagnetic fields.* CRC Press Boca Taton, Boston, London, New York, Washington DC.

[16] Quittan M., Schuhfried O., Wiesinger G. F., Fialka-Moser V.: *Klinische Wirksamkeiten der Magnetfeldtherapie – eine Literaturübersicht.* Acta Medica Austriaca 2000, 3, 61–68.

Adres do korespondencji:
Address for correspondence:
Krzysztof Spodaryk
Akademia Wychowania Fizycznego
al. Jana Pawła II 78
31-571 Kraków

Fundamental Research Using the BEMER Technology Clinical Studies on the Physical Stimulation of Flexible Arteriolar Wall Movement with Disturbed Autorhythmic and Centrally Cotrolled in Patients with Deficiencies in the Regulation of Blood Circulation of Organs

Dr. Rainer Klopp, Associate Professor Institute of Microcirculation, Berlin Objective

Detection of possible therapeutic effects of biorhythm-based physical stimulation in limited or malfunctioning flexible arteriolar wall movement for the therapeutic optimization of recognized preventive, rehabilitation and clinical treatment procedures.

PREFACE
Microcirculation is functionally the most important part of the human circulation system, which takes place in the smallest blood vessels and fulfils vital transport functions: it provides the tissues and organs with oxygen and nutrients and removes metabolic waste-products and supports the immune system. A limited or malfunctioning microcirculation is the cause of many conditions of poor health as well as illness, which leads to a faster aging of the cells.

SUPPORT FOR MALFUNCTIONING MICROCIRCULATION
An expensive research for an effective alternative for the treatment of limited or malfunctioning microcirculation using medicinal products was conducted in the Institute for Microcirculation in Berlin, headed by Dr. Klopp, which resulted in the development of a specific complex signal configuration allowing for a very effective stimulation of the regulatory processes of the malfunctioning microcirculation.

These researches were based on the BEMER devices developed earlier, which applies a particular pulsating electromagnetic field of low intensity. Its effects, already confirmed at that time, were very promising for a targeted development. New scientific fundamental knowledge gathered during years of intensive research constitutes a new starting point in the optimization of the therapy. This new BEMER system is not only a directly improved version of the earlier system, but it is also a quantitative and qualitative leap which has not been considered possible at the beginning of this research.

BEMER therapy system is now the most researched and most effective physical treatment method used in limited microcirculation! (Dr. med. R. Klopp, Institute for Microcirculation, Berlin)

In the case of the new BEMER systems the device improvements have been preceded by a significant gain in scientific knowledge. These discoveries involved the rhythmic processes in the small and big arterioles with different vibration characteristics, local (BEMER 3000 plus) and higher-level regulatory mechanisms of the artery walls, and above all, the distribution of mixture of plasma and blood cell as a result of all these processes in the capillary network.

Based on this new knowledge, a complex signal configuration was developed, determined by the biorhythm, to stimulate limited microcirculation, which is called the BEMER technology 2010.
The complex BEMER stimulation signal is represented by a composite waveform with the following particularities: different frequencies of the partial waves (local and higher-level regulation), specific envelope curve of the waveform, defined by the biorhythm, with a low-intensity pulsating electromagnetic field used as carrier.

Materials and methods
This randomized blind study was conducted on a nearly homogenous sample of a total number of 28 male rehabilitation patients (based on physiotherapeutic conditioning) aged of 55 to 65 years. The participants were randomly assigned to one of 3 subgroups: control group (n=14): treated using

physiotherapeutic conditioning according to standard practice, and treatment group (n=14): treated using physiotherapeutic conditioning according to standard practice + supplementary physical stimulation of the flexible arteriolar wall movement.

The BEMER system is used as a study device to stimulate the flexible arteriolar wall movement (a biorhythm-based stimulation signal, which is transmitted by a weak electromagnetic field with a specific flux). The treatment group received supplementary therapy using this device for 2 x 15 minutes per day. The duration of the treatment was 30 days; the duration of measurement was 40 days (10-days follow-up). Measurement points at identical intervals of 5 days (specific measurements with boundary conditions). Non-invasive measurement methods: macrocirculation (RR, Hf), intravital-microscopic examination unit with computer- aided secondary image processing (OLYMPUS, ZEISS, ARRI, and KONTRON systems), vital microscopic reflection spectrometry (SPEX system), combined white light spectroscopy and laser micro-flow measurement (LEA system).

The representative features of the functional status of the microcirculation, and the intracellular and humoral immune response of the subcutaneous and intestinal target tissue were evaluated: functional status of the flexible arterial wall movement
– AVM (area under the curve of the amplitude-frequency spectrum), number of nodes impregnated by blood cells in the microvascular network – nNP, oxygen use on the venule side – ΔpO_2, initial lymphatic volume flow – QL, number of leucocytes migrating in a specific tissue volume – nBC/V, ICA M-1 etc. Biometry: WILCOXON rank-sum test ($\alpha = 5\%$).

Results

During the 40 days of measurements, the following maximum changes in indicators were determined in two partial samples in the intestinal tissue to be accessed using the treatment:

Typical maximum % change compared to the baseline value on Day 0		
Features	Control group	Treatment group
AVM	8.6 (+/0 2.51)	29.7 (+/0 2.36)
nNP	4.4 (+/0 1.80)	32.8 (+/0 2.50)
ΔpO_2	3.1 (+/0 1.03)	29.3 (+/0 1.76)
QL	11.6 (+/0 2.56)	42.1 (+/0 3.61)
nBC/V	4.7 (+/0 1.47)	32.5 (+/0 2.60)

After the treatment is completed on Day 30, in the control group these values have returned to baseline by Day 40 unlike in the treatment group.

Conclusions

In addition to physiotherapeutic conditioning according to standard practice, using the BEMER system (physical stimulation of limited flexible arteriolar wall movement) in rehabilitation patients suffering from infection and stress leads to a clear increase in the therapeutic outcome (it improves the supply with nutrients of tissues and promotes the immune response).

Effect of BEMER Applications on the Formation of Biopolymers of Certain Bacterial Strains

Dr. Kesserű Péter, Ph.D., MSc
"Bay Zoltán" Foundation of Applied Research Director of the Bioremediation Department, Institute of Biotechnology (BayBio)

Chronic lung infections with mucoid Pseudomonas aeruginosa and the associated inflammation are the main cause of morbidity and mortality in patients with cystic fibrosis.

Removing the mucoid Pseudomonas aeruginosa from the lung tissue using classic therapy with antibiotics is rather difficult because the cells in the alginate biofilms have become increasingly insensitive to antibiotics.

There are a few new approaches to break the alginate exopolysaccharide structure to increase the efficiency of the therapy with antibiotics, such as inhalation of alginate lyases and aminoglycosides, or in vitro administration of antibiotics and weak electromagnetic fields (DC, 10-20 V, 20 mA, distance: 2.5 mm).

The 24-48 hours biopolymers of the Pseudomonas aeruginosa were evaluated during treatment with electromagnetic field using irradiation with extremely weak BEMER 3000 Signal Plus to examine the effect of the magnetic field on the alginate structure.

Direct application of the BEMER electromagnetic field (without distance) using 50 µT and 100 µT for 8 minutes (24 hours biopolymers) decreased by 55.5% and 58.3% the viscosity of the biopolymers studied, respectively. Setting the field strength to 100 µT, increasing the distance of the irradiation (5 cm) led to an increase of 65% in the destructive effect on the biopolymers. The efficacy of the therapy depends not only on the distance, but also by the duration and the continuously changing field strength (60-100 µT). Apparent viscosity has dramatically decreased in the case of all biopolymers (48 hours and well structured) treated using a field with a strength of 60-100 µT for 20 minutes.

Although the BEMER magnetic field broke the structure of the biopolymers, it had no negative effect on the viability of Pseudomonas aeruginosa cells. Based on this, the live cells (KbE 108) have reorganized the alginate after 24 to 48 hours which led to higher apparent viscosity. After a combination of ciprofloxacin (2 µg/ml) and magnetic field (60-100 µT, 20 minutes, distance: 5 cm), the full loss of the regeneration capacity of live cells was observed 24 hours after the irradiation. In such cases, 100% and 89% of the biopolymers examined lost their structure after 24 hours and turned into a Newtonian fluid after 96 hours, respectively. After administering Ciprofloxacin (2 µg/ml) alone 57% and 67% of the biopolymers examined 57%-a lost their structure after 24 hours and turned into a Newtonian fluid, respectively. After these experiments, 102 KbE was measured in the Pseudomonas aeruginosa for both treatments.

These results indicate that, in combination with classic antibiotic therapy, the BEMER 3000 Signal Plus electromagnetic field therapy, based on its capacity to destroy biopolymers, constitutes a gentle supplementary therapeutic option for patients with cystic fibrosis.

Preconditioning With Repeated Exposure to BEMER 3000 Signal Alleviates the Embryotoxic Effect of Cyclophosphamide

Jelínek, Richard, Bláha Jiři*

Charles University, 3rd Faculty of Medicine, *Geophysical Institute, Academy of Sciences of the Czech Republic, Prague, Czech Republic

Background: Several papers from the past decade signalized that short-term exposure to electromagnetic fields (EMF) might protect the progeny from the deleterious action of chemical teratogens. The present aim was to investigate whether a similar effect is observed with the wide band pulsed EMF in extreme low frequencies (BEMER 3000 signal) used for therapeutic purposes.

Method: The experimental system employed chick embryos treated under precisely controlled conditions. Fertile eggs were exposed to the BEMER signal 3 times daily for 20 minutes from the beginning of incubation. On day 4, the externally normal embryos were injected intraamniotically with increasing doses of a well-known teratogenic agent – Cyclophosphamide [CP]. The embryos incubated further in the normal geomagnetic field were harvested on day 9 and checked for malformations and other manifestations of embryotoxicity. Control groups comprised similarly treated embryos that were not exposed to the BEMER signal.

Results: Doses between 2 - 8 μg CP produced in the controls a typical dose effect, which in the CP-treated specimens appeared modified by a remarkable depression situated below the ED50. This phenomenon supports the hypothesis that exposure to BEMER prior to the teratogen administration beneficially modifies the embryotoxic effect in the lower segment of an overall dose-response curve.
Introduction

Extremely low, wide frequency range pulMsed electromagnetic (EMF) fields under BEMER 3000 signal configuration have been widely employed for therapeutic use in several indications (Kafka, 1998, 2000). Although many beneficial effects have been described, well-controlled clinical studies are still rare (Spodaryk, 2002). The action of EMF is gentle and moderate lacking acute and dramatic effects, so that very sensitive, complex, and sophisticated detection systems should be used. Such a system is offered by developing vertebrate embryos. Several papers have already documented that under specific conditions EMF protected the exposed progeny from the deleterious action of X-rays and several chemical teratogens (Patková, Jeřábek, 1994, Patková et al., 1996), and more recently even from the consequences of ischemia (DiCarlo et al., 1998). Basing upon our past experience we could expect that a similar effect might be exerted by the electromagnetic BEMER 3000 signal. However, working with embryos needs special knowledge, skills and experience concerning both exposure and assessment. Therefore we decided to start our paper with a brief Excursion in teratology

Modern teratology is a science dealing with poor pregnancy outcome. Poor pregnancy outcome comprises all phenomena other than a normal foetus delivered in term. To wit, from one hundred successfully fertilised human ova, only 30-50 healthy babies are born. The rest are either lost mainly during the first weeks of pregnancy, or develop abnormally, manifesting either intrauterine growth retardation (IUGR), or the least frequent event - developmental defect. Mechanisms of abnormal development can hardly be studied in humans. Many experimental models are therefore used – each for special purposes. Most difficulties arise from the fact that we deal with two biological units independent to a certain extent : the mother and the foetus. When a mammalian female is exposed to chemical agents (including drugs), the final outcome depends largely on the pharmacokinetic properties of the maternal organism. To avoid this complication, non-mammalian species (e.g. birds) are often used.

Investigations of such objects resulted in the past in the disclosure of several basic principles of teratology formulated concisely already by Wilson in 1977:

1. Susceptibility to teratogenic agents varies with the developmental stage at the time of the final manifestations of abnormal development (embryotoxicity phenomena) are death, malformation, growth retardation and functional disorder.

2. Manifestation of deviant development increase in degree as dosage increases from the no- effect to a totally lethal one.
   Two additional rules were added later (Jelínek, 1988):

3. To obtain the classical S-shaped dose-response curve, one must sum the manifestations of deviant development (at least malformation and death) into one parameter of embryotoxicity As a teratogen, such an agent should be labelled, which would significantly increase the overall incidence of embryotoxicity phenomena within the exposed population over their basal frequency present in an unexposed one. In the experiment, this basal frequency contributes to the so-called no-effect level.

Following our past experience with interactions other than those based on a chemical reaction between the teratogen and a modifying agent, the beneficial effect is regularly found only in doses that allow the majority of embryos to survive (Veselý, Veselá, Jelínek, unpublished).

Hypothesis

Respecting the principles mentioned above, we start to verify the hypothesis that if there exists any beneficial effect of the BEMER 3000 signal on embryotoxicity induced by a teratogen, we must search for it in doses affecting less than 50% of the exposed embryos above the no-effect level (real ED50).

Material and Method

An experimental system was developed with the aim to study the mechanisms of BEMER action (Janoutová et al., 1999). A pair of hot-air driven incubators - one placed in the BEMER magnetic field conditions and the second placed in the control system of magnetic field were developed. Air heating allows for entire non-magnetic construction. A special predictive logarithm for temperature control was developed to achieve the degree of precision of about $0.2°$ C. The actual temperature was recorded every 5 minutes. The wide band pulsed electromagnetic field in the extremely low frequencies as expressed by the formula $y = k(x)\ xa\ esin(x \wedge b)\ /c+d$, [e.g. $k(x)=l$, $x[0.4]$; $a=b=3$; $c=50$; $d=O$] - BEMER 3000® signal (Fig. I) (Kafka, 2000) - was induced by a coil situated at the bottom of one of the incubators.

Fresh laid eggs of random bred stock of White Leghorn Fowl purchased from the Institute of Molecular Genetics, Academy of Sciences of the Czech Republic were used. The experiment consisted of two phases. In the course of Phase I (1-4 days) the experimental (E) group was exposed to BEMER (step 10. 3 x 20 min per day, at eight-hour intervals). The flat circular coil was placed 10 cm below the shelf carrying about 34 eggs. The maximum intensity of the signal at the site of incubated eggs reached 20 µT above the natural background (Fig. 1). The rest of the experimental eggs (about twelve) were kept in the other half of the incubator where the intensity of BEMER-induced magnetic fields appeared negligible. Embryos kept in the latter compartment were added to the following control group.

The main control (C) group of approximately the same size was placed in the reference incubator without exposure. On day 4 the eggs were candled and opened using the conventional window technique (see, for instance, Jelínek, Peterka, 1983). Using an Olympus preparation microscope, the embryos were examined for normality and staged according to Hamburger and Hamilton (1951) - [HH stages].

By comparing the distribution of early embryonic death, abnormal specimens, and HH stages, we established information on the possible influence of BEMER during the first 96 hours of incubation. At the same time, we gained a starting point for Phase II in which the consequences of teratogen administration were studied in the BEMER exposed and unexposed groups. Altogether, 439 selected embryos in HH stages 22-24 were used. As a teratogen, cyclophosphamide (CP) (Endoxan®, ASTA Medica AG, Frankfurt, Germany) was chosen for establishing the standard dose-response relationships. One preliminary experiment served for establishing the no-effect level. In the main experimental series 2 to 8 □g of pure substance known to exert embryotoxic effects were injected intraamniotically to each embryo in both groups using a special glass canule. After moistening the vascular area with 0.7% saline and after closing windows in the shell with glass slides on paraffin frames, the eggs were put back to the appropriate oven. In the course of the 5-day re-incubation period, embryos were checked through windows and transparent walls of the incubators. Dead specimens were removed, inspected under the preparation microscope for visible malformation and probable cause of death and the findings were recorded. On day 9 of incubation the eggs were reopened, the embryos were harvested, weighed and checked for defects of the following organs: central nervous system, eyes, face, limbs, body wall and trunk. A routine dissection of the heart allowed us to include defects of great arteries and heart septation.

Every BEMER-treated group was compared with its relevant control group in any individual experiment. The STATISTICA® (Statsoft) software was used for the result evaluation that, besides the descriptive statistics, t-test for two dependent samples and Wilcoxon matched pair test, included a contingency table analysis. The 95% level was used as the arbitrary limit for statistical significance.

Results Phase I

The comparison of BEMER-treated (E) and non-treated (C) embryos on day 4 (Table 1, Fig. 2,) did not reveal any statistically significant difference. This applied both for the prevalence of non-developing (perhaps unfertilized) eggs (0), dead (D) and malformed (M) embryos (expressed as proportions P0, Pd and Pm, respectively), and in the individual organ affliction (malformation spectra) calculated as proportions of the surviving. The index of embryotoxicity, defined as (Pd+Pm) served for the comparison between the control (C) and BEMER-treated group in any individual experiment (Table 1). This comparison appeared insignificant, too.

We might conclude, therefore, that intermittent exposure to the BEMER signal of chick embryos until day 4, i.e. in the course of the main organogenetic period, did not interfere with their normal development.

Phase II

The initial experiment (No. 1) was focused on verifying the no-effect level, i.e. the basal incidence of embryotoxicity phenomena within the population of embryos used. We therefore incubated two groups of embryos without applying CP on day 4. The upper limit for the normal proportion of dead and malformed specimens occurring in the population of embryos that passed the procedure of windowing, sham intraamniotic administration, and re-incubation until day 9 reached 0.3. This has been considered a reference value (no-effect level) when using the Chick Embryotoxicity Screening Test (CHEST – e.g. Jelínek et al., 1985). The data for Experiment 1 (0.23 for both BEMER treated and untreated, see Table 2) fit the interval well and confirmed our first conclusion that intermittent BEMER exposure does not interfere with morphogenesis. Plotting the values (Pd+Pm) for the BEMER non-pretreated embryos in the rest of experiments (2-8), in which CP was administered in increasing dose yielded a positive dose-response curve (Fig. 3). A similar curve constructed for the BEMER pre-treated specimens exhibited a significant depression, situated below the point where cyclophosphamide adversely affected 50% of the embryos above the no-effect level (a real ED50). The difference was significant on the 0.05 level (Tab. 2), which means that the BEMER pre- treatment really has a beneficial effect on CP embryotoxicity. Thus, our hypothesis failed to be rejected.

Discussion

Finally, we will concentrate on the question of suitability of the chick embryo model for investigating the effects of EMFs on developing systems, which still remain controversial. According to Nguyen et al. (1995), the avian embryo does not represent a good model for mammalian teratogenesis. Omitting a long history of equivocal results starting in the seventies (Zervins, 1973, Krueger et al., 1975, Joshi et al., 1978 etc.), we are going to mention the study of Berman et al. (1990), which evaluated the results of experiments of six independent laboratories. The experiments were carried out under the same conditions (unipolar pulse 500 □s, 1 µT) for the first 18 h of incubation. Four of the laboratories found no statistical differences between control and experimental groups while the remaining two laboratories reported a significant increase in the incidence of malformed specimens at the end of incubation. A small but highly significant difference was the end result of pooling the data. Handcock and Kolassa (1992) undertook a statistical evaluation of these results. They confirmed the effect of exposure but demonstrated that undefined laboratory conditions were involved. This unwanted source of variation was active even in our experiments. We can see that one and the same dose produced a different effect in the controls (compare experiments 3, 4, 6) or even the lower dose could be slightly more effective than the higher one (see experiments 5 and 6). This uncertainty is by no means exclusive for the chick embryo model (Mevissen et al., 1994), and appears inherent in any complex system influenced by many variables. We became familiar with the problem when designing the aforementioned Chick Embryotoxicity Screening Test. As a consequence, while studying the dose-response relationships, we recommended administering doses differing by one order of magnitude (Jelinek, Peterka, 1983).

Apparently, this condition can hardly be fulfilled when examining weak factors to which EMFs undoubtedly belong. There appears to be a single solution – repeated experiments evaluated with respect to the relevant parallel controls. Repeat testing provides for greater confidence in the final interpretation of the results (Carr, Gorelicks, 1996).

Conclusion

A significant depression of the dose-response curve observed after administration of cyclophosphamide confirmed the hypothesis that exposure to BEMER beneficially modifies the embryotoxic effect in the lower segment of an overall dose- response curve.

References

1. Berman E, Chacon L, House D, Koch BA, Koch W, Leal J, Lovtrup S, Mantiply E, Martin AH, Martucci GI: Development of chicken embryos in a pulsed magnetic field. Bioelectromagnetics 1990, 11: 169-187
2. Carr GJ, Gorelicks NJ: A place for statistics in the generation and analysis of genetic toxicity data: a response to "rodent mutation assay data presentation and statistical assessment.". Mutation Res 1996, 357: 257-260
3. DiCarlo AL, Farrell, JM, Litovitz TA: A simple experiment to study electromagnetic field effects: protection induced by short-term exposures to 60 Hz magnetic fields. Bioelectromagnetics, 1998, 19: 498-500

4. Hamburger V, Hamilton HL: A series of normal stages in the development of the chick embryo. J Morphol. 1951, 88: 429-33
5. Handcock MS, Kolassa JE: Statistical review on the hen house experiments: the effects of pulsed magnetic field on chick embryos. Bioelectromagnetics, 1992, 13: 429-433
6. Janoutová J, Bláha J, Jelínek R: The absence of geomagnetic field does not influence the development of the chick embryo, Biologia (Bratislava) 1999, 54, Suppl. 6: 151-156
7. Jelínek R: The principles of teratogenesis revisited. Cong Anom. 1988, 28: S145-Sl55
8. Jelínek R, Peterka M: Method used in our laboratory in Prague for the Chick Embryotoxicity Screening Test (CHEST), pp. 599-602. In Neubert D, Merker H-J (eds) Culture Techniques: Applicability for Studies on Prenatal Differentiation and Toxicity, Walter de Gruyter, Berlin 1983
9. Jelínek R, Peterka P, Rychter Z: Chick embryotoxicity screening test – 130 substances tested. Indian J Exp Biol, 1985, 23: 588-595
10. Joshi VM, Khan MZ, Damle PS: Effect of electromagnetic field on chick morphogenesis. Differentiation 1978, 10: 39-43
11. Kafka WA: Device applying electric or electromagnetic signals for promoting biological processes. Europäische Patentanmeldung 98119944.1 v 21.10.98, 1998
12. Kafka WA: Extremely low, wide frequency range pulsed electromagnetic fields for therapeutical use (WFR-ELF-PEMS). Emphyspace Report.. Mediquant-Verlag, Sevelen 2000, pp. 20
13. Krueger WF, Giarola AJ, Bradley JW, Shrekenhamer, A: Effects of electromagnetic fields on fecundity in chick embryos. Ann NY Acad Sci, 1975, 247:391-400
14. Mevissen M, Buntenkoter S, Löscher W: Effects of static and time-varying (50 Hz) magnetic fields on reproduction and fetal development in rats. Teratology, 1994, 50: 229-237.
15. Nguyen P, Bounias-Vardiabasis N, Haggren W, Adey WR, Phillips JL: Exposure of Drosophila melanogaster embryonic cell cultures to 60 Hz sinusoidal magnetic fields: assessment of potential teratogenic effects. Teratology, 1995, 51: 273-277
16. Pafková H, Jeřábek J: Interaction of MF 50 Hz, 10 mT with high dose of X-rays; evaluation of embryotoxicity in chick embryos. Rev Environ Health. 1994, 10: 235-41
17. Pafkova H, Jeřábek J, Tejnorová I, Bednář V: Developmental effects of magnetic field (50 Hz) in combination with ionizing radiation and chemical teratogens. Toxicol Lett. 1996, 88: 313-6
18. Spodaryk, K: The effect of extremely weak pulsed electromagnetic field treatments upon signs and symptoms of delayed onset of muscle soreness; a placebo controlled clinical double blind study. Medicina Sportiva, 2002, 6: El9-E25
19. Wilson JG: Current status of teratology (General principles and mechanisms derived from animal studies) pp. 47-74. In Wilson JG, Fraser FC (eds), Handbook of Teratology, Vol. I. General Principles and Etiology. Plenum Press, N.Y., London, 1977
20. Zervins A: Chick embryo development in a 26 kHz electromagnetic field. Am Ind Hyg Assoc J, 1973, 34: 120-127

Figure Legends:

Fig. 1: (a) Characteristics of the BEMER signal measured magnetometrically within the area of exposure. Abscissa: time in milliseconds, Ordinate: magnetic flux density (B). (b) k(x)=l, x[0.4]; a=b=3; c=50; d=0], Ordinate arbitrary units; the dotted red line marks the 4th impulse at 19,062 nT (here at value 1.2); saturation occurs at the blue dotted line at 3.2 that is in the range of 19,062.00/1.2*3.2=50,832.00 Nt.

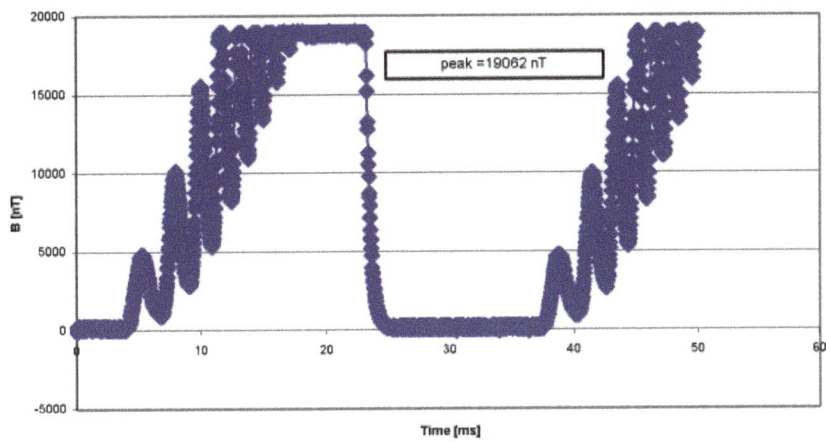

Figure 1a

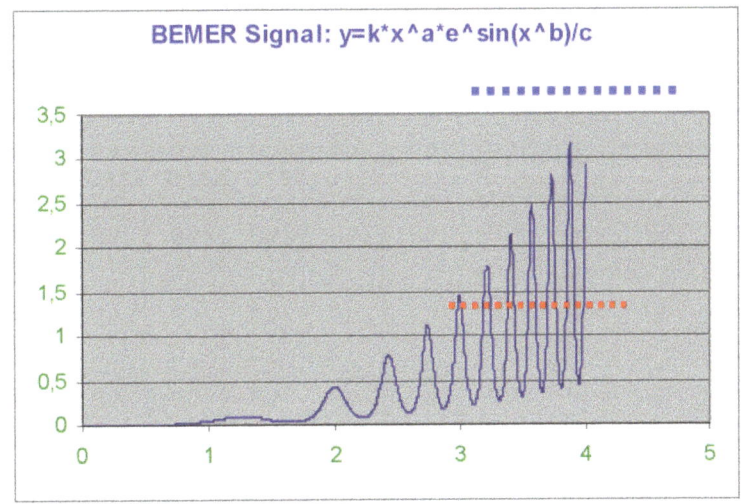

Figure 1b

Fig. 2: Effect of intermittent BEMER treatment during the first four days of incubation expressed as distribution of externally normal (N), dead (D), malformed
(M) and non-developing (possibly non-fertilized – 0) specimens. Sum of the eight experiments described in the Table 1. The resting columns depict the prevalence of organ affiction (malformation spectra) in the survivors. Abscissa: status of embryos and afflicted organs. CNS – central nervous system, B.W. – body wall. Ordinate: proportion of the total, Pc - control, non-exposed specimens, Pe - experimental specimens exposed to BEMER 3 times daily for 20 min.

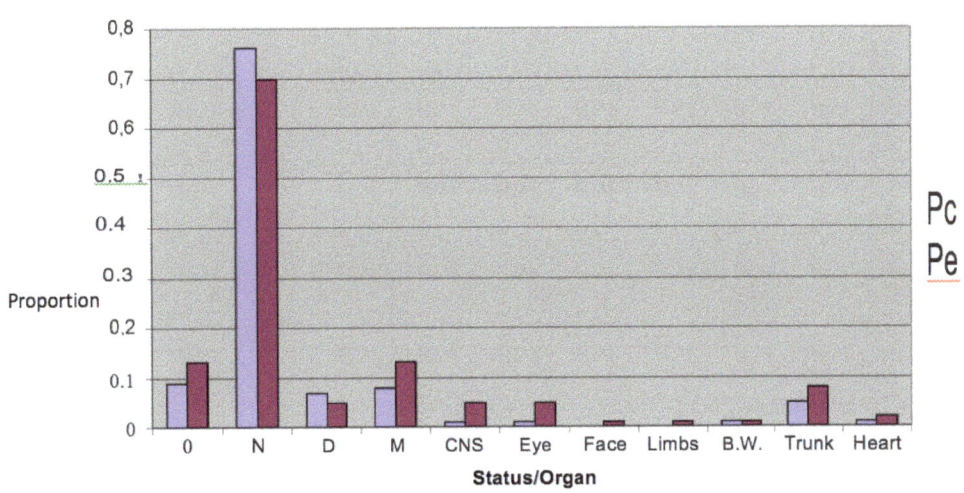

Figure 2b

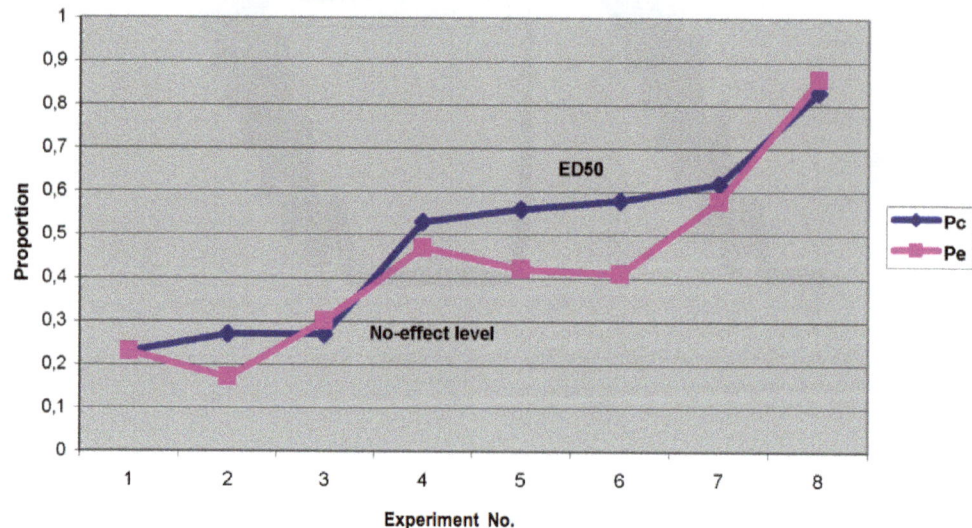

Figure 3 Table 1

Exp./Gr.	n	0	N	D	M	CNS	Eye	Face	Limbs	B.W.	Trunk
1/E	33	3	23	4	3	1					
1/C	45	1	34	5	5					4	2
2/E	45	5	34	2	4	3	4	2	2	2	3
2/C	44	5	34	1	4						2
3/E	32	9	19	2	2	1	1				2
3/C	39	4	29	3	3	1	1				1
4/E	32	6	18	1	7	3	3				1
4/C	49	5	33	4	7	2	2				4
5/E	34	2	28		4	1	1				3
5/C	45	4	36	5							
6/E	34	4	18	4	8	3	2				3
6/C	49	8	33	5	3	1					2
7/E	34	3	29	1	1						1
7/C	45	2	37	1	5	3					2
8/E	34	3	25		6						6
8/C	45	4	37	1	3						3
Sum C	361	33	273	25	30	4	3			4	16
Sum E	278	35	194	14	35	12	11	2	2	2	19
		0	N	D	M	CNS*	Eye	Face	Limbs	B.W.	Trunk
Pc		0,09	0,76	0,07	0,08	0,01	0,01			0,01	0,05
Pe		0,13	0,7	0,05	0,13	0,05	0,05	0,01	0,01	0,01	0,08
				p=0,13					p=0,14		

Embryotoxicity (Pd+Pm)	Individual comparisons							
	1	2	3	4	5	6	7	8
C	0,22	0,11	0,08	0,22	0,11	0,16	0,13	0,09
E	0,21	0,12	0,12	0,26	0,12	0,36	0,06	0,18

t-test dependent samples   p=0,216
Wilcoxon matched pair   p=0,207

Fig. 3. Proportion of the affected (malformed + dead) embryos observed on day 9 after Cyclophosphamide administration in increasing doses on day 4, ranked according the effect in control specimens (Pc) that were not exposed to BEMER. Pe– effect on BEMER pre-treated embryos. Abscissa: individual experiments (see Table 2). Ordinate: proportion of dead and malformed embryos.

Figure 3 Table 2

Exp./Gr.	Dose	n	N	D	M	CNS	Eye	Face	Limbs	B.W.	Trunk
1/E	0	30	23	4	3	1					
1/C	0	44	34	5	5					4	2
2/E	2	24	20	2	2					2	
2/C	2	44	32	4	8					1	
3/E	6	10	7		3	1		1			
3/C	6	22	16	3	3						
4/E	6	17	9	3	5	3	1	2	1		1
4/C	6	38	18	8	12			6			1
5/E	8	24	14	3	7	4		3	1		
5/C	8	34	15	6	13			6			
6/E	6	17	10	1	6						2
6/C	6	19	8	4	7			5			1
7/E	8	26	11	8	7	4		5	1		
7/C	8	34	13	6	15	6		8	1		
8/E	8	21	3	8	10	5		8			
8/C	8	35	6	17	12	5		10			
Total C		270	142	53	75	11		35	1	5	4
Total E		169	97	29	43	18	1	19	3	2	3

Embryotoxicity (Pd+Pm)	Individual comparisons							
	1	2	3	4	5	6	7	8
C	0,23	0,27	0,27	0,53	0,56	0,58	0,62	0,83
E	0,23	0,17	0,3	0,47	0,42	0,41	0,58	0,86
t-test dependent samples					p=0,042			
Wilcoxon matched pair					p=0,046			

Abbreviations:
Exp./Gr. - experiment/group, n - number of eggs, 0 - non-developing, possibly infertile, N - externally normal specimens, D - dead embryos, M - malformed embryos, CNS - central nervous system, B.W. - body wall defects, C - control, E - experimental Pc, Pe, Pd, Pm - proportions of the respective predicates

* The proportions of organ affliction are calculated for the total of survivors (N+M)

Oxidant Stress Clearance in Human Erythrocytes by Non-Invasive Stimulation with Extremely Weak (BEMER type) Pulsed Electromagnetic Fields: A Single-Blind, Randomized, Placebo-Controlled Study

Krzysztof Spodaryk* and Wolf A. Kafka** *Collegium Medicum of Jagiellonian University, 31-571 Krakow, ul. Kopernika 25, Poland

Preliminary version submitted to the Archives of Physiology and Biochemistry

**Internationa l Association on the Research of the Effects of Electromagnetic Fields under Normal and Extreme (Space) Conditions (EMPHYSPACE),

Johannishoehe 9 D-82288 Kottgeisering, Germany

Short title: *Weak Electromagnetic Stimulation and Free Radicals*

Abstract

The aim of this study was to investigate the effect of extremely weak pulsed electromagnetic fields on the status of lipid peroxidation and protein degradation of human red blood cells. Male volunteers (n=32; age 25-40, mean 28.3+/-7.8 years; weight 75.4+/-7.8 kg) were randomly divided into four groups of 8 subjects each under blinded conditions: control (C); sham- (S-T); verum- (Tl8) and verum- (T35). During the course of the 3 week-long experiments, all members of each group had to rest in supine position for a period of 20 minutes for 6 days a week. During this time all members, particularly those of group C, rested on mattresses (80x l70 cm) containing 6 equidistant arranged flat electrical applicator coils: four of them (beneath shoulders and back) were of circular shape (radius -15 cm) and two of them (below the legs) oval (22x50) shape.

Induced by a special designed generator system these coils were passed by defined currents so that members Tl8 were exposed for a period of 8 min with a 30 Hz pulsed mean magnetic flux intensity of 18 µT and those of T35 for a period of 20 min with a flux intensity of 35 µT, each pulse being characterized by a spectral wide banded flux density-time course y(x) according to $y=k(x)*x^a* esin(x^b)/c+d$, the so-called BEMER® signal. Blood samples were drawn from all subjects before (D0), on the ninth (D9) and the 2lst day (D2l) of the test period. The antioxidant status was tested by determining the red cell enzyme activities of glutathione S- transferase, glucose-6-phosphate dehydrogenase, 6-phosphogluconate dehydrogenase, NADPH-diaphorase, catalase and glutathione reductase and, to estimate the degradation red blood cell, the concentrations of glutathione (GSH), malonyldialdehyde (MDA) and alanine (AL). Whilst the enzyme activities and the concentration of peroxidation products of T18 do not significantly differ between those of S-T and C, they are significantly altered in T35 with higher enzyme activities and lowered lipid peroxidations. The results indicate that the BEMER pulsed 35 µT field effectively prevents oxidant stress in red blood cells.

Oxygen is the ultimate electron receptor in a closely linked electron flow system for the storage of chemical energy in the form of ATP. Under certain conditions, the electron flow may become disrupted and lead to the production of molecules or molecular fragments containing an unpaired electron, so-called free radicals, e.g. superoxide (O_2), hydroxyl (OH), peroxyl (RO_2), alcoxyl (RO), oxides of nitrogen (NO, NO_2) or sulfur (RS). Free radicals, (IO_2), hydrogen peroxide (H_2O_2), and hypochloric acid (HOCl) may additionally originate from reactive oxygen-containing species (ROS) during the processes of phagocyte activation, lipid and arachidon oxidation, autoxidation of catecholamines as well as from flavin, hemoprotein and iron-mediated reactions.

Free radicals are chemically very reactive and may thus strongly affect several biologically important functions, e.g. the defense of some strains of bacteria and fungi by phagocyte generated ROS, or O2 stimulated intercellular signaling and cell growth regulation. At higher concentrations, however, free radicals and ROS may initiate adverse, so-called oxidative stress reactions such as lipid peroxidation and protein degradation accompanied with harmful disruptions of membrane and cell functions (e.g. increased permeability, generation of lipid autoperoxidation and glycolysis, inactivation of enzymes, cross-linking or vulcanization of sulfhydryl rich proteins and even DNA damages (Chiu et al., 1989, Hayden & Tyagi, 2002, Oberley, 1988)). To reduce damage from free radicals, living aerobic organisms, from prokaryotes to complex eukaryotes, have developed elaborate sequences of adaptive feedback mechanisms to maintain a proper balance between anti- and pro-oxidants (redox homeostasis) (Hayden & Tyagi, 2002; Haddad, 2002; Knight, 2000).

In spite of this, certain exogenous and endogenous factors as for instance nutrition (food, alcohol, nicotine, metals), drug administration, physical and chemical stress (exhaustion, infection, heat shock, ethanol, radiation and presence of oxidants) or genetic conditions, might rule out these balancing mechanisms and initiate various processes of severe vital biological damage. Overdosed free radicals have even been implicated as contributing factors to aging and development of chronic diseases of heart and vascular system (Maytin, 1999), myalgias (Ninfali and Bresolin, 2002), diabetes, atherosclerosis presumably caused by hyperglycemia and a subsequent breakdown of the mechanisms controlling the glucose level (Hayden & Tyagi, 2002), oxygen signaling pathways (Haddad, 2002), chronic lung disease (Lunec, 1990), hemolysis (Saltman, 1989) as a consequence of a decreased rigidity and deformability of erythrocyte membranes (Srour et al., 2000; Van Der Berg et al., 1992), cancer (Costa & Moradas-Ferreira, 2001) and even Alzheimer's disease (Haddad , 2002).

A lot of attempts have therefore been undertaken to keep redox homeostasis balanced by means of various therapeutic methods e.g. drug administration, dietary nutrition, physical exercises and psychological methods (Hayden & Tyagi, 2002).

Because of the modest success, however, it still remains a challenging task to look out for further methods to effectively support those adaptive mechanisms and to minimize oxidant stress and prevent its harmful consequences.

Concerning the increased clinical acceptance for the therapy of pain, various etiologies, wound healing and inflammation of joints and muscle achieved by various non-invasive applications of pulsed, weak electromagnetic fields (Blank, 1993; Polk & Postow, 1996; Carpenter & Arapetyan, 1994; Quittan et al., 2000; Kafka 2000, 2001) and their possible involvement in the aforementioned processes, the present study is focused on the question of whether such electromagnetic stimulations might prove applicable also to support these redox-balance processes. <u>Especially on the basis of several hypotheses indicating that the primary site of interactions occurs at plasma membranes or, more precisely, adherent molecular or sub-molecular structures (Kafka, 2000), the electromagnetic stimulations were performed by application of a novel type of impulse form. Designed to tune the (charge/mass relation dependent) processes of molecular activation, these pulses are characterized by a special intensity/time course reflecting a wide spectral (so- called BEMER type) composition (Kafka, 2000).</u> Referring to the spectral composition these BEMER-pulses exceed the spectral power of sinus-, rectangular- or saw-tooth like pulses of conventional electromagnetic stimulations by more than a factor of 1,000, and have already proven effective in accelerated wound healing (Kafka and Preissinger, 2002), sedation processes (Michels-Wakili and Kafka, 2003), in- creased ATP synthesis (Spodaryk, 2001), delayed onset of muscle soreness (Spodaryk, 2002) and stress response activation against teratogens (Jelínek and Bláha, 2003).

Since mature red blood cells (RBCs) can be considered as metabolically active units whose functional capacity and integrity mainly depend on their metabolic activity, they may be treated as models well suited for the investigation of the influence of physical modalities on cell metabolism, especially as sensitive indicators of redox related effects as lipid peroxidation and protein degradation (Baker and Manwell, 1983; Scott et al., 1989; Richards et al., 1998). They lack a nucleus, ribosomal apparatus and mitochondria and have thus no ability to synthesize proteins or convert glucose to fatty or amino acids. Moreover, mature erythrocytes have a simple energy-producing metabolism (glycolysis) and most of its components, once damaged, cannot be replaced. The study was therefore designed to test this hypothesis referring to the oxidant status of mature RBCs under good clinical practice conditions by means of a randomized, blinded placebo- controlled investigation on human volunteers. To pilot even dose response relationships, the tests were performed at different magnetic flux intensities. signal generator unit (with manual adjusting time of exposure and intensity) and a mattress containing 6 (four circular, .Ø 25 cm and 2 oval 25/40) flat electrical coils as stimulus applicators. The stimulation was mediated via a sequence of extremely low frequent, wide-band pulsed weak electromagnetic fields, each pulse being characterized by the formula $y=k(x)*^1 xa* esin(x^b)/c+d$, [e.g. $k(x)=l$, $x[0,4]$; $a=b=3$; $c=50$; $d=O$] - BEMER 3000® signal (Fig. 1). The mean magnetic flux intensity of the signal at the surface of the mattress (0.7 x 1.7 m2) was either 18 or 35 µT. Its 3D spatial distribution is reflected in Fig 2. (The electrical components may easily be determined by the 1st derivative of $y(x)$ according to the Maxwell Equations).

Independent of the type of treatment all test persons had to rest in supine position for a period of 20 min each day, at 10 p.m., 6 days during the 3 week-long experiment. Individuals of group S-T, and T18 and T35 had to rest on the respective type of mattress. Within this resting period of resting they were treated according to their group affiliation.

Blood sampling

Venous blood samples were taken from each member of the individual groups (C, S-T, T18 and T35) by vein puncture at three intervals: one day before the start of the experiments (D0), before the ninth exposition on the 9th day (D9) and the day following the last exposition (D21) each between 7:30 a.m. and 9:00 a.m.

Preparation of red blood cell suspensions

The samples were drawn into a heparinized plastic vacutainer and after centrifugation (1,000 g for 10 min at 4°C), separated from plasma. To minimize contamination with leukocytes, the erythrocytes were carefully sampled from the bottom of the tubes, washed (three times) in a cold sodium chloride solution, lysed by the addition of a β-mercaptoethanol EDTA stabilizing solution (Beutler, 1984) and after vigorous vortex-mixing stored on ice for 10 min.
Laboratory methods

The determination of the erythrocyte enzyme activities (glucose-6-phosphate dehydrogenase (G-6-PD), 6-phosphogluconate dehydrogenase (6-PGD), NADPH- diaphorase (ND), catalase (CAT) and glutathione reductase (GR), glutathione S- transferase (GST) and the concentration of reduced glutathione (GSH) were performed spectrophotometrically (LKB Ultraspec 2, at 340 nm for G-6PD, 6-PGD, ND, GST, GR, 230 nm for CAT or 412 nm for GSH) according to the methods of Beutler (1984).

Malonyldialdehyde (MDA) was colorimetrically determined as concentrations (nmol/gHb) as a measure of lipid peroxidation according to the method of Stocks and Dormandy's (1971) by adding TBA to the trichloroacetic acid (TCA) extraction of MDA (from erythrocyte suspension) giving a pink colored complex (absorption max 532 nm).

---

1 * A sham-effect of ~ 5 µT might be induced via the coils by ambient electromagnetic fields

Alanine (AL) was determined in nmol/gHb as a measure of protein degradation according to Davies and Goldberg (1987).

Hemoglobin (Hb) was measured in g/L by the cyanmethemoglobin method (Dacie and Lewis, 1995). Enzyme activities are expressed in International Units (IU/gHb). The relevant coenzymes, enzymes and substrates stemmed from Sigma (St. Louis, MO) and Boehringer (Mannheim, Ger- many). Analytical-grade chemicals were obtained from Merck (Darmstadt, Germany).

Statistical analysis

Data are expressed as means and standard deviations (±SD). A two-way analysis of variance with repeated measures was used to assess significant variations during the experimental procedure. Relationships between selected vari ables were evidenced by a Pearson's correlation analysis for each point in time and for maximal variations. The p value was obtained by transforming Pearson's r into Fisher's z.

Statistical significance level was set at $p<0.05$.

Results

The precision of measurements was assessed by a repeated assay of pools of hemolysates that were stored at -40 °C. The coefficients of variation for within-day and day-to-day reproducibilities ranged between 3.7% and 7.8% for the various enzyme activities.

The activity of the enzymes, determined for (D0), (D9) and (D21) are presented in Tab (1) and Figures (3-5) for all four groups (C, S-T, T18 and T35) inclusive means and ± SD.

There are no statistically significant differences of enzyme activities and other intraerythrocytic compounds to be seen between the four experimental groups at (D0) and even numbered ones between groups C and S-T at (D9) and (D21).

Concerning the period between D0 and D21 the activities of GR (10.5±0.9 and 11.6±0.8 IU/ gHb), CAT (1.37±0.09 and 1.92±0.09 mg/gHb) and MDA (0.92±0.23 and 0.65±0.14 IU/gHb)of group T18 however significantly differ from those ones of group C and S-T and even indicate a slight but statistically significant decrease in the MDA concentration between D0 and D21. Significant changes of else enzyme activities or AL concentrations were not observed within T18. Except GST, significant increases of enzyme activities during D0 and D21 were also observed for T35. For some of them the activities significantly increased already between D0 and D9: 6-PGD (from 7.52±0.34 to 8.29±0 .37 IU/gHb; p<0.03); CAT (from 1.25±0.06 to 1.75±0.09 mg/gHb, p<0.05) . The concentration of AL, however, significantly decreased between D0 and D9 from 663.2± 176.3 to 534.5± 178.9 nmol/gHb; p<0.05.
In T35 the activities of investigated enzymes, except GST, significantly increased from D0 to D21: G-6PD (from 12.3±0.8 to 13.5± 1.1 IU/gHb; p<0.04); 6-PGD (from 7.52±0.34 to 8.99±0.86 IU/gHb; p<0.02); GR (from 10.0±0.8 to 11.8±0.5 IU/gHb; p<0.05); CAT (from 1.25±0.06 to 2.02±0.11 mg/gHb; p<0.01); ND (from 2.0±0.2 to 2.9±0.5 IU/gHb; p<0.05). During D0 and D21 a significant decrease was found for GSH (from 2.28±0.21 to 1.76±0.16 mg/gHb; p<0.04); MDA (from 1.01±0.28 to 0.69±0.14 mg/gHb; p<0.05);AL (from 663.2±176.3 to 497.3±198.1 mg/gHb; p<0.05).

Discussion

As far as we know, there are no reports published concerning the influence of pulsed electromagnetic field as a physiotherapeutical modality on the oxidant status of red blood cells. The present work was concerned with the antioxidant effect induced by BEMER 3000-type electromagnetic fields at stimulations (doses) differing in time and in magnetic flux intensity . An exposure to a 35 µT pulsed electromagnetic field was found to prevent the oxidant stress of the red cell which can be taken as to be proven both by the increasing rates of enzyme activities (involved in protecting cells from the negative effects of oxygen radicals) and as the decreasing concentrations of lipid peroxidation products found after electromagentic whole body exposures.

Glucose-6-phosphate dehydrogenase, a NADP-dependent enzyme, the initial and rate-limiting enzyme of the hexose monophosphate pathway catalyses the dehydrogenase of glucose-6-phosphate to 6-phosphogluconate. The next oxidative step is catalyzed by 6-phosphogluconate dehydrogenase, which also requires NADP as a hydrogen receptor, to produce the pentose, ribulose-5-phosphate.
Ribulose-5-phosphate is converted back to the main stream of glycolysis by transketolase and transaldolase. NADPH, provided from the hexose monophosphate pathway, reduces oxidized glutathione (GSSG) to reduced glutathione (GSH), catalyzed by glutathione reductase (GR). In turn, GSH removes oxidants, such as superoxide anion (O_2-) and hydrogen peroxide (H_2O_2), catalyzed by glutathione peroxidase. This reaction is important because the accumulation of oxidants may decrease the life span of the red blood cells by increasing the rate of oxidation of protein, that is, hemoglobin, cell membrane and enzyme protein. Since G-6-PD is sensitive to H_2O_2 and to the sulfhydryl group oxidizing agent, this enzyme plays a major role in the defense mechanism against oxidative stress (Fuji and Miwa, 1999). Among the different ROS scavengers, the glutathione dependent system is heretofore also of great importance: This system does not only work as a peroxide scavenger, but also as a regulator of the redox state within the red blood cells. While scavenging the ROS, GSH is oxidized and forms glutathione-protein mixed disulfides. Thus by supporting the red blood cell's reducing or synthesizing abilities, GSH turns out to play the major role in managing oxidative stress situations. The antioxidants present in the red blood cells, such as glutathione and vitamin E (α-tocopherol) are able to prevent oxidation of iron in the hem group and labile (sulphhydryl) groups as well as on the hemoglobin molecule and the erythrocyte cell membranes. Oxidized protein sulphhydryl groups can be reactivated by glutathione-mediated reduction and thus in turn prevent irreversible damage of erythrocytes (Luzzato, 1995).

While it is well recognized that erythrocytes possess mechanisms for combating oxidative stress, it has so far not been considered that they might provide a free radical detoxification system even for the whole body (Papas, 1996; Richardas et al., 1998). Our study indicates that stimulation by magnetic flux intensity of 35 µT has protective influence on red blood cells. Since the potential damage is considerably lessened by the ubiquitous presence of erythrocytes competing with other tissues for scavenging the free radicals, we may therefore speculate that this physiotherapeutical stimulus (modality) effectively prevents oxidative damage in other tissues of the body. This hypothesis is supported by increased activity of GST as determined in T35. GST serves to clean the blood from xenobiotics to which the red cell membrane is permeable. This enzyme could conjugate such substances to glutathione, and thus render the disposal of these thusly detoxified conjugates out from the red blood cells (Jakoby, 1978; Halliwell and Gutteridge, 1999). Further investigations are however needed to test the effect of this physical modality on different kinds of cells. Since the brain is especially susceptible to oxidative damage, and, furthermore, antioxidant enzymes dysfunctions may lead to neurodegenerative processes including cell death, motoneuronal diseases and axonal injury (Mates et al., 1999), studies concerning the oxidant stress within neural cells would be of high interest. Despite a high rate of ROS production due to a highly active oxidative metabolism and an abundance of polyunsaturated fatty acids- these cells are characterized by a relatively weak antioxidant defense system. (Within the brain they might be protected by astrocytes, highly against oxidative stress resistant neuroectodermal matrix cells).

The suppression of the oxidation of cellular oxidizable substrates by antioxidants is an essential process in all aerobic organisms. Several biologically important compounds have been reported to have antioxidant functions. These include vitamin C (ascorbic acid), vitamin E (α-tocopherol), vitamin A, β-carotene, coenzyme Q-10, flavonoids, cysteine and many others (Mates, 2000). Meanwhile their therapeutical use either in the form of naturally occurring or completely synthetic antioxidants gathered considerable interest. There is already some evidence that some clinically applied drugs may exert part or all their effect via antioxidant mechanisms. Antioxidant enzymes, small molecules, genes and proteins are geared towards modern molecular biology. Many groups, studying antioxidant therapy even use adenovirus-containing manganese superoxide dismutase (SOD) or infusions of SPD in liposomes (Halliwell & Gutteridge, 1999).This enzyme has an anti-inflammatory effect in animal models of acute inflammation, because it can decrease the number of neutrophils entering the sites of inflammation. However, little is known about effects of physiotherapeutic modalities on antioxidant enzymes and lipid peroxidation in tissues, plasma and erythrocytes. In view of the results reported here, the application of specially tuned electromagnetic fields turns out as a most promising method to effectively support antioxidant protection of the organism, minimize oxi- dant stress and prevent its harmful consequences for maintaining good health.

Regarding the process of several weeks necessary to monitor the aforementioned significances induced by T35, the lack of significant metabolic modifications achieved for TI8 must not necessarily be referred to as ineffectiveness of the corresponding lower magnetic flux density of 18 µT. Instead they may depend on the duration of the applications, meaning that elongated periods of stimulation would turn out effective as well. This study demonstrates a dose dependent protective influence on oxidative damages of red blood cells. The exposure to BEMER 3000 type pulsed electromagnetic fields can thus be treated as a beneficial antioxidant modality for living organisms. On account of the specially designed, spectrally wide-band stimulus signals focused at the energetic processes of diversified molecular activations - and thus relieving the start of a wide scale of metabolic processes - these results are restricted to the BEMER 3000 system and may therefore not be taken as valid for other electromagnetic therapy systems either. Clinical studies are in progress for a refined understanding of the antioxidant status after such physiotherapeutic electromagnetic BEMER 3000 interventions.

References
1. Baker CMN, Manwell C. (1983) Electrophoretic variation of erythrocyte enzymes of domesticated mammals. In: Red Blood Cells of Domestic Mammals. Eds. Agar NS, Board PG. Elsevier, Amsterdam
2. Beutler E. Red Cell Metabolism: A Manual of Biochemical Methods. (1984) New York, Grune and Stratton
3. Blank E. (1993) Electricity and Magnetism in Biology and Medicine. San Francisco: San Francisco Press
4. Chiu D., Kuypers F., Lubin B. (1989) Lipid peroxidation in human red cells. Semin Hematol 26:257-276
5. Carpenter DO., Aryapetyan S. (1994) Biolo- gical Effects of Electric and Magnetic Fields: Sources and mechanism (Vol 1); Beneficial and Harmful Effects (Vol 2); Academic Press, San Diego, New York, Boston, London, Sydney, Tokyo, Toronto
6. Costa V., Moradas-Ferreira P. (2001) Oxidative stress and signal transduction in Saccharomyces cerevisiae: insights into ageing, apoptosis and diseases Molecular Aspects of Medicine 22:217-246
7. Dacie JV, Lewis SM. (1995) Practical Haematology. Edinburgh: Churchill Livingstone
8. Davies KJA, Goldberg AL. (1987) Proteins damaged by oxygen radicals are rapidly degraded in extracts of red blood cells. J Biol Chem 262:8227-8234
9. Fuji M, Miwa S. (1999) Red blood cell enzymes and their clinical application. Adv Clin Chem 33:1-54
10. Haddad JJ. (2002) Oxygen-sensing mecha nisms and the regulation of redox- responsive transcription factors in development and pathophysiology. Respir Res 3:26-53
11. Halliwell B, Gutteridge JMC. (1999) Free Radicals in Biology and Medicine. 3rd ed.n, Oxford, University Press, NY
12. Hayden MR, Tyagi SC (2002) Intimal redox stress: Accelerated atheroscleroscis in metabolic syndrome and type 2 diabetes mellitus. Atheroscleropathy. Cardiovascular Diabetology 1: Diabetology I:3-30
13. Jakoby WB. (1978) The glutathione S-transferase: a group of multifunctional detoxification proteins. Adv Enzymol 46, 383-414

14. Jelínek R, Bláha J (2003) Preconditioning with repeated exposure to BEMER 3000 signal alleviates the embryotoxic effect of cyclophosphamide, Bioelectromagnetics , in pressi presss
15. Kafka WA. (2000) Extremely low, wide frequency range pulsed electromagnetic fields for therapeutical use. Emphyspace 2:1-22
16. Kafka WA. (2001) Device applying electric or magnetic signals for promoting biological processes. Europäisches Patent Nr 0995463 (16.08. 2001)
17. Kafka WA., Preißinger M. (2002) Verbesserte Wundheilung durch gekoppelte, BEMER 3000 typisch gepulste, Elektromagnetfeld- und LED-Licht-Therapie am Beispiel vergleichender Untersuchungen an standardisierten Wunden nach Ovarektomie bei Katzen (felidae). In: Edwin Ganster (editor) Österreichische Gesellschaft der Tierärzte (ÖGT) Kleintiertage-Dermatologie 02.-03. März 2002,
18. Salzburg Congress 72-7
19. Knight A. (2000) Review: Free radicals, antioxidants and the immune system. Ann Clin Lab Sci 30:145-158
20. Lunec J. (1990) Free radicals: their involvement in disease processes. Ann Clin Biochem 27: 173-182
21. Mates JM, Perez-Gomez C, De Castro IN. (1999) Antioxidant enzymes and human diseases. Clin Biochem 32:595-603
22. Mates JM. (2000) Effects of antioxidant enzymes in the molecular control of reactive oxygen species toxicology. Toxicology 153:83-104
23. Melvin R.H., Suresh CT. (2002) Intimal redox stress: Accelerated atherosclerosis in metabolic syndrome and type 2 diabetes mellitus. Cardiovascular Diabetology 1:3-30
24. Michels-Wakili S, Kafka WA (2003) Bemer 3000 Type Pulsed Low-Energy Electromagnetic Fields Reduce Dental Anxiety: A Randomized Placebo- Controlled Single-Blind Study. 10th International Dental Congress on Modern Pain Control IFDAS June 2003, Edinburgh, Scotland, in press
25. Ninfali P, Bresolin N (2002) The role of glucose-6-phosphate dehydrogenase in the clearance of oxidant stress products in muscle during exercise Favism Res Papers 12:l-3 (rialto.com/favism/ninfali2.htm)
26. Oberley LW. (1988) Free radical and diabetes. Free Radic Bio Med 5:113-124
27. Papas AM. (1996) Determinants of antioxidant status in humans. Lipids 31 (suppl): 77-82
28. Polk C., Postow E (1996) Handbook of Biological Effects of Electromagnetic Fields, CRC
29. Press Boca Taton,Boston, London, New York, Washington, DC
30. Quittan M., Schuhfried 0., Wiesinger GF., Fialka-Moser V. (2000) Klinische Wirksamkeiten der Magnetfeldtherapie - eine Literaturübersicht. Acta Medica Austriaca 3:61-68
31. Richards RS., Roberts TK., McGregor NR., Dunstan RH., Butt HL. (1998) The role of erythrocytes in the inactivation of free radicals. Medical Hypotheses 50:363-367
32. Saltman P. (1989) Oxidative stress: a radical view. Semin Hematol 26:249-256
33. Scott MD, Eaton JW, Kuypers FA, Chiu DT, Lubin BH. (1989) Enhancement of erythrocyte superoxide dismutase activity: effects on cellular oxidant defense. Blood 74: 2542-2549
34. Spodaryk K (2001) Red blood metabolism and hemoglobin-haemoglobin oxygen affinity: Effect of electromagnetic fields on electromagnetic field in healthy adults. In: Wolf A Kafka (editor) 2nd Int. World Congress Bio-Electro-Magnetic- Energy-Regulation, Emphyspace 200l; 2:15-9
35. Spodaryk K (2002) The effect of extremely weak electromagnetic field treatments upon signs and symptoms of delayed onset of muscle soreness: A placebo controlled clinical double blind study. Medicina Sportiva 2002; 6:19-25
36. Srour MA, Bilto YY, Juma M, Irhimeh MR. (2000) Exposure of human erythrocytes to oxygen radicals causes loss of deformability, increased osmotic fragility, lipid peroxidation and protein degradation. Clin Hemorheol Microcircul 23: 13-2l
37. Stocks J, Dormandy TL. (1971) The autooxidation of human red cell lipids induced by hydrogen peroxide. Br J Haematol 20:95-111
38. Van Den Berg JJM, Op Den Kamp JAF, Lubin BH, Relofsen B, Kuypers FA. (1992) Kinetics and site specificity of hydroperoxide induced oxidative damage in red blood cells. Free Rad Biol Med 12:487-498

Healing and Quality of Life:
Our Experiences with the BEMER Application at the Matyas Health Center

Lecture at the Budapest Congress 03.27.2011

Dr. György Seress

SUMMARY: We believe that BEMER is changing the assessment of health-illness by promoting the capacity to regenerate already hardwired into us and that BEMER application is changing quality of life even for seemingly healthy people.

Our health center opened in April 2009. We can summarize our experiences as follows:
The advantage of the health center is: We strive to look at patients who come or are referred to us as a whole, or – to use the current word in fashion – holistically. And that is why, when establishing case history, accompanying illnesses of a psychosomatic nature can be assessed separately. With these points in mind, the BEMER program can be tailored to the individual. The program requires the current and basic illness to be monitored, as the changes are individual and can be varied in illnesses associated with injury. You also cannot work from your medical handbook. The contribution to therapy management of a well-educated doctor is a real advantage, whereas a half-educated specialist is a serious disadvantage, because the credibility of the procedure may be cast into doubt. The health center can look at a person as a whole and take on the role of organizing a team for treatment. Traditional academic medicine becomes not an alternative, but complementary.

We believe that BEMER is changing the assessment of health-illness by promoting the capacity to regenerate already hardwired into us and that BEMER application is changing quality of life even for seemingly healthy people.

It is opening up the possibilities of traditional therapy and helping to achieve outcomes after an operation not only more quickly, but with a much better final outcome. It is therefore a new possible therapy for such chronic illnesses as Sudeck's disease (Sudeck dystrophy).

Today we are able to confirm, from our own experiences, that the BEMER application have changed the possibilities of medicine fundamentally.

Its application cause a change in the quality of life even in the case of seemingly healthy people. It opens up the possibilities of conservative treatment, and outcome following surgical treatment is not only faster, but it comes with a much better final result. In the process it means having a new treatment option for diseases such as pain syndrome (reflex sympathetic dystrophy syndrome, Sudeck) in the case of such chronic diseases.

Today we can claim based on our own insights and experiences that the BEMER application fundamentally changed the abilities of medicine.

Bemer Therapy in Rehabilitation

Dr. Kovács Matild, chief physician

"Jahn Ferenc" Hospital in South Pest, "Weiss Manfréd" Department in Csepel

According to current definition, rehabilitation is a process in the health, mental hygiene, educational, training, retraining, occupational and social systems which aim at developing and maintaining the abilities of disabled persons, facilitating their participation in social life and independent life style (Act XXVI of 1998).

Objective

We have been using the first generation BEMER devices at our Rehabilitation Department since 2003. In June 2010 we purchased a BEMER Professional therapeutic system, and we evaluated the efficacy and efficiency of the therapy based on the experiences with this system in patients admitted to our department for multimorbid rehabilitation.

Patients and methods

We analyzed the data of patients admitted to the Rehabilitation Department between August 1, 2010 and January 31, 2011, who were treated using the BEMER Pro system. These patient data were retrospectively analyzed. Status scales (Barthel index, VAS, FIM, FNO) were used at admission and discharge to evaluate the results.

110 patients were included in this study. All patients were admitted to the Rehabilitation Department during the abovementioned period for treatment for their conditions requiring rehabilitation. The Rehabilitation Department is part of a public hospital that ensures care for non-specialized conditions where all diseases are addressed, which cause damages to the musculoskeletal function and disability.

Therefore, a wide spectrum of applications could be evaluated such as in post- treatment traumatic injuries, degenerative musculoskeletal disorders, conditions after cerebrovascular lesions and chronic neurological syndromes, internal diseases, immunological syndromes, peripheral vascular diseases, metabolic disorders and tumors.

Distribution of patients involved in the study			
By gender:	Women: 74	Mean age	Women: 68.3 years (33098 years)
	Men: 36		Men: 71.5 years (38090 years)

For the purposes of this analysis, patients were stratified based on the disease currently leading to hospitalization, that is, the so-called "main diagnosis".
The distribution of the patients included is as follows:

Degenerative joint diseases	Total	By gender	
Spondylarthrosis, discopathia	25 patients	women: 20	men: 5
Primary coxarthrosis, gonarthrosis	10 patients	women: 8	men: 2

Disc herniation, radiculopathia	10 patients	women: 7	men: 3
Post-traumatic status	12 patients		
Hip fracture	7 patients	women: 4	men: 3
Hip and knee prosthesis	5 patients	women: 4	men: 1
Osteoporosis	5 patients	women: 4	men: 1
Neurological syndromes			
Post-stroke status with paralysis on one side	15 patients	women: 20	men: 5
Syndromes associated with dizziness	16 patients		
Vertebrobasilar insufficiency, vertigo	13 patients	women: 7	men: 6
Sclerosis multiplex	3 patients	women: 2	men: 1
Lower limb vasoconstriction	7 patients	women: 3	men: 4

Characteristics of the patients included in the analysis: multimorbidity – the diagnostic classification was done based on the syndrome currently requiring hospital care and the main symptoms for all patients. Each patient has more than 3 comorbidities; some of them even had 6-8 conditions.

In 20% of the patients treated the underlying disease was associated with mood disorders requiring moderate and severe medication.

Therapeutic procedures used: medication for the status and condition of the patients, and rehabilitation procedures according to the injuries or disabilities, such as physiotherapy, therapeutic massage, ergotherapy and therapy administered using the BEMER Professional device.

The patients treated with the BEMER Professional device in this analysis were not administered electrotherapeutic treatments. Using the BEMER therapy

Individual programs according to each condition: the duration of one treatment session is minimum 16 minutes and maximum 36 minutes.

Frequency: once a day, in acute cases twice a day.

Number of treatment sessions – mean number: 15 sessions – 5 times a week, the shortest: 10 sessions – 3-5 times a week, the longest: 30 sessions – 5 times a week.

Results:
Changes in pain based on the VAS 10 Scale

Degenerative joint diseases	At Admission	At Discharge
Spondylarthrosis, discopathia	9 (6-10)	4 (1-5)
Primary coxarthrosis, gonarthrosis	8 (5-10)	4 (1-5)
Disc herniation, radiculopathia	8 (5-10)	2 (1-5)
Post-traumatic status		
Hip fracture	7 (6-10)	2 (1-5)

Hip and knee prosthesis	9 (6-10)	4 (1-5)
Osteoporosis	9 (6-10)	4 (1-5)
Lower limb vasoconstriction	9 (6-10) Walking distance 50 m	Walking distance 400 m

Changes in the Barthel-index based on the 100-point scale.

Degenerative joint diseases	At Admission	At Discharge
Spondylarthrosis, discopathia	30	95
Primary coxarthrosis, gonarthrosis	30	85
Disc herniation, radiculopathia	20	100
Post-traumatic status		
Hip fracture	15	75
Hip and knee prosthesis	20	80
Osteoporosis	50	100
Lower limb vasoconstriction	65	100
Neurological syndromes		
Post-stroke status with paralysis on one side	20	80
Syndromes associated with dizziness		
Vertebrobasilar insufficiency, vertigo	60	100
Sclerosis multiplex	15	55

Changes in the FIM and FNO scores that measures self-sufficiency: these scales quantify how much assistance is needed in personal hygiene, eating and self care.

The BEMER therapy provides support in becoming self-sufficient in case of deficiencies in self care associated with all conditions as follows:

	At Admission	At Discharge
Degenerative joint diseases	requires help to a moderate extent	self-sufficient
Post-traumatic status	requires help	self-sufficient
Neurological disorders	requires help to a great extent	self-sufficient

Summary

Similarly to the previous first and second generation therapeutic systems, the BEMER Professional device can be used in rehabilitation with good results as an independent therapy. It can improve the efficacy of the health care.

Effects used in therapy

Analgesic effect: increased production of endorphins; anti-inflammatory effect: harmonization of the vegetative nervous system, improvement of the oxygen supply of cells, dilatation of capillaries, increasing the permeability of blood vessels and promoting the absorption of different fluid accumulation by increasing the permeability.

It helps the integration of calcium into the bones by improving circulation. It improves the metabolic processes, increases the reactivity of the conduction of peripheral motor nerves, promotes the regeneration of neurons and improves the intensity of muscle contractions. It accelerates wound healing, and stimulates melatonin secretion, and thus helps physiological sleep and regulates the sleep-wake cycle.

Benefits of the therapy

It is a non invasive procedure. There is no age limit: it can be used both in elderly and children. There are no known adverse effects so far. It can be well combined with traditional and alternative treatments. A patient-friendly treatment. It allows achieving a symptom-free (complaint-free) state, improves patient compliance, self- sufficiency, improves the quality of life and accelerates rehabilitation. The treatment can be easily repeated and is simple to maintain the state achieved. It is cost- efficient and shortens hospitalization. It does not expose the body to chemicals.

When the body reacts, the energy delivered solves not only the symptoms of the diseases, but also influences or improves the changes of other organ systems.

Effects of Physical Stimulation of Spontaneous Arteriolar Vasomotion in Patients of Various Ages Undergoing Rehabilitation.

Klopp RC, Niemer W, Schulz J.
J Complement Integr Med. 2013;10(Suppl):S13-9. doi: 10.1515/jcim-2013-0032.

Abstract

In two samples of rehabilitation patients of different age groups (approx. 38 years and approx. 51 years), via a placebo-controlled study series using representative features of microcirculation, the complementary therapeutic success of additional treatment complementing the biorhythmically defined physical vasomotion stimulation was determined. The results showed that in older rehabilitation patients the amounts of characteristic microcirculatory changes were greater than in younger persons undergoing rehabilitation, but they would subside faster after termination of the additional treatment than in the younger group.

PMID:24021602 [PubMed - in process]

Treatment Results of Patients Who Were Treated with Electromagnetic Fields that the BEMER 3000 Device Generates.

Stryla W; Knapczyk M; Zurawski P; 2004

Chair and Rehabilitation Clinic at the Medical Academy in Poznan; Poznan Center for Rehabilitation and Orthopaedics "PozCeRO" in Poznan

SUMMARY: Out of 811 enrolled patients, 497 were evaluated who have experienced a consecutive treatment of at least one daily application with the BEMER 3000 devices over at least 2 weeks. The patients were divided into 3 main indication groups: 1. Patients with painful spinal syndromes, 2. Patients who have experienced trauma (resulting from fractures, sprains, and overloading of joints and soft tissues), 3. Patients with pain symptoms in the hips, knees or shoulders. No significant changes were observed in neurological examinations. Orthopaedic examinations showed an increase in the mobility of the examined joints. In conclusion, the following resulted: The BEMER 3000 device is suitable for the rehabilitation of patients with musculoskeletal pain.

In view of the positive results of the work, it is appropriate to continue the examinations and expand patient groups with a control group.

Introduction

The magnetic field therapy occupies a significant place among the physiotherapy methods used in contemporary medicine. In rehabilitation, it is one of the most commonly recommended measures. Despite its proliferation, indications and contraindications for the use of the electromagnetic field have not yet been described enough in the accessible literature.

The electromagnetic field is determined by such parameters as frequency, pulse shape and amplitude. There are differentiated opinions among researchers on the biophysical effects of different frequencies. For our examinations we chose the BEMER 3000 device that exudes electromagnetic fields with a frequency of about 200 Hz.

Objective

The research project is scheduled to research the effects of magnetic field therapy in the treatment of patients with various pain disorders of the musculoskeletal system in the period from April 2001 to January 2004.

Object of research

This work contains the results of treatment of patients in the Poznan "PozCeRO" Rehabilitation and Orthopaedics Center where magnetic field therapy was applied using the BEMER 3000 device from April 2001 to December 2001.

BEMER 3000 is also constantly used on patients who are hospitalized at the rehabilitation clinic. We tried our best to include the patients in the research. However, the application of the electromagnetic field as the only physiotherapy method is not practically possible under the conditions of the physiotherapy clinic, thus the examinations had no scientific value.

The magnetic field therapy was indicated to 811 patients of the Poznan "PozCeRO" Rehabilitation and Orthopaedics Center. This figure does not include the patients who had interrupted treatment for various reasons, or had not reported for a check-up. 497 patients were qualified for the examinations with pain symptoms of the spine and other joints based on degeneration and strain injuries and consequences resulting from trauma. BEMER 3000 magnetic field therapy was used on patients as the only physiotherapy measure. Because of the preliminary nature of the examinations, patients who used kinetic therapy and pharmacotherapy were not excluded.

Stimulation density took place once daily for 15 consecutive days, no Saturdays, Sundays or holidays. In contrast, in the remaining 314 outpatients magnetic field therapy in conjunction with other physical measures was applied, which excluded the usefulness of the evaluation of these patients for scientific research. It was assumed that patients with pain symptoms of the knee, cervical spine and shoulder locally use magnetic field therapy with an applicator with the remainder of them being treated lying on the mat. The attending "PozCeRO" physician determined the nature of the applicable program. The patients were divided into three main groups:

- Patients with painful spinal syndrome
- Patients who have experienced trauma – resulting from fractures, sprains, and overloading of joints and soft tissues.
- Patients with pain symptoms in the hips, knees and shoulders

A separate form was used for all subjects, which was presented to the course for methodology of scientific research, organized and accepted by the Medical Academy in Poznan in March 2001.

No significant changes were observed in neurological examinations. Orthopaedic examinations showed an increase in the mobility of the examined joints. The results obtained were shown in tables.

Table I shows the intensity level of pain according to the visual analog scale (VAS) in all patients before and after magnetic field therapy. Tables II - IV show pain assessment in the individual patient groups in the VAS scale before and after magnetic field therapy.

Table 1 All patients

		Result After										Patients
	VAS	0	1	2	3	4	5	6	7	8	9	
Result Before	1	1	0	0	0	0	0	0	0	0	0	1
	2	1	3	0	1	0	0	0	0	0	0	5
	3	4	12	2	1	1	0	0	0	0	0	20
	4	4	30	14	6	8	5	1	1	0	0	69
	5	1	22	38	23	17	7	3	0	0	0	111
	6	1	15	28	29	15	9	14	7	2	1	121
	7	0	8	21	15	8	11	8	6	2	1	80
	8	0	4	8	7	8	4	11	7	2	1	52
	9	0	5	5	6	2	1	3	7	7	1	37
	10	0	0	0	0	0	0	0	1	0	0	1
Patients		12	99	116	88	56	37	40	29	13	4	497

Table II
Group 1

		Result After										Patients
	VAS	0	1	2	3	4	5	6	7	8	9	
Result Before	1	1	0	0	0	0	0	0	0	0	0	1
	2	1	3	0	1	0	0	0	0	0	0	5
	3	4	11	1	1	1	0	0	0	0	0	18
	4	3	22	7	5	8	5	1	1	0	0	52
	5	1	13	27	17	15	7	3	0	0	0	83
	6	0	10	19	22	11	7	11	7	1	0	88
	7	0	6	12	10	6	6	8	6	1	0	55
	8	0	4	3	6	6	1	7	5	2	1	35
	9	0	4	2	5	1	0	2	4	7	1	26
	10	0	0	0	0	0	0	0	1	0	0	1
Patients		10	73	71	67	48	26	32	24	11	2	364

Table III
Group 2

		Result After										Patients
	VAS	0	1	2	3	4	5	6	7	8	9	
Results Before	3	1	0	1	1	1	0	0	0		0	1
	4	5	3	7	5	8	5	1	1		0	9
	5	3	2	27	17	15	7	3	0		0	8
	6	0	5	19	22	11	7	11	7		0	10
	7	1	2	12	10	6	6	8	6		1	9
	8	0	3	3	6	6	1	7	5		0	7
	9	1	1	2	5	1	0	2	4		0	7
Patients		11	16	8	6	4	2	3	1		2	51

Table IV

Group 3

	VAS	0	1	2	3	4	5	6	7	8	9	Patients
Results Before	3	0	0	1	0	0	0	0	0	0	0	1
	4	1	3	4	0	0	0	0	0	0	0	8
	5	0	6	9	4	1	0	0	0	0	0	20
	6	1	5	4	4	3	2	2	0	1	1	23
	7	0	1	7	4	1	2	0	0	1	0	16
	8	0	0	2	1	0	2	4	1	0	0	10
	9	0	0	2	0	0	1	0	1	0	0	4
Patients		2	15	29	13	5	7	6	2	2	1	82

As a major improvement after application of magnetic field therapy, the results 0 or 1 were recognized on the VAS scale. In all patients approximately 20% of these results were obtained. Over 30% significant improvement was achieved in the IL group, which included patients with post-traumatic symptoms. The exact results of significant improvement are shown in Table V. Due to the differences in the results of the VAS scale before and after magnetic field therapy, a separate scale of treatment effectiveness was determined, which is presented in Table VI.

Table V

	0 VAS After	%	1 VAS After	%
Group I (364)	10	2.7	73	20.1
Group II (51)	11	21.6	16	31.4
Group III (82)	2	2.4	15	18.3
All patients (497)	12	2.4	99	19.9

Table VI
Before and After differences on the VAS scale

	Significant improvement	Improvement	Minimal improvement	Unchanged	Worsening
VAS change	> or = 3	= 2	= 1	0	< 0
Group I	190	64	52	36	22
Group II	34	12	3	1	1
Group III	54	18	5	2	3
All patients	278	94	60	39	26

For the statistical examinations, the Wilcoxon test was used to assess therapy efficacy. The difference between the result distributions before and after magnetic field therapy is statistically highly significant (p<0.000001). The median before magnetic field therapy was 6, afterwards 3, which is presented in Table VII. In the individual groups, a similar result distribution was achieved, which is presented in tables VIII to X.

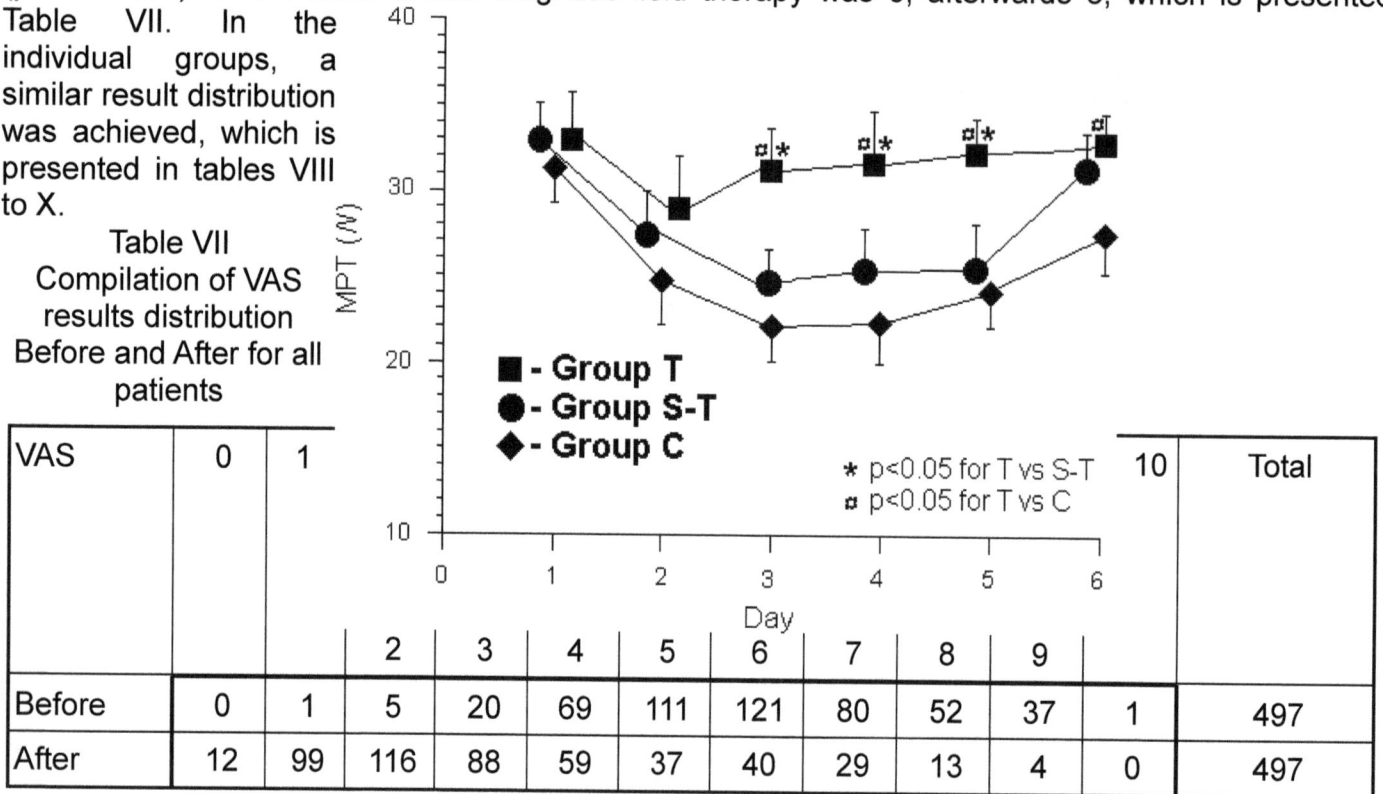

Table VII
Compilation of VAS results distribution Before and After for all patients

VAS	0	1	2	3	4	5	6	7	8	9	10	Total
Before	0	1	5	20	69	111	121	80	52	37	1	497
After	12	99	116	88	59	37	40	29	13	4	0	497

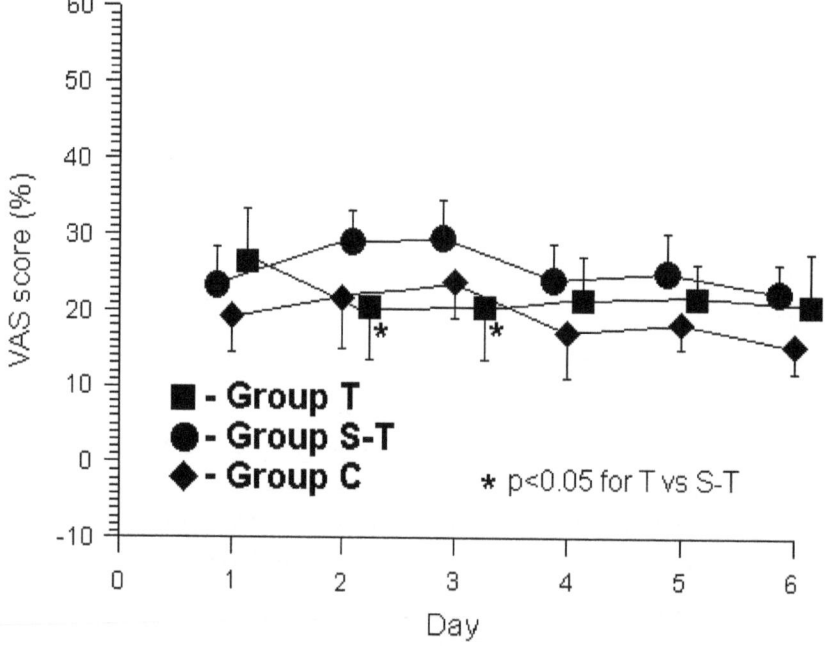

The difference between the result distributions BEFORE and AFTER is statistically highly significant (Wilcoxon-Test: p<0.000001).

The median for BEFORE is 6, the median for AFTER is 3

Apart from the visual analog scale, the effectiveness of the therapy of the subjective evaluation was evaluated by the patients upon completion of the therapy cycle. The results are shown in Table XI.

Table XI
Subjective evaluation by the patients

	Worsening	Unchanged	improvement	Symptom-free	Total
Group I	13	87	210	54	364
Group II	3	0	45	3	51
Group III	5	1	64	12	82
All patients	21	88	319	69	497

Statistically, the assessments of the effectiveness of the therapy were compared, which were subjectively determined by VAS. In the chi-square test, $p < 0.001$, a statistically significant dependence was determined between the good subjective assessments that correlate with the good assessments of the difference in the VAS scale.

Conclusions
The BEMER 3000 device is suitable for the rehabilitation of patients with musculoskeletal pain. In view of the positive results of the work, it is appropriate to continue the examinations and expand patient groups with a control group.

Stamp:
Chair and Department of Rehabilitation at the Karol-Marcinkowski Academy ul. 28. czerwca 1956r. No. 135/147 61-545 POZAN Tel. 831-02-17, 833-39-48. Fax 831-01-73 signed Prof. Dr. hab. med. Wanda Stryla Specialist for medical rehabilitation 60-615 Poznan ul. Podolska 4 Tel.: (0-61) 848-05-29
Translated from Polish by Mgr. Ludwik Kozlowski

Bemer Therapy Applied to Sports Medicine

Influencing Recovery Time by Using the BEMER 3000 Electromagnetic Field in Professional Sports - Examinations of the CK Elimination Curve

Möbes K, Michaelis H, Villinger B

A placebo-controlled, cross-over, double-blind study as part of the diploma course DTLG 1 Elite 02 / 03 of the coach's training by Swiss Olympic

SUMMARY: The significant earlier decrease in CK levels in the active treatment group compared with the placebo group shows a clear, positive effect of the BEMER 3000 electromagnetic field on the athlete.

Study design; *Working hypothesis, preliminary examinations*

Through their own investigations, the authors were aware that a pulsating electromagnetic field can affect several physiological features, such as blood microcirculation. The studies of Jellinek suggest that there could be an activation of the so-called HSP 70 proteins, thereby positively influencing the regeneration processes.

Working hypothesis:
Under the influence of a suitable electromagnetic field, the regeneration time of an athlete's stressed muscles can be shortened.

Regeneration means that a damaged structure is restored. "In the regeneration phase, equilibrium (homeostasis) disturbed by stress-strain regulation is restored to the body's functions. Constructive (anabolic) processes begin in the regeneration period (recovery)." [Neumann, Pfützner, Berbalk. 2001].

Intense or prolonged athletic activity leads to microtrauma in the muscles. As a result, the CK value increases in the blood. The increase of the CK value is attributed to the permeability of damaged cell membranes. Since this value usually increases over the course of hours and only slowly decreases, the CK trajectory is also considered as a parameter for muscle damage. Assuming that the electromagnetic field can positively affect the stabilization of the cell membrane structure, e.g. expedite the "repair" of the cell membrane, this means that the CK value increases over a relatively shorter period of time, the maximum value is lower and the CK values fall quickly back to baseline levels.

Task
Does the CK value on the trajectory change in terms of its maximum and/or temporal course under the influence of the BEMER 3000 electromagnetic field system?

Test equipment
BEMER 3000, INNOMED International AG (FL 9495 Triesen).

Subjects, sample
17 athletes, professional and recreational athletes between the ages of 17-46 who compete and train and sometimes train very hard and extremely long. (i.e. preparation for crossing Alaska, the 100 km Biel Ultra marathon, Ironman, etc.), 7 women and 10 men in the following sport categories: Cycling, mountain biking, running, climbing, mountaineering (ice climbing), triathlon, cross-country skiing. half pipe snowboarding, canoeing.

Exclusion criteria
Recent illnesses or injuries, inadequate training conditions for passing the standing requirements in the Proprio Dynamics Test (strong local overacidification in the thigh muscles), as well as mental problems

Sample
Each athlete must complete the test twice. He or she receives an active treatment device and placebo device once whereby the order is determined by lot (cross- over). The time between the two tests for an athlete is at least one week.

The devices are provided with a code by the manufacturer, which is announced only after all tests are completed (double-blind).

Procedure, method of measurement
Each athlete will fill out a questionnaire on personal circumstances upon arrival.

A venous blood sample is taken before starting the test to determine CK-output value. The CK values are always determined in the same manner in the Viollier, Bad Ragaz laboratory using the Integra 400 device.

The stress test takes place after an adequate warm-up phase: 6x 2 min on the Proprio Dynamics (made by Georg Hagmann).

Proprio Dynamics simulates the movements such as those in downhill skiing, where the slope profile (lift height) and the speed (intensity) can be set. For the test, the lift height shall be 14 and the speed shall be 3. Athletes hold a rod weight in their hands in the downhill position (90-degree target knee angle) for stabilization support.

After initial stress lasting 2 minutes, the athlete has a 2 min break, but must remain on the device and may not carry any regenerative measures. During this break, the lactate is determined in order to estimate the intensity of the stress. Lactate is determined using the lactate per device of Axon Lab AG. In addition, the subjective stress assessment is enquired according to the Borg scale (scale 1-20). Then the next two-minute stress is run with subsequent two minute break, etc. A total of six stresses of two minutes each are performed.

Immediately after the last stress, the subject lies on the coil mat of the BEMER 3000 system. Level 3 is activated, which lasts 8 minutes and operates with an average intensity of 10.5 micro tesla. Next, the coil cushion is placed on the athlete's thigh and program P 4 is applied. This lasts 20 minutes and the flux density gradually increases from level 6 to 10 (intensities of 60 to 100 micro tesla). Four hours later, the BEMER 3000 System is used again as described.

Six hours after the end of the test, the first blood test is performed. Then blood is taken venously after 8h, 10h, 12h and 18h and the BEMER 3000 System is applied as described above. The athletes are monitored at least 18h after the test and may not do any physical work nor conduct a training workload.

Statistical methodology
Data collection and calculation was performed on the computer using the Microsoft spreadsheet and graphics program Excel. Standard deviation and standard deviation error of the mean (SEM = Standard deviation error of mean), and the significance are calculated for the statistical calculation of the arithmetic mean.

The following values shall apply in this work for the significance p > 0 05 = 0 not significant, p <= 0.05 = significant, p <= 0.01 = highly significant.

Result

Subjects in the group that were treated with the BEMER 3000 System show a highly significant early decrease in CK levels compared to the placebo group. In the active treatment group, the "point of deflection" comes after 7.2 hours and after 9.2 hours (p = 0.025) in the placebo group.

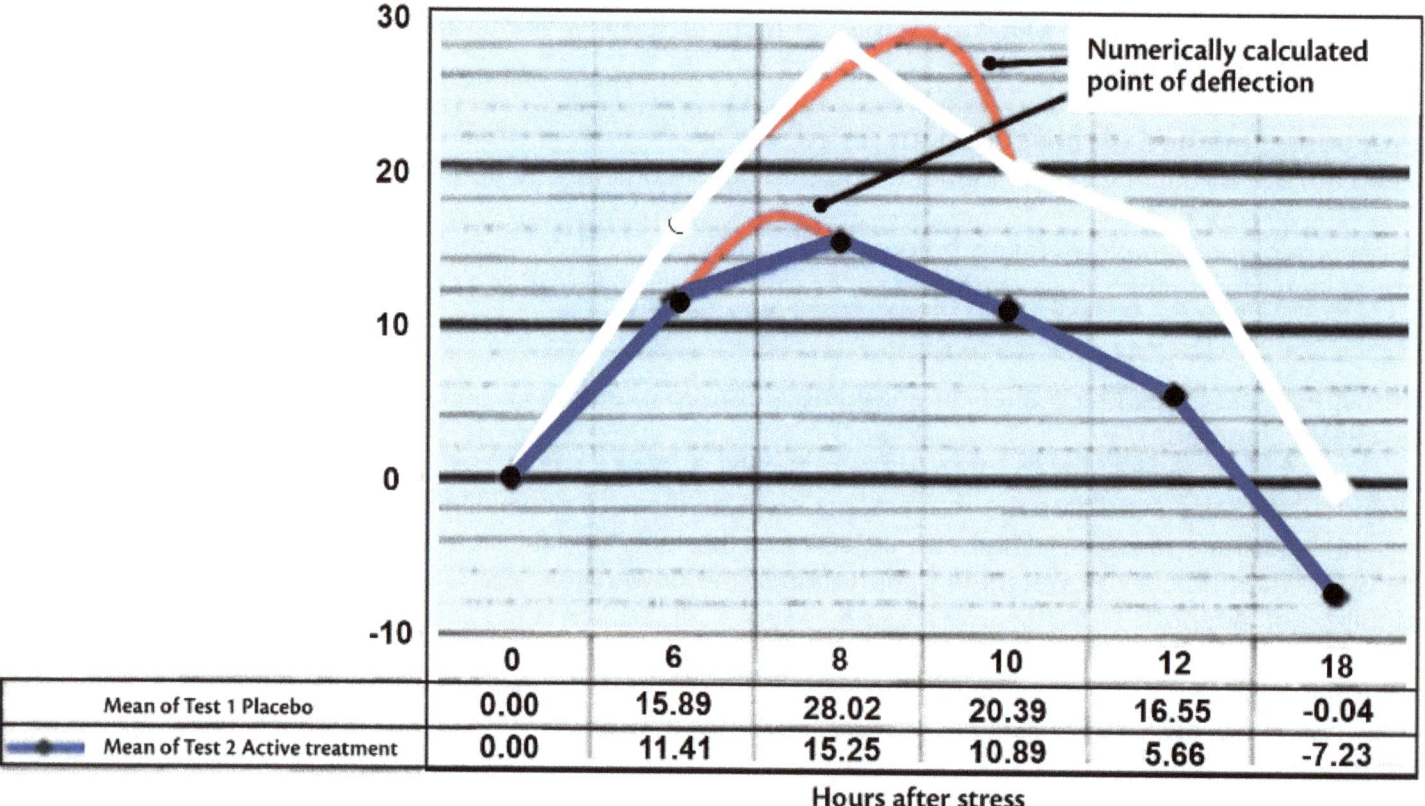

Points of deflection (PD) of creatine kinase (CK)-degradation curve in hours after stress:
Subjectively, the results of the evaluation of Dorg scale stated that the athletes had less muscle pain and not as "heavy legs" after application of the active treatment device as they did after using the placebo device.

Discussion and conclusions

The significant early decrease in CK levels earlier the active treatment group compared with the placebo group shows a clear, positive effect of the BEMER 3000 electromagnetic field on the athletes. However, the result allows for different interpretation methods. It is possible that activation of repair proteins (HSP 70) causes the cell membrane to regenerate more rapidly (reduction in permeability) and therefore less CK enters the blood, that lactate is removed faster by proven improvement of blood microcirculation in connection with the BEMER 3000, through which damage from subsequent stress is reduced and less CK is released into the blood and/or that the electromagnetic field promotes CK elimination from the blood, because of which the value does not rise so high and drops more quickly. In order to answer these questions clearly, further studies are necessary.

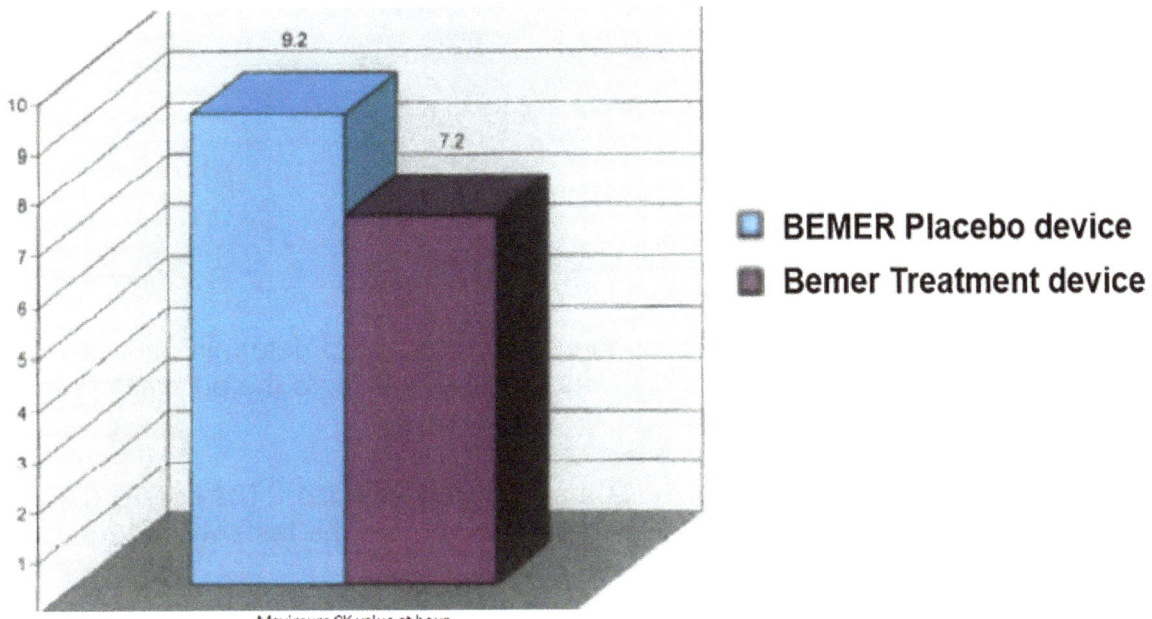

Maximum CK value at hour

- BEMER Placebo device
- Bemer Treatment device

SUMMARY: The aim of this examination was for the authors to clarify whether treatment with low-frequency pulsed electromagnetic fields may have an impact on the physical fitness of athletes and if so, whether there are correlative changes to certain parameters. 12 athletes were divided into 2 groups during a 3-week training camp and included in the study with a randomized, double-blind design.

The results show a significant superiority in the improvement of physical performance in athletes in the group of those actually treated compared to the group of those not treated.

The Effect of Magnetic Field Therapy on the Performance Capacity of Athletes and on certain Physiology Indicators of Performance.

J. Malomsoki; E. Babindák.
National Institute of Sports Medicine, Budapest.

ABSTRACT

This study investigated low-frequency pulsed magnetic field therapy to determine if it has an effect on performance capacity and, where any such effect was found, to elucidate the parameters that correlate with that effect.

Twelve tennis players participated in the study (9 males and 3 females). They were divided into two groups: treated and untreated, on a double-blind randomized basis,. The tests were performed during a three-week training camp.

Each of the test subjects received eight minutes of low-frequency pulsed magnetic field therapy everyday, for five days out of seven, with no therapy given on Saturday and Sunday. The magnetic field intensity used for treatments was between 10.5-21.0 µT (The BEMER 3000 equipment at levels 3, 4, 5 and 6).

A treadmill was used to measure performance. Running speed was increased at two minute intervals, and performance was characterized by the distancecovered.

The test also measured the following: anaerobic threshold (Conconi test), lactic acidosis, a number of oxygen status parameters, blood sugar levels and blood gases analysis (Astrup).

From these data it was ascertained that the performance of the treated group improved by almost 440 m (15.0%) at time of testing, while the performance of the untreated group improved by 166 m (5.4%). The treated group performed better, increasing their anaerobic threshold with a running speed of 1.5 km/h (9.5%), while the anaerobic threshold of the untreated group increased by less than 0.5 km/h (0.4%). It was also ascertained that compared to the untreated group, the treated group's performance was attained with higher lactic acidosis; however, the treated group compensated faster for lactic acidosis than the untreated group. The performance improvement observed in the treated group can be also explained by beneficial changes in a number of oxygen status parameters and reduced physiological shunting. It is proposed, and literature data also point to the possibility, that the beneficial effect experienced by those who had pulsed electromagnetic field treatment can be attributed partly to an improvement in microcirculation, and to the hypocoagulation of red blood cells.

The authors also hypothesize that the rise in blood sugar levels in the treated group signifies activation of the neurohumoral system, while in the untreated group it could be a sign of fatigue.

The authors also point out that pulsed magnetic field intensity and treatment duration correlate closely with physiological effects.

The use of magnetic fields for therapeutic effects has gained prominence among the paramedical treatments that have appeared in recent decades. There are numerous reports that set out the beneficial effects of magnetic therapy [8] and recommend its use. However, some of these reports comprise summarized congressional lectures (i.e. works published in non-peer-reviewed periodicals); and do not mention ineffective treatments and why they are ineffective – they make no attempt at analysis. In practice, research on magnetic therapies and the evaluation of its results are directed by Professor A. Sieron (The Silesian University of Medical Science, Bytom, Poland – developer of Viofor device) and by Professor W. A. Kafka (developer of BEMER therapy equipment – Euroinstitut für Bioenergetische Medizin [European Institute of Bioenergetic Medicine], Dornbirn).

The beneficial physiological effects of magnetic fields are attributed to the effects exerted by magnetic fields on polarized molecules. As for polarized molecules, the magnetic field affects the structure of electron shells controlling the molecules' spatial arrangement and, thus, may influence the course of chemical/biochemical reactions. In addition, it is worth highlighting the results of vital microscopic studies [2]. These studies aim to prove that the magnetic field's effect results in improved capillarization, i.e.– microcirculation. The increase in blood supply could facilitate oxygenation which, for example, in athletes could increase performance capacity.

In the present study we tried to answer the following questions on the systematic use of magnetic fields, or rather — magnetic stimulation:
- Do they affect performance capacity?
- If they do and there is change in performance capacity, with which performance-physiology parameters do they correlate; which physiological processes produce the change?

Test Subjects

Twelve tennis players from the IDOM tennis club were enrolled onto the study (9 male, 3 female). Age range was 13–24 years, height ranged from 144–166 cm and weight ranged from 44–65 kg. Measurements and observations were made during routine fitness tests. The subjects and their parents were informed in writing about the aim of the study and its course, they consented to the tests. Following double- blind procedure, the athletes were split into two groups. One group received the magnetic treatment, while the other group received sham treatment.

Test Procedures

We subjected the athletes to exercise stress test on a treadmill. We increased the running speed every two minutes and the exercise was repeated under the same conditions both before and after the start of the magnetic therapy period. Initial running speed was 7 km/h and 9 km/h respectively. The study used an all-out exercise (vita maxima) stress test. Evaluation was based on the distance covered. All the athletes took part in the planned training camp that was being held the same time as the study, as expected.

We used BEMER 3000 system for the magnetic therapy. In essence, this system transmits a pulsed electromagnetic field to the whole body. The field intensity varied between 10.5 and 21.0 µT. The person being treated lay down on a mattress containing magnetic field generating coils. Each treatment lasted for 8 minutes (using BEMER 3000's basic level 3-4-5-6 program). The program gradually increased field intensity, and then gradually decreased it at the end of the treatment sequence. Treatment was given on five days out of seven, with no treatment given on Saturday and Sunday. The test subjects received 27–30 treatments each.

Using arterialized capillary blood we determined a number of parameters, before and after exercise stress, with respect to the acidosis that arises during exertion: blood lactate levels, pH, negative base excess (–BE), pCO_2, and current bicarbonate levels (AB); as well as a few oxygen status indicators: pO_2, alveolar- arterial pO_2 difference ($aADpO_2$, the difference between the oxygen partial pressures of alveolar air and of arterial blood), oxygen tension at 50% saturation ($p50$, indicating hemoglobin oxygen affinity), and the oxygen extraction tension of arterial blood (px). Additionally, we measured the physiological shunt fraction (% shunt), the mixed venous blood shunted to the arterial blood, at a constant, 2.3 mmol/l, arterial-venous oxygen concentration difference. In every case we determined blood sugar levels before and after exercise. (RADIOMÉTER 520 apparatus and DEEP PICTURE system were used to carry out blood gas analysis and oxygenation measurements) [7].

Heart rate was monitored continuously before, during and after the exercise test (using a POLAR tester) and anaerobic threshold was determined (Conconi) [4].

In our statistical calculations, we used the one-sample t-test, and baseline values for the variables were given as percentages. This process is justified partly by the large dispersion of values due to the diverging age classes of the test subjects, and partly because it helps the demonstration of the physiological characteristics of the variables.

Results

Figure 1 shows that the performance of both the treated and untreated groups improved during the observation period. The treated group attained a performance increase of 440 m, which, compared to baseline value, equals 15%; while the untreated group attained an increase of 166 m, which signifies a 5.4% improvement. Figure 1 also shows that the treated group's better performance was achieved with the anaerobic threshold speed increase of more than 1.5 km/h, showing a 9.5% improvement from baseline; whereas the untreated group attained an anaerobic threshold speed increase of less than 0.5 km/h, corresponding to a 0.4% improvement. The graph also shows that the treated group attained a greater performance increase with a far greater rise in lactic acid levels; in contrast to the untreated group's more modest performance, and smaller performance improvement.

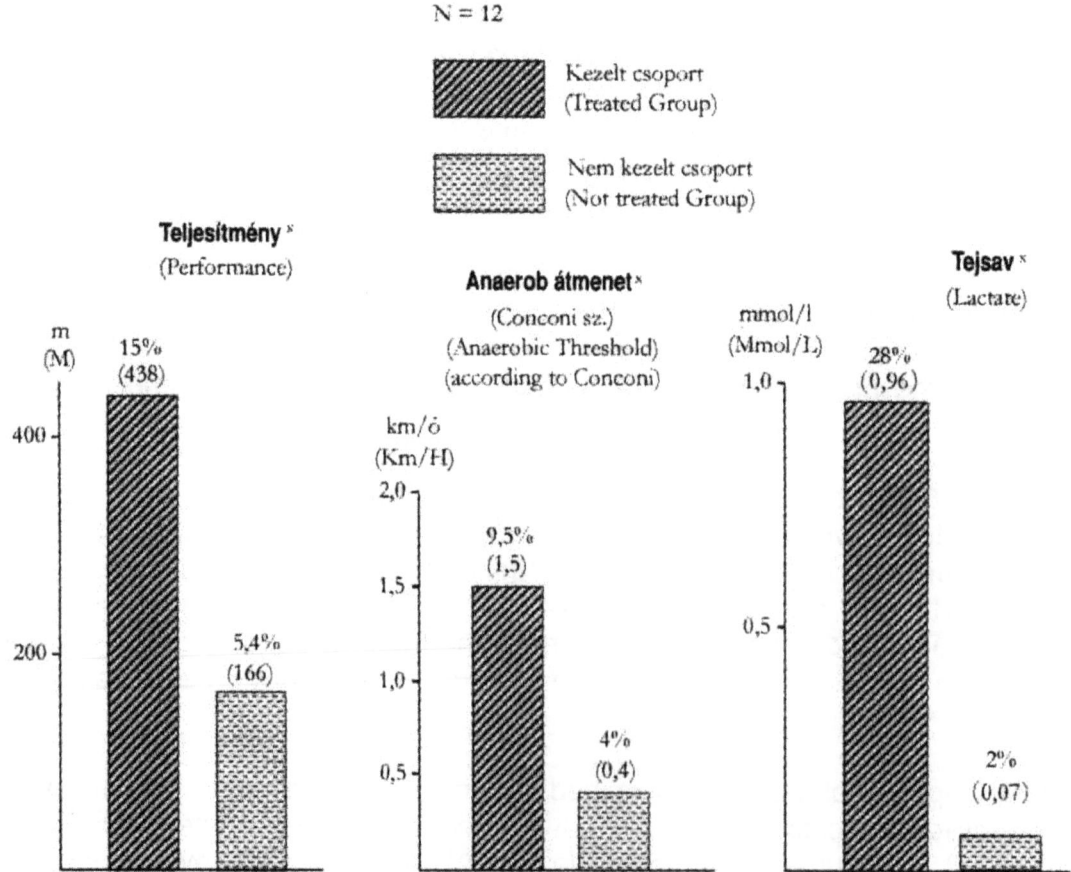

Figure 1.
Performance, anaerobic threshold and lactate changes in magnetic field treated and untreated groups. (x = change at 5% significance level)

Figure 2 shows that despite the higher lactate levels found in the treated group, the changes in pH values in both treated and untreated groups did not present any difference; however, the change in the treated group was smaller in comparison to baseline than in the untreated group (25% and 35% respectively). The larger AB and more modest pCO2 changes measured indicate that the higher amount of lactic acidosis generated was compensated more rapidly already during the exercise than in the untreated group. This statement is also proven by the smaller – BE decrease measured in the treated group. Furthermore, the blood sugar change shown in Figure 2 indicates that while in the treated group there was a 39% increase compared to baseline, in the untreated group a 16% decrease was observed.

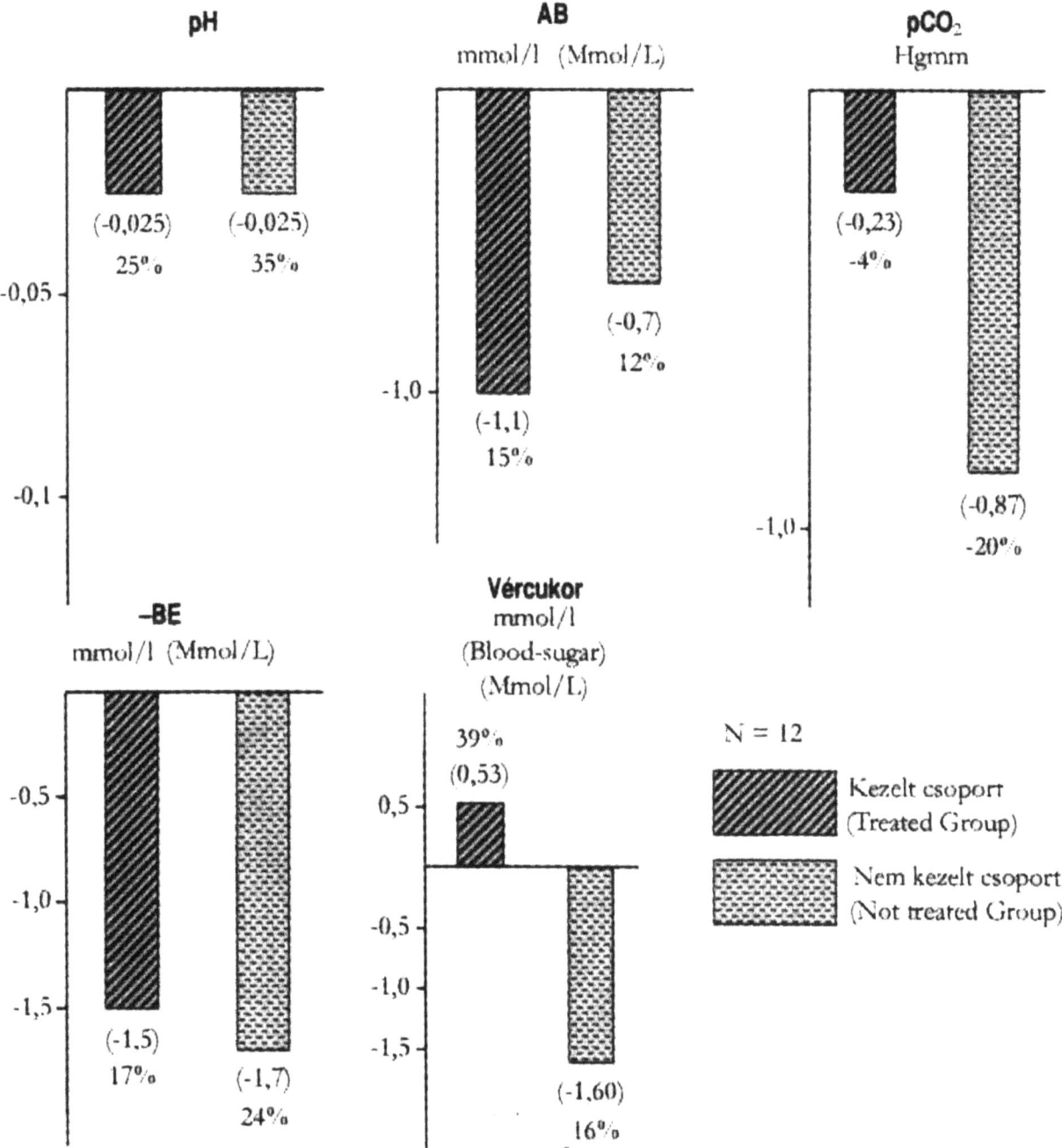

Figure 2. Changes in pH level, actual bicarbonate level (AB), CO2 partial pressure (pCO2), negative base excess and blood sugar level in magnetic field treated and untreated groups.

Figure 3 shows changes in oxygen status and selected oximetric data for the magnetic treatment's effect:
- The aADpO2 decreased in the treated group, while in the untreated group it rose, albeit to a very small degree
- The p50 also decreased in the treated group to a small degree, while in the untreated group it practically showed no change.
- The px value followed a similar trend. The physiological shunt fraction (shunt %) decreased in the treated group, while in the untreated group it practically showed no change.

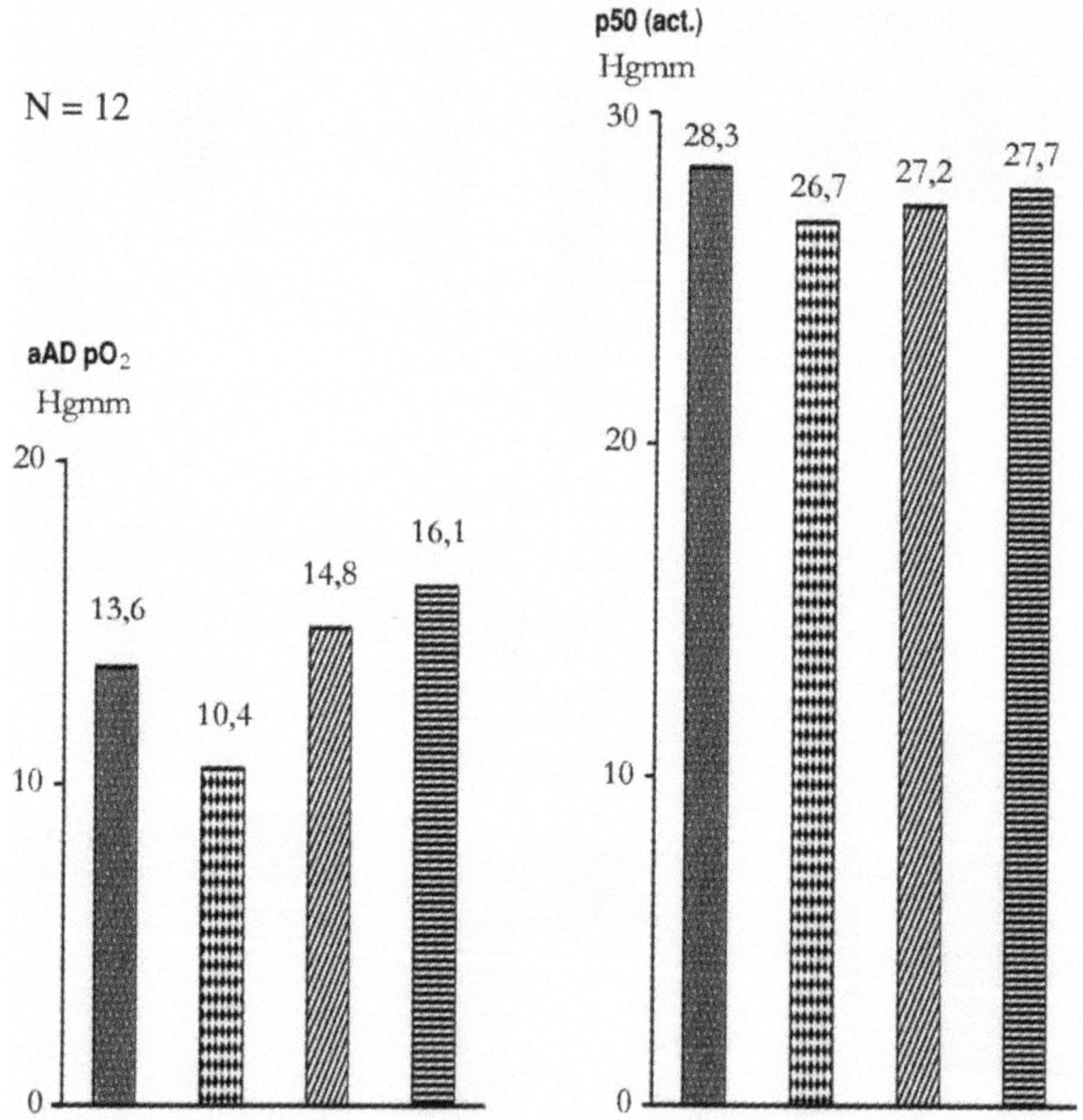

Figure 3. The effect of magnetic treatment on the pO2 difference between alveolar air and arterial blood (aADpO2), onpO2 at 50% saturation (p50), O2 extraction tension of arterial blood (px) and on the physiological shunt in treated and untreated groups.

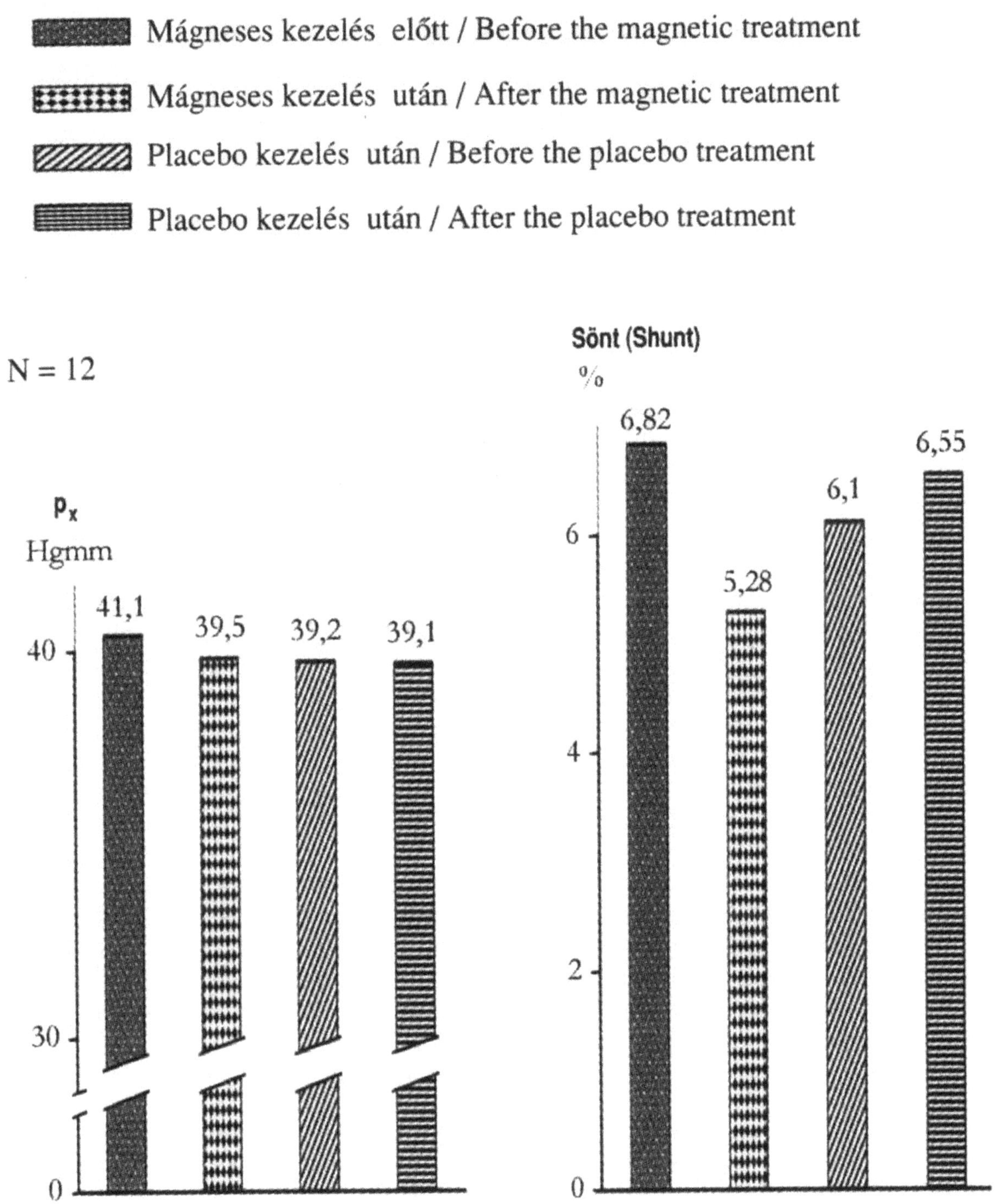

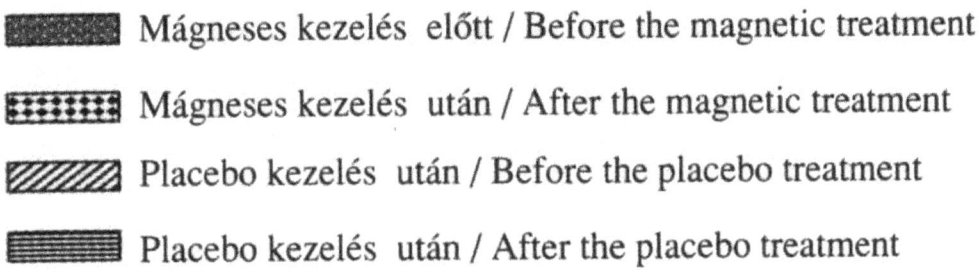

Figure 3 (cont.) The effect of magnetic treatment on the pO2 difference between alveolar air and arterial blood (aADpO2), on the pO2 in the blood at 50% saturation (p50), the O2 extraction tension of arterial blood (px) and the physiological shunt, in treated and untreated groups.

Discussion

On evaluation of the data, it can be established that the performance of athletes who received pulsed magnetic treatment improved to a greater degree during the routine fitness camp than it did in those who did not receive treatment. The treated athletes attained a greater improvement in performance with greater anaerobic, lactic acid exertion and with the formation of a more beneficial threshold of the sort described by Conconi. On evaluation of blood pH and blood gas data, it appears that the treated group could compensate more rapidly for the lactic acidosis arising from exertion, than the untreated group. The beneficial effects of pulsed magnetic treatment are well demonstrated by the tendency of the parameters that characterize oxygen status: decreased alveolar-arterial pO2 difference; hemoglobin-oxygen affinity, and decreased arterial blood oxygen extraction tension which may result in a decreased physiological shunt. These changes clearly point to the fact that athletes who received pulsed magnetic treatment had better tissue blood supply than those who did not receive treatment. In addition, the changes are in accordance with and can be explained by previous observations made in animal experiments. According to these, the change in the properties of red blood cell membranes under the effect of magnetic fields results in decreased red blood cell aggregation, which, consequently, results in increased active surface for oxygen transport. However, it should be noted that in animal experiments (and often in clinical application too) pulsed magnetic treatments, in most cases, use greater magnetic intensity and longer treatment duration than the treatments used by us (10.5–21.0 µT) [1][3][5][8].

The increase in performance capacity can be explained well by the magnetic treatment induced increase in microcapillarization and vasodilation, as well as by the acceleration of cell respiration, which many authors have reported primarily about tests on animals [2][8].

With respect to blood sugar levels, our results and other published reports are not in such close agreement. Many authors found that blood sugar levels decreased during magnetic treatment, while according to our own measurements, blood sugar levels rose during treatment, and we experienced a decrease only in the untreated group. Presumably the discrepancy can be attributed to more intensive magnetic field application as well as to the use of extended treatment time. In male guinea pigs, after treatment over many months with a large inductive magnetic field, it was possible to demonstrate Islets of Langerhans hypertrophy, increase in insulin levels and considerable drops in blood sugar levels. [8] Evaluating our own data, with regard to the effects of the magnetic field, it appears that hypothalamus-pituitary-adrenal system activity increased and this had beneficial effects on performance-physiology parameters and increased performance capacity.

These assumptions are in accordance with the experiences of other authors [8]. In their own animal experiments, they call attention to the system's exhaustibility: on the one hand—with structural changes in the adrenal glands, and increase in cortisol level; on the other—with increased pulsed magnetic field intensity and treatment duration and with decreased pituitary activity and adrenal steroidogenesis. It cannot be ruled out that the decreased blood sugar levels in the untreated athletes can be attributed to this; and that it was a sign of the athletes' fatigue.

Summary
In the course of the three-week training camp, the performance of the athletes who received pulsed magnetic field treatment improved to a greater extent than that of the untreated athletes. The treated group improved more, with greater lactic acidosis than the untreated group, developing a more favorable anaerobic threshold (Conconi) and also compensated acidosis faster. The performance-physiology parameters and improved performance in the treated group can be explained by the better oxygenation measured and decreased physiological shunt.

Comparing the effects of pulsed magnetic field treatment to data from other publications, it can be presumed that the basis for the favorable changes recorded are improved microcirculation and red blood cell hypercoagulability.

Acknowledgements

The authors are first and foremost grateful for the athletes who took part in the study for their cooperation and they would like to thank their parents for tolerating the additional troubles the tests may have caused.

Thanks are due to Dr Adam Gödry and Gábor Juhász, the directors of IDOM Sportclub, who ensured the completion of the series of tests, and also to trainers Levente Rácz and Gábor Punyi for conducting the training camp.

The authors thank Éva Dankó for carrying out the magnetic treatments, Mária Jeney for the assistance provided in obtaining literature data, and also Imre Szanyi for carrying out the blood gas analysis.

Finally, particular thanks are owed to Professor Dr Lajos Kullman, Chief Medical Director of the Hungarian National Medical Rehabilitation Institute (OORI), and also to Dr Lajos Ary, Chief Financial Officer at OORI, for allowing us to use the Radiometer 520 blood gas analyzer at their institute.

Bibliography

1. Barnothy M. F., Sumegi I.: Effects of the magnetic field on internal organ and the endocrine system of mice. In: Barnothy (Ed.) Biological effects of magnetic fields. Plenum Press, New York. 1969. Vol. 2.
2. BEMER-Terápia: Új tudományos eredmények. Innomed International AG. BEMER Medicintechnika Kft. Budapest 2006.
3. Blank M.: Biological effects of environmental electromagnetic fields: molecular mechanisms. 35, 175-178. 1995.
4. Bourgois J., Vrijens J.: The Conconi Test: A Controversial Concept for the Determination of the Anaerobic Threshold in Young Rowers. Int. J. Sport Med. 19. 553-559. 1998.
5. Diemiecki A. M.: Ekspierimientalnoje obosnowanije primienija isskustwiennych magnitnych polej w chirurgii. Vopr. Kurortol. Fizioter. Lech. Fiz Kult., 1 , 43-46. 1981.
6. Reiter R. J.: Static and extremely low frequency magnetic field exposure: reported effects on the circadian production of melatonin. J. Cell Biochem. 51,394-403. 1993.
7. RADIOMETER A/S, Dánia: A Vérgáz Analízis Kézikönyve. The DEEP PICTURE, 16-17. 1997.
8. Sieron A. és mtsai: Mágneses terek alkalmazása az orvostudományban. II. kiadás. Budapest, 2004.

Address:
Malomsoki Jenő
Országos Sportegészségügyi Intézet [National Institute of Sports Medicine] H-1123 Budapest, Alkotás utca 48.

The Use of BEMER Therapy in Sports Medicine
Lecture

Abstract for the Freudenstadt Consensus Conference 10.02.2010

Univ.-Prof. Dr. med. Klaus Jung, Sports Medicine, University of Mainz

SUMMARY: *Several primary studies have now demonstrated the accuracy of the theoretical conclusions and thereby have documented the extensive applications in sports medicine. It is now well-known that low-energy pulsed electromagnetic fields trigger many healing effects in the body. However, for a long time experts doubted that such effects could be so comprehensive and profound. The BEMER therapy was therefore viewed as an additional natural healing procedure, with good success in prevention, therapy and rehabilitation, as an additional preparation and follow-up therapy, as a means of supporting other therapeutic procedures and as a means of alleviating side effects.*

The foundational investigations by Klopp (1) were the first to demonstrate the physiological aspects with ubiquitous and universal application, such as the changes in distribution of the plasma/blood cell mixture in microvascular networks; the changes in perfusion at the node points, in vasomotion and in tone; the increased reticular production of white blood cells in persons exposed to infection and stress; the increase in venular outward flow; the local increase in NO concentration with actively extending effect on the vessel wall.

Four aspects in particular seem of primary interest for successful application in sports medicine:

- Improvement of oxygen supply
- Activation of the immune system
- Influence on protein synthesis
- Stabilization of the oxidative balance.

Several primary studies have now demonstrated the accuracy of the theoretical conclusions and thereby have documented the extensive applications in sports medicine.

Spodaryk (2) demonstrated the delayed initiation of muscular fatigue under load and with simultaneous BEMER 3000 local therapy with the intensive applicator in a placebo-controlled clinical double-blind study ($p< 0.05$). There was also a statistically significant fall in limitation on movement.

In a further clinical placebo-controlled double-blind study, Kafka and Spodaryk (3) pointed to the fact that the degree of effort experienced at the aerobic/anaerobic threshold, the primary point of exertion in endurance sport, was reduced to a statistically significant extent, despite increased performance, when BEMER 3000 was applied.

The working group led by Babindak (4) confirmed these results. In another placebo-controlled, double-blind study of tennis players, there was a greater increase in performance with regard to distance run (15 percent; 5.4% in the control group) and with regard to the running speed at the aerobic/anaerobic threshold (9.5%; control group 0.4%) when BEMER 3000 was applied simultaneously. The effects of such increase in performance despite a subjectively and objectively lower perception of exertion (lower exertion-related change in O2 status in the BEMER-treated test group) are readily explained by improved microcirculation and hypocoagulation of erythrocytes.

Möbes (5) similarly came to the unambiguous conclusion in his placebo-controlled double-blind study with 17 healthy athletes that the increase in CK values (the recognized parameter for muscular stress) was not as great and the fall in CK values began earlier under the influence of the BEMER 3000 electromagnetic field. This points to less muscle damage and accelerated regeneration, which can be explained by the modified (BEMER-induced) permeability of cell membranes.

Numerous athletes use BEMER 3000 and have reported good experiences. These responses similarly report accelerated regeneration (associated faster resumption of training after competitions and more and/or more intense training sessions are possible), optimum preparation for competitions thanks to energy-saving warming (partial replacement of warm-up with comparable effect), accelerated healing of sporting injuries and strains, as well as reduction in the risk of injury (statement by the German University Sports Federation).

Hence, a daily 8-20 minutes of regeneration on a BEMER mat was as much part of the daily program as warming up on the mat before a competition for many Swiss athletes in the 2004 Swiss Olympic Team in Athens – and with most success alongside massage and other special therapies. The relaxing effect and the accelerated healing of acute and chronic injuries and strains were also popular indications (Villiger) (6).

Claudia Pechstein (7), ice speed skating world champion and Olympic champion in 2002, has reported using the BEMER 3000 system for years, primarily for accelerated regeneration after training. She experiences a stabilization of her performance and immune system, as well as a reduced risk of injury and a significant reduction in fatigue symptoms. She believes BEMER 3000 has a meaningful place in sport.

In my own opinion (active long-distance runner, in particular with mountain running training sessions), I have experience significant benefits from using BEMER 3000 in the form of accelerated regeneration times, a reduction almost to zero of fatigue symptoms (such as muscle cramps), and I am almost free of colds over the winter as an indication of a stable and active immune system. I experience almost no deficit in energy, despite great physical exertion. I love to use BEMER 3000 as a preventative between rounds in the sauna and in situations where O2 utilization and O2 supply are high.

Literature:
1. Klopp, R.- Ch.: „Mikrozirkulation", Mediquant-Verlag, Triesen 2008
2. Spodaryk, K.: „The effect of extremely weak pulsed-electromagnetic field treatments upon signs and symptoms of delayed onset of muscle soreness; a placebo controlled clinical double blind study", Medicina Sportiva Vol. 6: E 19 – E 25, 2002
3. Kafka, W. A., Spodaryk, K.: "The influence of extremely weak, Bemer 3000 type pulsed, electromagnetic fields on ratings of perceived exertion (RPE) at ventilatory threshold", Kafka-Spodaryk-Ratings-Exertion abstract.doc, o.J.
4. Malomsoki, J., Babindak, E.: "The effect of magnetic treatment on the physical fitness and certain exercise-physiological parameters of athletes", Hungarian Review of Sports Medicine 47/2 – 3/2006
5. Möbes k (2003); Verkürzung der Regenerationszeit im Spitzensport anhand der Veränderung der CK – Eliminationskurve durch Einsatz der BEMER 3000 – Therapie nach Prof. Dr. W.A.Kafka. Diplom arbeit im rahmen des dtlg 1 elite 02/03, ehsm magglingen(ch)
6. Villiger, B.: Bundeswehr- Sportmagazin 6,2 (2002)
7. Pechstein, C.: Bundeswehr- Sportmagazin 6,2 (2002)

The use of Bio-Electro-Magnetic-Energy-Regulation (BEMER) in Sports Competitions: Swimming, Triathlon, Marathon, Football and Light Athletics.
Lecture at the 2nd BEMER World Congress in Bad Windsheim 2001

Armin Dirschauer; Lecturer in Sports Physiotherapy, German Sport University, Cologne, Germany

SUMMARY: *A significant reduction in sport-specific fatigue complaints in athletes was identified at sports events after using BEMER 3000 systems.*

Swimming: German Open Swimming Championships 2000 (Berlin), German Championship in the Dortmund-Ems Canal (Münster), 24 Hour Swim 2000 (Braunschweig).

Individual athletes of both genders from GVO Oldenburg receive sports physiotherapy after warming up (running, stretching and swimming) and after competitions and games. They then lay on the electromagnetic (BEMER 3000) field for a further 20 minutes to recover and regenerate muscle and fibrous tissue in joints.

Subjectively, the subjects reports tingling, warmth and relaxation (no sense of weight, but almost a sense of floating). Objectively, the "tingling" (range of sensitivity) was localized solely in the sport-specific areas of exertion. The tone regulation of the muscles was checked before and after the application by palpation (= physical investigation with one or more fingers, including with both hands) of the body surface and accessible body cavities to determine consistency, elasticity, flexibility, sensitivity to pain etc. and muscle function. In general, tone regulation was confirmed.

Compared to the previous year (1999), there was a significant reduction in sport-specific fatigue symptoms in athletes at the same sport events.

Use of BEMER Therapy in Musculoskeletal Sports Injuries for Regeneration and in the Post-Operative Phase

Dr. med. L. Weisskopf, Racetrack Clinic [Rennbahnklinik], Basel, Switzerland

Abstract for the BEMER Symposium at the Freudenstadt ZAEN Congress 04.01.2011

SUMMARY: As Olympic physician for Vancouver 2010, I can strongly recommend electromagnetic field therapy as a safe, extremely beneficial, complementary therapy for acute musculoskeletal injuries, in particular for bruises, muscle tendon injuries and bone fractures. The therapy also provides chondroprotection and improved bone metabolism, which is beneficial when treating arthrosis. The BEMER therapy's promotion of wound healing should also be highlighted once again.

The Muttenz Racetrack Practice [Praxisklinik Rennbahn Muttenz, Switzerland] has relied on the supporting effect of electromagnetic field therapy for many years, primarily for musculoskeletal injuries and for regeneration in athletes, in particular after operations.

As specialist clinic for hamstring pathologies, we apply the BEMER magnetic field mat in particular as part of the post-operative protocol to reduce anticipated disruptions to wound healing in this poorly supplied areal. Reduction has demonstrably been achieved. Similarly, swelling reduces more quickly and patients generally recover more quickly after, in some cases, complex hamstring reconstruction. The scientifically demonstrated effect, which promotes wound healing (Steven et al. 2008) and circulation, is therefore regularly and successfully applied in everyday practice for the benefit of the patient.

In addition, the doctors at the practice also use the electromagnetic field therapy to treat and care for top athletes and national teams as a therapy for very frequent bruises as well as bone and cartilage injuries. The effects in these cases are also astonishing, with extremely good healing rates and reduced tendency for complications to occur. Thanks to close cooperation with BEMER, the handball national team was also equipped with BEMER mats and acceptance among the athletes was enormous thanks to the faster regeneration time.

Over what is so far a relatively short period of observation, the number of fatigue symptoms/injuries has also been reduced by electromagnetic field therapy. A more accurate analysis of a longer period is planned and will give a better indication of any general prevention of injuries as a result of faster tissue recovery and improved blood flow.

As Olympic physician for Vancouver 2010, I can strongly recommend electromagnetic field therapy as a safe, extremely beneficial, complementary therapy for acute musculoskeletal injuries, in particular for bruises, muscle tendon injuries and bone fractures. It should also be mentioned that there is good evidence in the scientific literature for the therapy as a supporting treatment in arthrosis (Ganesan K et al. 2009), in particular to improve the level of pain and to inhibit inflammation. The therapy also provides chondroprotection and improved bone metabolism, which is beneficial when treating arthrosis. The BEMER therapy's promotion of wound healing should also be highlighted once again: In our opinion, there is great potential for significantly reducing post-operative rates of complication with disruption of wound healing and general subsequent infections.

The Effect of Extremely Weak Pulsed Electromagnetic Field Treatments on Signs and Symptoms of Delayed Onset of Muscle Soreness; a Placebo-Controlled Clinical Double-Blind Study

Krzysztof Spodaryk

Jagiellonian University and Academy of Physical Education, Krakow, Poland

ABSTRACT

The effect of pulsed weak electromagnetic fields on experimentally induced delayed onset of muscle soreness (DOMS) was assessed in a placebo-controlled clinical double-blind study. DOMS was induced in 36 volunteers and the elbow flexors of the non-dominant arm were used for a standardized eccentric exercise regime. Subjects were randomly allocated to one of the three groups: control (C, n=12), sham-treated (S-T, n=12) and treated with a special kind of pulsed electromagnetic fields (T, n=12) by applying the BEMER 3000 local therapy intensive applicator. Volunteers from group T were electromagnetically stimulated each day with a magnetic field of 86 mT. Subjects from the sham-treated group were treated by deactivated BEMER 3000 systems. One-way analysis of variance (ANOVA) demonstrated significant effects of electromagnetic field treatment on retarding pain intensity as measured by visual analogue scale (VAS) ($p<0.05$). According to standard methods of goniometrical measurements statistically significant differences in the range of movement between the control-, sham-treated- and electromagnetic treated groups were further found on the second day of the experiments. Within the conditions of the current experiments the pulsed electromagnetic (BEMER 3000) field treatment exerts clear-cut and favorable effects upon the cardinal signs and symptoms of DOMS.

The poor standard of research design and analysis in many studies concerning the efficacy of electromagnetic therapy systems published to date precludes any definitive conclusions regarding its efficacy. It could even be argued that many of these reports rather serve to fuel the controversy surrounding electromagnetic field therapy. Distinguished by its scientifically and technically well designed concept of research, however, therapies applying the extremely weak BEMER 3000 type pulsed electromagnetic fields (8, 9, 10), gain exceptionally increasing clinical acceptance, especially for the alleviation of pain of various etiologies, inflammation, sweating, and other pathologies of soft tissues. The analgesic effects of physical modalities using delayed onset of muscle soreness (DOMS) as a model of clinical myogenic pain treatment have been assessed by a number of researchers but experimental conditions varied significantly concerning the induction of muscle pain (1, 3). Many of the reports furthermore do not fulfill the accepted minimum requirements for adequate experimental design of clinical research studies, such as placebo conditions, blinding procedures, crossover designs, etc. Despite controversy surrounding its pathophysiology, the development of a standardized DOMS-induction protocol could thus convey to a useful laboratory model for the investigation of musculoskeletal pain.

DOMS typically occurs in untrained subjects particularly after eccentric exer-cise. Under these circumstances pain is delayed, occurring between 6 and 12 h post exercise, peaking at between 48 and 72 h and persisting for up to 7 days after exercise (1). Although the underlying pathophysiology remains a matter of debate, its progression and multifaceted presentation reveals DOMS as a useful laboratory model for assessing the efficacy of different modalities applied for the relief of musculoskeletal pain and the associated dysfunction.

In view of the above, a randomized, double blind, placebo-controlled study was performed both to assess the putative efficacy of experimentally induced myogenic pain and dysfunction of movement to investigate the beneficial (pain relieving) effects of one of the few modalities used in physiotherapy by applying the well designed (Fig. 1) extremely low pulsed weak electromagnetic fields (BEMER 3000) mentioned above.

Materials and Methods
Experimental conditions and screening procedure

Subjects for the trial experiments consisting of 36 healthy male student volunteers, aged 18-22 years, were requested to attend the experiments on seven subsequent days. They were randomly allocated to one of the following groups under blind test conditions: Control group (C) - subjects allocated in this group rested supine for a period of 20 min. Sham-treated group (S- T) - subjects in this group received pseudo- treatment of electromagnetic field (equipment was deactivated).

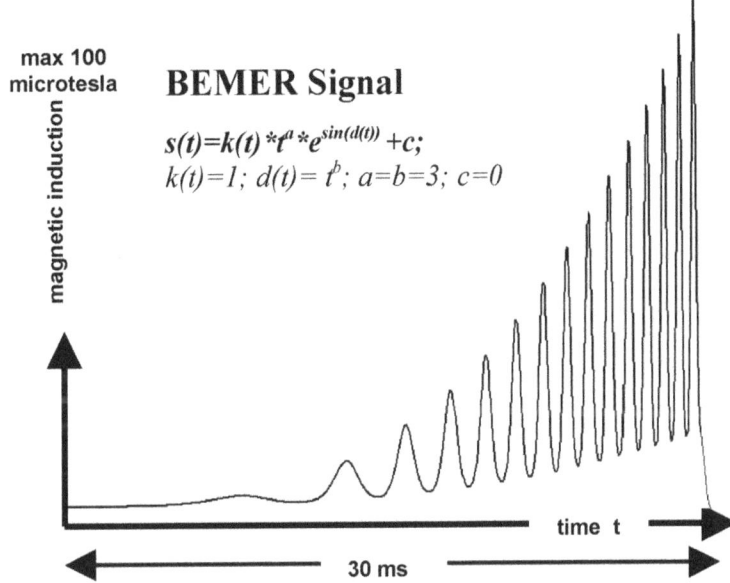

True treated by electromagnetic field group (T) - subjects in this group received 86 mT on the elbow. All subjects were screened for current injury or pain, ingestion of any form of drugs, any hematological diseases, diabetes, asthma, weight-training, and participation in a similar experiments within the past year. All were instructed to avoid any form of exercise for the duration of the study. Subjects were requested to attend the tests for a full working week on consecutive days (Monday-Friday, i.e. 5 days in total).

Tenderness

Once the screening procedure was completed, mechanical-pain threshold (MPT) measurements were performed over the biceps brachii muscle of the non-dominant arm as a correlate of tenderness as described by Barlas et al. (2). The measurements were accordingly performed on eight equidistant points on the flexor of the subjects' brachius, each marked with semi-permanent ink. These points were standardized by first identifying the intersection of the biceps brachii on the radius and marking this as the first point. The next seven points were then marked at 3 cm intervals proximal to the first one on a line joining the insertion of the biceps brachii (on the radius) and the acromion. Pressure was applied through the spherical ending (1 cm diameter) of a pressure algometer (Electronic Force Gauge, Salter, West Bromwich, UK) with increasing force for periods of 1 to 10 s, until either the subject reported the sensation to be painful, or the exerted pressure reached 40 N (used as a cut off value to avoid bruising).

Range of movement

After assessment of MPT, ranges of movement (ROM) were measured using a standard universal goniometer. For this, two anatomical points were marked with a semipermanent ink as reference points: the styloid process of the radius and a point corresponding to the greater tuberosity of the humerus. A total number of three measurements were taken, all in the erect position: elbow flexion (FANG), elbow extension (EANG), and elbow relaxed angle (RANG) according to standardized procedures used in rehabilitation (3).

Induction procedure DOMS was induced in the non-dominant arm using a dumb-bell and free weights. For the DOMS induction procedure, the subject sat on a custom-made apparatus (Preacher's bench), and the greatest amount of weight that the subject could lift concentrically on a single occasion was determined (i.e. one experimenter lifted the pre-determined weight to the point of FANG, and the subject was instructed to lower the weights as slowly as possible). This continued until the subject was no longer able to lower the weights under control. A 30 s rest interval was then allowed and the procedure repeated twice more (with further intervening 30 s rest periods), to ensure exhaustion of the elbow flexors. Pain measurement After completing the DOMS induction procedure, the subjects rated their current level of pain on a computerized visual analog scale (VAS). Briefly, a customized program was used, whereby VAS could be displayed on a computer monitor at 30 s intervals. A line anchored with "No pain" and "Maximum pain" at either end appeared on the screen in random orientation. With the help of a mouse control, subjects were able to move a marker along the scale and, using the integral switch of the mouse, mark a point to indicate their current level of pain. The distances of the marker along the scale, representing individual current-pain intensity scales, were stored automatically as percentages of the total length of the line. VAS scores were obtained for all subjects for each attendance: the mean values of four pre-treatment and four post-treatment (respectively) scores were used as the basis of analysis.
Statistical analysis

All results are expressed as the mean ±SEM of individual observations. Statistical analysis was performed with one ANOVA factor. The statistical significance level was accepted at 95%. For the purposes of statistical analysis, all data were standardized (for each subject) as differences from the individual baseline by subtracting the values of the pre-induction measurements from those obtained during subsequent attendances.

Results

Mechanical pain threshold (MPT) Figure 2 shows an increase in tenderness or sensitivity in all groups as a result of the induction procedure. There are consistent patterns of differences between groups. Analysis of these data using repeated ANOVA measures showed a significant change in MPT over the 5 days of the experiment, reflecting the effects of the induction procedure. The reduced values of MPT represent an increase in tenderness or worsening of the condition. The mean values of all eight points spanning the length of the biceps brachii were calculated in order to monitor the effects of treatment along the whole muscle. Figure 2 shows an increase in tenderness in all groups as a result of the induction procedure, as well as a partial recovery on the final day of the experiment. Significant ($p<0.05$) differences (effects) between the groups S-T vs. T and C vs. T were found from the 3rd onwards.

Visual analogue scale (VAS)

The graphs in Figure 3 represent the values of the mean pain intensity pre-treatments on any day in reference to those which were calculated on day one as a baseline. ANOVA analysis revealed a significant difference in the VAS values over the experimental period and a significant interactive effect, indicating significant differences between the test groups over time. Further analysis of VAS difference values using one-factor ANOVA (with relevant Fisher tests) revealed isolated significant differences (pre-treatment) on the second day between the control group and other experimental groups (S-T placebo and T treatment group).

Range of movement (ROM)

The values deriving from the measurement of the range of movement reveal a clearcut effect of DOMS induction upon ROM during the 5 days of testing and render a significant statistical difference between the relevant groups. ANOVA revealed not only a significant effect over time but also showed well separated differences between the individual test groups. Increasing EANG values reflect the inability of subjects to fully extend the arm. Decreases in FANG represent loss of flexion owing to swelling, and increased RANG reflects lack of extension, thus resulting in the conclusion that the ranges of movement of subjects treated by the pulsed electro- magnetic (BEMER 3000) fields were already enhanced at the second day of the experiment (Fig. 4).

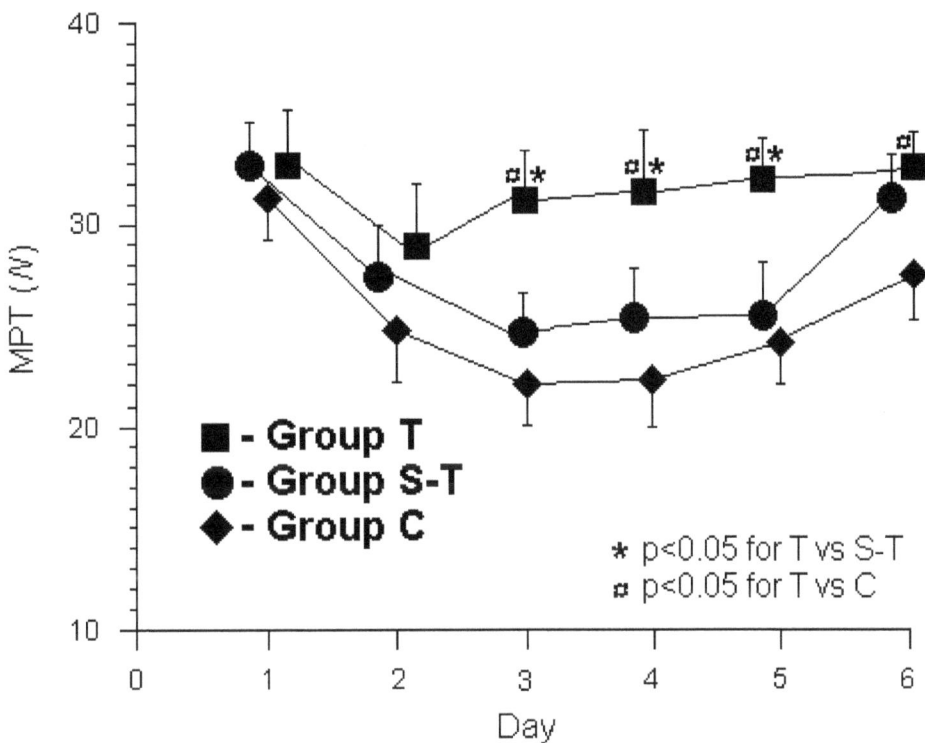

Fig. 2. *Mechanical pain threshold (MPT) as mean values for all eight points on the biceps brachii muscle. Decreasing values represent a decrease in MPT and thus an increase in tenderness or worsening of the condition.*

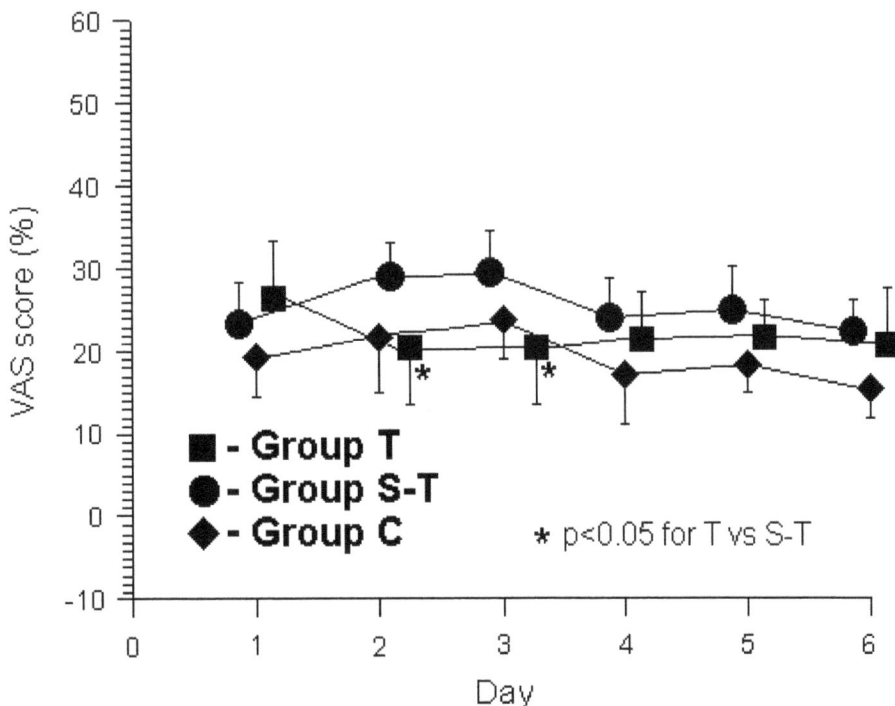

Fig. 3. *Visual analogue scale scores (VAS) as the mean pain intensity pre-treatment on any day (%; mean ± SEM)*

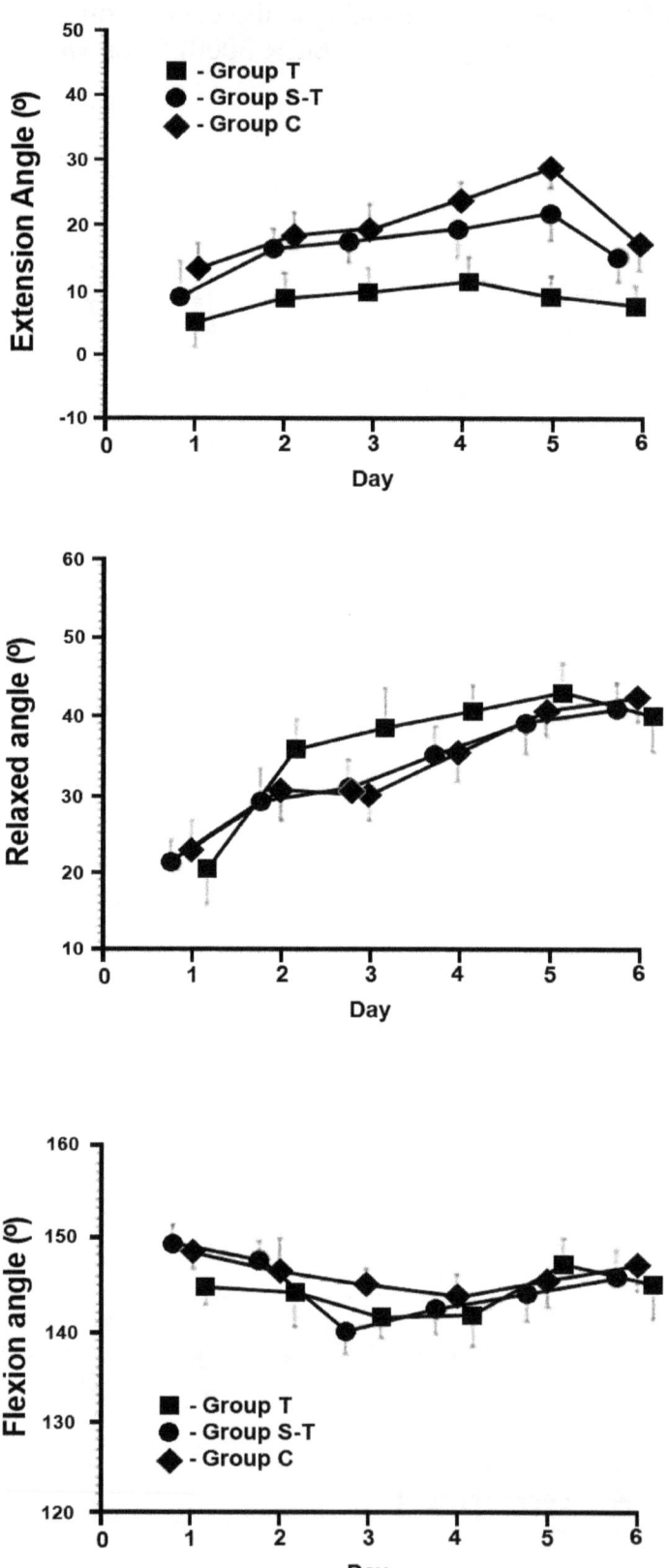

Fig. 4. *The ranges of movement scores (degrees; mean ± SEM) pre-treatment on any day. (Upper graph: mean values for EANG, middle graph mean values for FANG and lower graph mean values for RANG). Increasing EANG values reflect the inability of the subjects to fully extend their arm; decreasing FANG values represent loss of flexion due to swelling; increasing RANG values reflect a lack of extension at rest. The statistical significant differences between the groups are not shown.*

Range of movement (ROM)

The values deriving from the measurement of the range of movement reveal a clearcut effect of DOMS induction upon ROM during the 5 days of testing and render a significant statistical difference between the relevant groups. ANOVA revealed not only a significant effect over time but also showed well separated differences between the individual test groups. Increasing EANG values reflect the inability of subjects to fully extend the arm. Decreases in FANG represent loss of flexion owing to swelling, and increased RANG reflects lack of extension, thus resulting in the conclusion that the ranges of movement of subjects treated by the pulsed electro- magnetic (BEMER 3000) fields were already enhanced at the second day of the experiment (Fig. 4).

Discussion

The aim of this study was to investigate the effects of the BEMER 3000-type electromagnetic field upon experimentally induced muscle pain and motor dysfunction (the standardized DOMS-induction protocol) under randomized, double- blind, placebo-controlled conditions. Measurements of the elbow range of movement (flexion, extension, relaxed angle), and pain as well as visual analogue scores (VAS), and tenderness (using a pressure algometer) were employed to indicate the treatments'effectiveness. Measurements of the elbow range of movement and tenderness were made prior to DOMS induction on the first day, and repeated post- treatment on subsequent days. Pain intensity was assessed using visual analogue scales post-induction and post-treatment each day of the whole treatment. The results indicate a clearcut beneficial effect induced by the applied physical modality of the BEMER 3000-type electromagnetic stimulation.

Significant differences of pain levels were furthermore found between the intergroups (C vs. T and S-T vs. T). Non significant differences were observed between the control and sham-treated group. The intergroup difference in VAS scores were found on the second day of the experiments. Some authors have assessed the assumed analgesic effects of physical modalities using DOMS as a model of myogenic pain. However, results and conclusions are often conflicting. The benefit of physical modalities such as transcutaneous electrical nerve stimulation and ultrasound were reported by Denegar et al. (5) and Hasson et al. (7) but others have failed to demonstrate any such effects (4, 11). Too small numbers of test persons and the lack of control and sham-treated groups cause both reasons for such discrepancies. In the case of this study, care was taken to address these issues to ensure the validity of the findings. The comparison of existing studies regarding electromagnetic field as an analgesic modality is confounded by the wide variety of induction measurements and doses used, but, in common with previous research in this area of physiotherapy (electromagnetic field therapy), precludes replication on account of the lack of detailed description of the experimental setup and procedures. The presented clinical methods of experiments of this paper, however, were based on the rules of Good Clinical Practice and design according to Barlas et al. (2).

Significant differences in the range of movement were found between the intergroups (S-T vs. T and C vs. T). The ANOVA showed a significant effect over time and significant differences were detected between the groups in all of the ROM measurements. The beneficial effect of the BEMER 3000-type electromagnetic field on ranges of joint movement can be explained by the retarded pain intensity during the periods of exposition on this therapeutic modality. The implication of muscle receptors can be the proposed mechanisms of action of this modality. On the other hand, in accordance with the findings of incre ased rate of synthesized ATP in red blood cells (12) changes in metabolism in skeletal muscle tissue must be taken into consideration as well. BEMER 3000 stimulation might also be effective in activating endogenous-opioid systems as it exists for example in acupuncture (6) but this hypothesis requires further exploration.

References

1. Armstrong R.B. Mechanisms of exercise-induced delayed onset muscle soreness: a brief review. Med. Sci. Sports Exerc. 16: 529-538, 1984
2. Barlas P., Robinson J. et al. Lack of effect of acupuncture upon signs and symptoms of delayed onset muscle soreness. Clin. Physiol. 6: 449-456, 2000
3. Clarkson H.M., Gilewich J.B. Musculoskeletal Assessment Joint Range of Movement and Manual Muscle Strength. Williams & Wilkins, Baltimore, 1989
4. Craig J.A., Cunningham M.B., Walsh D.M., Baxter G. Lack of effect of transcutaneous electrical nerve stimulation upon experimentally induced delayed onset muscle soreness in humans. Pain 67: 285-289, 1996
5. Denegar R.C., Penin D.H., Rogol A. Influence of transcutaneous electrical nerve stimulation on pain, range of motion and serum cortisol concentration in females experiencing delayed onset muscle soreness. J. Orthop. Sports Phys. Ther. 11: 100-103, 1989
6. Han J.S., Wang Q. Mobilisation of specific neuropeptides by peripheral stimulation of identified frequencies. News Physiol. Sci. 7: 176-180, 1992
7. Hasson S., Mundorf R., Bames W. et al. Williams J. Effect of pulsed ultrasound versus placebo on muscle soreness perception and muscular performance. Scand. J. Rehabil. Med. 22: 199-205, 1990
8. Kafka W.A. Device applying electric or electromagnetic signals for promoting biological processes. Europäische Patentanmeldung 98119944.1 v 21.10.98, 1998
9. Kafka W.A. Reference Database: Biological effects of electromagnetic fields. Emphyspace 1: 1-10, 1999
10. Kafka W.A. Extremely low, wide frequency range pulsed electromagnetic fields for therapeutical use. Emphyspace 2: 1-20, 2000
11. Nussbaum E.L., Gabison S. Rebox effect on exercise-induced acute inflammation in human muscle. Arch. Phys. Med. Rehabil. 79:1258-1263, 1998
12. Spodaryk K. Red Blood Metabolism and Haemoglobin Oxygen Affinity: Effect of Electromagnetic Fields on Healthy Adults. Emphyspace 3:15-19, 2001
13.

Received: December 10, 2001 Accepted: February 1, 2002

Address for correspondence: Prof. Dr. hab. med. K. Spodaryk Academy of Physical Education Al. Jana Pawla II 7831 571 Krakow, Polandirspodar@skok.awf.krakow.pl

BEMER Therapy Applied to Dentistry

Objectives of BEMER Therapy in Current Dentistry
Presentation of concomitant therapeutic uses

Zehner P; DHZ (3)1-3, 2007

SUMMARY: The Bio-Electro-Magnetic-Energy-Regulation (BEMER) system from the Liechtenstein-based manufacturer, Innomed Int. AG, was used as concomitant therapy to improve blood flow characteristics against a background of painful symptoms caused by odontogenic disease in 35 patients with 39 cases of disease in a 13-month trial. The positive outcome in the form of clinically demonstrated, faster alleviation of pain confirms the claim by the study performed by the Institute for Microcirculation in Berlin.

BEMER Type Pulsed Low-Energy Electromagnetic Fields Reduce Dental Anxiety – A Placebo-Controlled, Randomized Double-Blind Study

Michels-Wakili S; Kafka W; 10th International Dental Congress on Modern Pain Control; Edinburgh; 2003

SUMMARY: Blood pressure, heart rate and anxiety in patients are significantly reduced by an 8-minute application of the BEMER 3000 intensive applicator over the area of the solar plexus in a dentist waiting room.

BEMER Therapy Applied to Veterinary Medicine

Using BEMER Therapy in Some Domains of Veterinary Medicine

Dr. Mezősi László Veterinarian

I have been using the BEMER 3000 Vet device for more than 4 years. This is a classic first generation device. The vast majority of the animals treated (in total 117) were dogs (91). The rest were cats, horses and 3 other animals. Although this number of cases cannot be compared with the rehabilitation department of a hospital using this method, it allows for a statistical evaluation of the procedure. Based on this, it can be unequivocally stated that the BEMER therapy (as a procedure free of adverse effects) can be successfully used in veterinary medicine. At this Conference I want to talk not about the most common indication (late posterior weakness in dogs which usually occurs at an advanced age), but about a condition that is very rare and is a curiosity because of the species it affects or the form of the diseases.

Siberian chipmunk (Boeroendoek) – posterior paralysis
Siberian chipmunks are becoming increasingly popular among pet owners because they can be kept in apartments. A 3 years old female was brought to the practice because she had 6 puppies and suddenly she was unable to use her hind legs. The owner is an experienced breeder, so the animal was provide everything she needed. Her rearing conditions were very professional, as well. The animal was extremely agile and corky so it was impossible to perform a thorough examination. These animals are highly sensitive to stress.

We decided against performing the examination with the animal put to sleep.

Based on experiences in other animals, I administered BEMER therapy for 12 minutes at intensity level 2. After the third session she drew her legs beneath her and started to walk a little.

I treated the animal 5 times in total when her control over her limbs normalized, the only change being that she was a bit slower than before.

Berni, the watch-dog with elbow bursitis
A three-month old puppy was brought by the owner because of the inflammation of the bursa of the elbow.

This is a relatively rare condition usually caused by a mechanical impact (mainly a blow) on the elbow. As a result there is a fluid accumulation in the enlarged sac of the bursa which can lead to swelling to the size of an egg. The enlarged bursa is not painful and is only an esthetic problem.

Surgical removal of the bursa is recommended.

Reading the materials of previous BEMER Conferences, I found the lecture of dr. Babindák Elvira on sport medicine, in which she reported the successful use of the BEMER therapy in athletes for olecranon bursitis.

The owner of the dog consented to the treatment. I started the treatment using an intensive applicator; however, after a couple of days, the bursa on the other side became inflamed, as well. Subsequently, I used the pillow so as to administer the therapy to both sides at the same time. In addition to this treatment, I have drained the bursa and injected Aloe First or dexamethasone on several occasions. After drainage, I tried to apply a flexible bandage on the elbow, but the distal limb swelled every time and the bandage had to be removed.

The owner had the possibility to treat the dog at home for 2x1 weeks for 3x20 minutes at intensity level 2. After all, the success rate was 50% since the first bursitis completely disappeared, but the second one remained. As a matter of fact, I did not succeed to determine why the other side did not heal after the same therapy was administered. But I think it is success that the problem was solved with a single surgery instead of two.

German Shepherd – bilateral masseter muscle atrophy, mouth disorder
Both masseters of a 2.5 years old dog were completely atrophied. The animal was able to eat, but his or her appetite was decreased and was unable to open his or her mouth to take his ball.

The history showed that a tick was found on the animal so it was supposed that these symptoms indicative of head nerve injury might be caused by Lyme disease. The positive serology test confirmed this hypothesis.

At the beginning, the dog was very agitated, but as the treatment progressed the animal became calmer and his/her mood was improved, as well.

In total, the treatment was administered 6 times for 20 minutes.

After the treatment, the animal's appetite and mood was good. The function of the mouth fully normalized and now the dog can continue his/her passionate ball game.

I believe that in all three cases the cause was the Lyme disease based on the fact that the head nerves were affected. In one case the big masseter muscles of a 1 year old Hovawart dog atrophied one after the other. Although the animal was able to eat, but his or her appetite was decreased. After the administration of the BEMER therapy, the animal's appetite was normalized and was able to fully open his/her mouth.

In two other cases (a 6 years old Belgian Shepherd and a 14 years old hybrid dog) salivation and the interesting movement of the tongue was observed. The eating and drinking functions were not perfect. The Lyme test was negative for the older hybrid dog, while this test was not performed for the other two dogs. After the BEMER therapy, the mouth function and appetite of all three animals were normalized.

Five year old rabbit – posterior paralysis
According to the owner, the rabbit has not used properly his/her posterior part of the body and finally the animal was completely paralyzed. When the animal was examined no pain sensation was observed in the hind legs. The X-ray confirmed spondylosis of the lumbar and thoracic spine.

The owner brought the pet twice a day for three consecutive days for treatment sessions of 20 minutes at intensity level 2.

After the third day, the leg of the animal regained pain perception. The animal almost jumped out from the box and his/her movement was reestablished. The human aspect in this story is remarkable because the owner brought the rabbit from a village near Győr and spent several days in Budapest for the animal. There was no other veterinary practice closer to the owner's residence that provides the BEMER therapy.

Comparative Clinical Chemical Studies Demonstrate the Reduction of Bovine Herd Fertility Problems Thanks to Special (BEMER 3000 Typical) Low-Intensity Pulsed Electromagnetic Fields

Preissinger M; Kafka W; Austrian Society of Veterinarians, German Veterinary Medical Society (ÖGT-DVG) Congress; Fertility and Neonatology 2001

Maximilian Preißinger* And Wolf A. Kafka**
* Veterinary practice, Keltenstr. 17, D-86825 Schlingen, Germany
** EMPHYSPACE, Johannishöhe 9, D-82288 Kottgeisering, Germany wolf.kafkas@t- online.de

SUMMARY: *Electromagnetic BEMER stimulation clearly activates metabolism in the liver. In particular, preventative treatment of cows in the first 6 weeks post partum creates the best conditions for a subsequent pregnancy. As positive side effect, there is also a liver cell stabilization effect in cases of sub- clinical ketosis in high-performance cows. Comparative quantitative clinical chemical analyses indicate the reduction of bovine fertility problems due to stimulation with extremely weak, BEMER 3000 type, pulsed electromagnetic fields.*

Introduction and Statement of Issue

Supported by the physical properties of electromagnetic fields, the effect of electromagnetic field therapy can be explained by the physical and chemical activation stimulated by the direct or indirect energetic impact on atomic or molecular electron shells (I). Owing to the varying molecular masses of the relevant charge carriers, their structure and their interactions, the latter primarily as a result of their inertia in response to mechanical acceleration, the temporal intensity curve of the active fields plays a decisive role in this case. They spectral breadth and intensity establish the conditions for potential energetic activations and thereby also determine the sequence of physical and chemical interactions. The potential effects of the typically narrow-band sinusoidal, trapezoidal or sawtooth-shaped stimulation signals commonly used in traditional therapy devices are limited to relatively small ranges of molecular masses and are therefore severely limited in effect. Their application relies on more or less empirically determined frequency adjustments that are typically not sufficiently supported by experiments. Only once a special signal shape (2) characterized by a particular high bandwidth is developed and realized technically in the BEMER 3000 can this problem by principally considered solved (studies, therapeutic interventions and database (3-13)).

Thanks to its high number of different frequency components, the BEMER (BEMER = Bio-Electro-Magnetic-Energy-Regulation) 3000 system can reactivate a broad band of potentially disrupted chemical mechanisms, which are typically the point of origin of metabolism-related and, therefore, health-related impairments.

On the basis of these terms of reference, we planned to evaluate quantitatively to what extent the BEMER 3000 therapy system also gives rise to significant and, in particular, positive effects in the herd treatment of bovine fertility disorders via comparative clinical chemical analyses, initially on a small scale, but under strict compliance with a stringent experimental test protocol, taking the phases of recurrent pregnancy as our example – first to second week post partum (p.p.) until renewed pregnancy, i.e. in a period of four weeks. Detailed therapeutic analysis was therefore not the main focus of interest.

Materials and methods Experimental animals and holding

The experimental animals were 14 high-performance cows (Holstein-Friesian, annual performances of up to 11846 kg of milk) from an agricultural holding in Schlingert, Unterallgäu, Germany. Of these, 7 animals were treated with the BEMER 3000 therapy device over a period of 4 weeks at intervals of 2 days. The remaining 7 animals were left untreated and used as control group (control). The BVD/MD-vaccinated holding had additional problems in the previous 2 years with genital catarrh.

Feed
With reference in each case to 650 kg live weight, basic feed of 2,700 kg hay/cobs, 1,000 kg aftergrass, 9,000 kg grass silage and 18,000 kg corn silage including fresh mass. Calcium carbonate, livestock salt, soybean meal, animal feed R18, grain mix and a special blend put in automatic feeders depending on performance were used as balancing feed. The need-based feed rationing was calculated by the responsible Office of Agriculture and Food (AfLuE), Mindelheim, Germany.

Stimulation
Electromagnetic stimulation was applied in accordance with the instruction manual (INNOMED International AG, Triesen. FL., www.bemer3000.com) by simply placing and attaching the therapy mat to the back of the animals and start one of the freely selectable intensity or intensity/time programs. In this experiment, an intensity of constant 30 microteslas was selected for all stimulations. Stimulation was performed every other day for 12 minutes over a period of 4 weeks after the last calving.

Sampling - Qualification - Chemical diagnostics
Sampling (tail vein) and blood analysis was performed at intervals of 8 days. The blood analysis was carried out by MEDPHARM, Gesellschaft für Analytik, Diagnostika und Consulting mbH, Augsburg. Analysis involved quantitative diagnostic measurement of the following blood parameters typical for these types of investigation:

Urea (URINE): The serum content is used to assess protein supply. Urea is produced, inter alia, in the liver from excess ammonia (NH_3) formed during protein degradation in the rumen and is excreted from there via the blood through the kidneys.

Total cholesterol (CHOL): Increased and reduced contents of total cholesterol are associated with ovarian disorders and abortions.

Total bilirubin (BILI): This is a sensitive indicator for incipient liver disorders due to lack of energy (subclinical ketosis). Glutamate oxaloacetate transaminase (GOT): Increased GOT values are associated with genital catarrhs and endometritis. During herd investigations, GOT values are reliable indicators for feed-related damage to liver cells. Glutamate dehydrogenase (GLDH): This increases in the event of comprehensive damage to the liver cells as the result of long-term feed errors. It has been found that higher values occur between 6-8 weeks p.p.

Standard values (13):

		at the lactation stage
Urea	10-45 mg/dl	peripartum 18-30 otherwise 25-35
Total cholesterol	70-150mg/dl	up to 2 weeks p.p. 85+/-25 after 3 weeks 160+/-15
Total bilirubin	up to 0.4 mg/dl	
GOT	10-50 U/l	
GLDH	1-8.0 U/l	

Results
The results of diagnostic analysis are summarized separately for the untreated and treated animals in Table 1 a, b individual values, Table 2 a, b mean values and normalized mean values including standard deviation, Table 3 Difference of the normalized average values and Figure 1 a, b and c. Normalization (division by the corresponding first mean value from Table 2) was performed to simplify graphical comparison and relates to the mean values at the start of the trial on 07.06.01.

Comparison of the group block charts of the normalized mean values (with x- coordinate as time) shows significant changes after initial values were at comparable levels. The different development in the two animal groups is conspicuous.

Compared to the standard values, this is reflected in particular in a trend for lower GLDH and GOT values. Cholesterol, in contract, tends towards higher values. The values for bilirubin and urea largely remain constant. This relationship is clarified in Figure 1c by calculating the normalized differences in mean values.

Discussion
Statistical evaluation and significance of the results:

The significance of the differences shown here was tested by testing the pair differences (Wilcom test) of the blood values measured for each set of 7 animals at the four same points in time. Taking into account the initially relatively small number of just 14 animals (small for the reasons given above), a modification proposed by Duckworth and Wyatt (sign test) was used to test the null hypothesis (the diagnostic data populations of the treated animals do not show any difference) (see L. Sachs "Statistische Methoden", Springer Verlag, 1984). The following significances were determined using the values from Table 1 a and b, largely confirming the trend indicated by the tables of mean values:

Urea   Difference not significant $p>0.10$, probably only when $p=0.2$
Cholesterol Difference not significant $p>0.10$, probably only when $p>0.2$
Bilirubin   Difference not significant $p>0.10$, probably only when $p>0.2$
GOT   Difference significant $p<0.10$
GLDH $p>10$, estimated difference significant probably only when $p=0.2$

Table 1 a and b: Comparative clinical analytical measurements of fertility-relevant parameters in cows (Holstein-Friesian). a: Untreated animals (control). b:Animals stimulated electromagnetically using BEMER 3000 (LC - last calving; see above for other abbreviations. The values for urea, cholesterol and bilirubin are in mg/dl. The values for GOT and GLDH are in U/l).

a: Animals without stimulation (control) b: Animals with BEMER 3000 stimulation Sample

a: Animals without stimulation (control)
Sample
LC (last calving): 06.14.01 07.06.01   07.13.01   07.20.01   07.27.01

Urea	16.00	14.00	9.00	14.00
Cholesterol	84.00	92.00	90.00	90.00
Bilirubin	0.30	0.30	0.40	0.20
GOT	44.00	50.00	60.00	36.00
GLDH	3.80	4.90	2.60	3.20

LC (last calving): 06.25.01

Urea	26.00	31.00	23.00	22.00
Cholesterol	117.00	102.00	88.00	85.00
Bilirubin	0.20	0.20	0.20	0.10
GOT	28.00	23.00	20.00	47.00
GLDH	6.60	6.10	5.30	6.40

LC (last calving): 04.23.01

Urea	20.00	16.00	13.00	14.00
Cholesterol	179.00	173.00	170.00	179.00
Bilirubin	0.30	0.20	0.20	0.20
GOT	37.00	32.00	35.00	37.00
GLDH	5.70	6.10	8.30	7.30

LC (last calving): 06.19.01

Urea	16.00	15.00	18.00	21.00
Cholesterol	84.00	94.00	149.00	85.00
Bilirubin	0.50	0.30	0.90	0.40
GOT	49.00	29.00	14.00	55.00
GLDH	13.20	9.80	8.40	13.30

LC (last calving): 06.19.01

Urea	27.00	17.00	31.00	31.00
Cholesterol	279.00	267.00	272.00	290.00
Bilirubin	0.20	0.20	0.20	0.20
GOT	42.00	36.00	35.00	39.00
GLDH	9.20	9.20	11.50	9.60

Urea	26.00	23.00	43.00	26.00
Cholesterol	176.00	171.00	178.00	179.00
Bilirubin	0.20	0.20	0.20	0.20
GOT	38.00	32.00	36.00	39.00
GLDH	6.30	5.70	6.40	7.20

Urea	25.00	16.00	24.00	23.00
Cholesterol	151.00	155.00	149.00	163.00
Bilirubin	0.30	0.20	0.20	0.20
GOT	340.00	32.00	33.00	34.00
GLDH	6.80	6.80	6.40	6.70

a: Animals without stimulation (control)

Sample
LC (last calving): 06.29.01 07.06.01 07.13.01 07.20.01 07.27.01

Urea	27.00	19.00	22.00	22.00
Cholesterol	112.00	138.00	167.00	194.00
Bilirubin	0.20	0.20	0.20	0.20
GOT	40.00	32.00	34.00	44.00
GLDH	13.40	7.50	11.20	6.00

LC (last calving): 03.24.01 (Ketosis on 07.05) annually 11846 kg milk

Urea	31.00	20.00	20.00	27.00
Cholesterol	228.00	217.00	218.00	225.00
Bilirubin	0.20	0.20	0.30	0.20
GOT	40.00	33.00	35.00	41.00
GLDH	7.60	8.00	11.70	9.30

LC (last calving): 05.02. 01

Urea	22.00	18.00	29.00	20.00
Cholesterol	229.00	241.00	251.00	252.00
Bilirubin	0.20	0.20	0.30	0.20
GOT	41.00	33.00	31.00	39.00
GLDH	18.10	14.10	15.20	16.00

LC (last calving): 08.07.00

Urea	33.00	32.00	32.00	29.00
Cholesterol	56.00	115.00	112.00	109.00
Bilirubin	0.30	0.20	0.20	0.30
GOT	32.00	23.00	24.00	30.00
GLDH	4.70	4.90	3.70	3.50

LC (last calving): 12.07.00

Urea	25.00	21.00	36.00	32.00
Cholesterol	144.00	150.00	151.00	133.00
Bilirubin	0.20	0.20	0.20	0.20
GOT	40.00	44.00	36.00	32.00
GLDH	9.10	7.90	6.10	5.70

Urea	28.00	25.00	31.00	26.00
Cholesterol	99.00	98.00	104.00	97.00
Bilirubin	0.20	0.20	0.20	0.20
GOT	44.00	37.00	34.00	37.00
GLDH	4.50	4.40	3.40	4.70

Urea	28.00	24.00	39.00	33.00
Cholesterol	185.00	182.00	190.00	184.00
Bilirubin	0.20	0.20	0.20	0.20
GOT	40.00	32.00	34.00	44.00
GLDH	6.90	5.80	6.50	7.60

Table 2 (means from Table 1)
a: Animals without stimulation (control) b: Animals with BEMER 3000 stimulation

a: Animals without stimulation (control)

Urea	25.00	18.86	23.00	21.57
Cholesterol	150.21	150.57	156.57	153.00
Bilirubin	0.25	0.23	0.33	0.21
GOT	39.21	33.43	33.29	41.00
GLDH	8.28	7.39	6.99	7.67

Standard value				
	4.99	6.09	11.45	6.13
	66.49	62.56	62.20	74.65

	0.09	0.05	0.26	0.09
	5.31	8.32	14.58	7.42
	4.05	2.02	2.79	3.12

b: Animals with BEMER 3000 stimulation

Urea	27.71	22.71	29.88	27.00
Cholesterol	150.43	162.71	170.43	170.57
Bilirubin	0.21	0.20	0.23	0.21
GOT	39.57	33.43	32.57	38.14
GLDH	9.19	7.51	8.26	7.54

Standard value				
	3.64	4.82	6.91	4.83
	66.42	53.15	53.78	59.07
	0.04	0.00	0.05	0.04
	3.64	6.29	4.08	5.52
	4.95	3.25	4.49	4.18

Summary and future perspective

Despite the relatively small number of experimental animals, the data strikingly illustrate the significant biochemical effect on metabolic activity induced by a special electromagnetic stimulation signal (BEMER 3000) within the relatively short experimental period of just 4 weeks. Measured against the standard values presented above, the trend of electromagnetically induced changes confirms in particular the positive impact on fertility behavior:

1. **Urea:** BEMER 3000 group: The treatment reduced the urea content in 73% of experimental animals. Control group: A total of 57% of the animals demonstrated an increased in urea content.
2. **Total cholesterol:** BEMER 3000 group: The treatment led to no significant changes, taking account of the number of animals. Control group: There was a slight increase above the standard value of 150 mg/dl in 73% of the animals.
3. **Total bilirubin:** There were no characteristic changes in either group.
4. **GOT:** BEMER 3000 group: Treatment led to a fall in GOT values in all animals (100%). Control group: The GOT value increased in 57% of the animals.
5. **GLDH:** BEMER 3000 group: The treatment lead to a fall in GLDH value in 57% of the animals. Control group: The GLDH value increased in approx. 57% of the animals.

In the present case, the electromagnetic BEMER 3000 stimulation clearly causes activation of the metabolism in the liver. In particular, preventative treatment of cows in the first 6 weeks post partum creates the best conditions for a subsequent pregnancy. As positive side effect, there is also a liver cell stabilization effect in cases of sub-clinical ketosis (which unfortunately occurred very frequently in the investigated holding) in high-performance cows. It also appeared anecdotally to be the case that estrous symptoms also improved. As treatment was performed without special technical alterations to the device, the results confirm in particular the physical mechanisms of broadband molecular activation of physiological response mechanisms, quoted significantly more generally in the introduction.

References:

Kafka W A (1999) Extremely low, wide frequency range pulsed electromagnetic fields for therapeutical use (WFR-ELF-PEMS) International Organization for the Research of the physiological effects of electromagnetic fields under normal and extreme (space) conditions (Emphyspace), Emphyspace-Report 2: 1-20

Kafka W A (2001) The physical and physiological Basis of the BEMER 3000 Signal. In: (WA Kafka ed) II World Congress on Bioelectromagnetic Energy Regulation. Emphyspace Report 1, 2001, Mediquant Verlag, Triesen pp. 9-14

The BEMER 3000 signal has a least a 1000x broader spectral band of possible applications and was awarded the silver medal in 1998 at the IENA inventions trade fair in Nuremberg and the gold medal in 1999 at the International Exhibition of Inventions in Geneva (developed by Wolf A Kafka)

Härtling H (2001) The treatment of various orthopedic symptoms using BEMER 3000. (Behandlung verschiedener orthopädischer Krankheitsbilder mit dem BEMER 3000.) In: (WA Kafka ed) II World Congress on Bioelectromagnetic Energy Regulation.
Mediquant Verlag, Triesen pp37-38

Homoky M (1999) Independent clinical opinion on the efficacy of the BEMER 3000 (Unabhängiges Klinisches Gutachten über die Wirksamkeit des BEMER 3000) (translated from Hungarian), Szent András Állami Reumatológiai és Rehabilitációs Kórház, Hévíz fürdő, Hungary

Kafka WA (1999) EMPHYSPACE Database: Biological effects of electromagnetic fields, pp. 1-1286

Kafka WA (1998) Vasodilatory effects induced by extremely low rates of specially shaped, extremely low-energy electromagnetic pulses (internal publication)

Lütge N (1999) Electromagnetic field therapy (Magnetfeldtherapie), Bio 3; 25-30

Spodaryk K Red Blood Metabolism and Hemoglobin-Oxygen Affinity: Effect of the electromagnetic BEMER 3000 field on Healthy adults In: (WA Kafka ed) II World Congress on Bioelectromagnetic Energy Regulation.

2001 Mediquant Verlag, Triesen pp. 15-19

Jelinek R (2001) Electromagnetic (BEMER 3000) fields, Stress Proteins, Teratogens. In: (WA Kafka ed) II World Congress on Bioelectromagnetic Energy Regulation.

Emphyspace Report 1, 2001, Mediquant Verlag, Triesen pp. 33-36

Michaelis, H (2000) Results of the medical user study of a device comparable to the BEMER, AFB Academy for Bioenergetics, AFB 14032000

Preißinger M (2001) BEMER 3000 Vet: Beneficial application of pulsed electromagnetic fields in veterinary practice.

(WA Kafka ed) II World Congress on Bioelectromagnetic Energy Regulation Emphyspace Report 1, 2001, Mediquant Verlag, Triesen pp. 38-41 Grünert Eberhard und Berchtold Max (1982) Infertility in female cattle (Fertilitätsstörungen beim weiblichen Rind), Paul Parey Verlag Berlin and Hamburg

BEMER History

The Technological Development History and Current Significance of the "Physical BEMER® Vascular Therapy" in Medicine

Dr. med. Wolfgang Bohn

DOI 10.1515/jcim-2013-0036 J Complement Integr Med. 2013; 10(Suppl): S1–S3

Editorial

The history of BEMER technology, whose preliminary highlight is the development of the signal configuration that is currently used in therapeutic systems to apply the "physical BEMER® vascular therapy", began in 1998. The basis for this was the development of a specific base signal, which differed from all signal forms used in nonspecific electromagnetic field therapy until that time due to a particular mathematical formula and the physical signal form resulting from it.

However, the initial considerations on the development of this special signal were still dominated by the idea that the transfer of electromagnetic energy – in a way like a catalyst – could be used to intervene in, and activate, certain biomolecular processes in an organism. Today we can say that, in light of the small amount of energy transferred, this fact is not the decisive determinant of effectiveness. Instead, it is particularly the rhythm of the signal configuration, that is, the selection of repetitions (frequencies) and vascular-specific allocation, that is of greater importance.

Initial scientific studies on the fundamentals of the working mechanism in and after 2004 done at the Institute of Microcirculation in Berlin by means of intravital microscopy (a technically complex process to represent and measure microcirculatory processes) revealed that the use of this special physical signal produced in healthy, younger test subjects who were disposed to stress and infections positive changes in microcirculatory characteristics, such as vasomotion, capillary blood distribution, venular outflow and oxygen utilization, of such magnitude as had never been achieved before in the numerousstudies of the Institute by means of any of the drugs administered. This fact piqued the interest of researchers, and was the start of new, targeted research and development efforts with respect to this technology. It also marked the definitive departure from the conventional, non-specific "magnetic field therapy" or "electromagnetic field therapy".

In the process of this scientific work, some essential processes were discovered regarding the particularly important regulatory mechanism of blood distribution with respect to precapillary and postcapillary microcirculation. This also included observation of different repetition rates of vascular vasomotion depending on the caliber of vessels. Minuscule precapillary arterioles, as well as postcapillary venules, were characterized by around 3–5 vasomotions per minute under regular circumstances. The vascular sections upstream and downstream, which are only slightly bigger, had only one vasomotion per minute.

These vasomotions essentially determine the distribution of the blood and its components in the capillary network according to the respective requirements of the tissue and cells that depend on this network. The researchers also discovered that the more rapid vasomotion of the smallest vessels was autorhythmic, while the slower vasomotion of the slightly bigger vessels was subject to central, humoral or neural control. The clear objective of further development was, therefore, to optimize the effect through more precise addressing and frequency-based differentiation in the signal configuration, thus creating effect-relevant synergy in the different vasomotions of the various vascular sections.

The autorhythmically controlled vasomotions of the smallest precapillary and postcapillary vessels, discovered first, with a repetition rate of around three times per minute were the reason why, in the first development step of the signal configuration, 5 pulses with a flux density about a third higher than in the rest of the pulse sequence were inserted into the signal sequence at the time at 20 s apart. This 2007 signal configuration came to be known as the "plus" signal. It already produced a first, significant increase in the characteristic changes of microcirculation.

The researchers also found that the frequency of vasomotion decreased relative to age and/or severity of an illness. Thus, in seriously ill, older patients, only one vasomotion per 10 min was detected in the precapillary and postcapillary vascular sections. Such vasomotion frequency is absolutely inadequate for adjusted blood distribution in the capillaries, that is, the sufficient circulation of the dependent cellular tissue. Even if this is not the cause of the illness, it is still a serious negative factor in the progression of the illness or even in the patient's recovery.

When the new BEMER technology was applied to such patients, it was found that the frequency of the vasomotion, and also the other microcirculatory characteristics, such as capillary perfusion, venular outflow or oxygen utilization, improved significantly. The patients treated described these positive changes in most cases as feeling better.

The further development of the technology depended on finding the right time-based distributions and the specific addressing to the appropriate vascular sections, also recognizable by the organism, in the signal configuration. The frequencies and frequency components as well as their time-based distribution in the signal were examined. Using intravital microscopy, it was possible always to measure and evaluate the effects of the changes on the microcirculatory characteristics immediately. This approach, commonly called "trial and error" in the scientific community, produced better and better results and, finally, resulted in the signal configuration that proved to be the most effective in these experiments and that today is used in the current systems applying the technology.

This signal configuration, set to 120 s run time, also includes two stimulation areas that are separated from each other by intervals of 3 s. These intervals allow the organism to recognize that each stimulation is allocated to a different address (vascular section). The signal section for stimulating the smallest precapillary vascular sections via autorhythm runs over 83 s at a frequency of 30 Hertz (Hz). The stimulation section of the somewhat bigger vascular sections, which are subject to central, humoral or neural control, runs over 31 s at a frequency of 10 Hertz (Hz).

Further research dealt with the redistribution of the organic tissue-perfusion centers in the relaxation and resting phases, as opposed to the activity phases in the circadian rhythm of an organism. In this case, the results led to the development of an additional, special signal configuration that is to support regeneration and immunological processes in the rest/sleep phases of the organism. This additional treatment option is to benefit primarily patients suffering from sleep disorders, frequently those who are multimorbid and/or older patients who, due to their sleep disorders, often experience or develop deficits in regeneration and with respect to their immune system.

Today, the BEMER technology and its use via special application systems represents an effective, targeted, physical treatment method for dysfunctional microcirculation. Since therapeutic-pharmacological interventions, especially in the small-caliber arteriolar area and its autorhythmic vasomotion, are very limited, it thus currently represents virtually an unprecedented treatment option and should be used in medical practice widely as a complementary basic therapy to improve impaired microcirculation. Considering that impaired microcirculation has been recognized as the cause of a number of diseases, and substantially more conditions are affected adversely by impaired microcirculation, the fundamental importance of this new complementary physical therapy becomes clear and makes sense in many areas of medicine.

Patients suffering life-threatening shock are an especially impressive example, because impaired microcirculation plays a decisive role in the prognosis in these cases. If the regulation of endogenously released messenger substances of cells involved in the immune system and their subsequent processes, such as inflammation or changes in blood coagulation, no longer function due to flawed distribution in microcirculation, this will ultimately lead to organ dysfunction and, eventually, organ failure because of the pathophysiological mechanisms triggered by this. This is complicated further by the fact that pharmacological active ingredients applied can no longer reach the intended site of action in sufficient levels of concentration for that same reason and that the prognosis for the patient becomes severe due to this vicious circle. The use of effective stimulation of microcirculation, which is fully unaffected by the actual impairment, and its improvement through direct, physical means, that is, the "physical BEMER® vascular therapy", is thus
urgently needed for the patients affected, and can be crucial to their survival.

In summary, it bears emphasizing again that, thanks to intensive and complex research and development, the "physical BEMER® vascular therapy" in its current form has absolutely nothing in common with the conventional "magnetic field therapy" anymore, except for the fact that an electromagnetic field is used for the transmission of the effective stimulus for economic and practical reasons.

www.ingramcontent.com/pod-product-compliance
Ingram Content Group UK Ltd.
Pitfield, Milton Keynes, MK11 3LW, UK
UKHW051351180426
11947UKWH00014B/878